ECG Signal Processing, Classification and Interpretation

Adam Gacek • Witold Pedrycz
Editors

ECG Signal Processing, Classification and Interpretation

A Comprehensive Framework of Computational Intelligence

Springer

Editors
Adam Gacek
Institute of Medical Technology and Equipment
Roosevelta 118
41-800 Zabrze
Poland
adam.gacek@itam.zabrze.pl

Witold Pedrycz
Department of Electrical and Computer Engineering
University of Alberta
116 Street 9107
T6G 2V4 Edmonton Alberta
Canada
pedrycz@ece.ualberta.ca

ISBN 978-0-85729-867-6 e-ISBN 978-0-85729-868-3
DOI 10.1007/978-0-85729-868-3
Springer London Dordrecht Heidelberg New York

British Library Cataloguing in Publication Data
A catalogue record for this book is available from the British Library

Library of Congress Control Number: 2011938277

Printed on acid-free paper

Springer is part of Springer Science+Business Media (www.springer.com)

Preface

ECG signals are one among the most important sources of diagnostic information. There has been a great deal of progress in the area of signal processing, classification, and interpretation in terms of the underlying signal acquisition technology itself as well as a variety of algorithmic and system developments supported by advanced information technologies. In the past decades, Computational Intelligence (CI) has emerged as a highly synergistic, computationally appealing, and conceptually unified framework supporting intelligent system design and analysis. Computational Intelligence promotes synergy. The key contributing technologies of CI – neurocomputing, fuzzy sets (or information granules and Granular Computing, in general), as well as evolutionary and population-based optimization – exhibit well-focused yet highly complementary research agenda. Neural networks are about learning and constructing nonlinear mappings. Fuzzy sets are concerned with the representation and organization of domain knowledge in terms of information granules – semantically meaningful entities, which are perceived and processed when describing and classifying real-world phenomena. Evolutionary computing is about forming a comprehensive optimization framework where structure and parameters of the system under design can be effectively developed.

From the perspective of ECG signal processing, classification, interpretation, and integration, the settings of Computational Intelligence bring forward a number of conceptually and computationally appealing and unique opportunities. The nonlinear nature of signal processing is well captured through neural networks. Information granules and their processing is essential to offer a significant level of interpretability of automatic classification systems. Information granules helps acquiring domain knowledge existing in the area. Evolutionary optimization becomes critical in supporting a structural development of classifiers.

As we are witnessing vigorous pursuits along this line of research and applied developments, we are also becoming aware of a very scattered nature of the material encountered in the literature. It becomes evident that there is a genuine need for a volume, which could offer a comprehensive, fully updated, and systematic exposure to the subject matter, addressing concepts, methodology, algorithms, and case studies/applications. This edited volume intends to fill the gap. Our ultimate objective is to provide the reader with an in-depth, comprehensive material on the conceptually appealing and practically sound technology of Computational Intelligence and its use in the realm of ECG signal analysis, synthesis, classification, and interpretation.

With this objective in mind, the volume strives to articulate several focal points. We offer a systematic exposure of the concepts, design methodology, and detailed algorithms. Likewise, we stress a self-contained nature of the volume to enhance the exposure and readability of the material. We provide the reader with all necessary prerequisites and, if necessary, augment some parts with a step-by-step explanation of more advanced concepts supported by a significant amount of illustrative numeric material and some application scenarios to motivate the reader and make some abstract concepts more tangible. In particular, we offer a concise yet in-depth and well-focused exposure to Computational Intelligence as well as ECG signals themselves. The medical perspective at the ECG diagnostic content is offered as well. The systematic, well-organized flow of the presentation of the ideas is directly supported by a way in which the material is structured (with details presented in the next section of this book proposal). In general, we adhere to the top-down strategy by starting with the concepts and their underlying motivation and then proceeding with the detailed design that materializes in specific algorithms and representative applications and case studies. The individual chapters come with a clearly delineated agenda and a well-defined focus.

In what follows, we briefly highlight the main features of the chapters.

The opening chapter ***An Introduction to ECG Interpretation*** authored by J. Wasilewski and L. Poloński brings an important generic medical material. It offers an essential perspective at ECG signals regarded as an important source of vital diagnostic information and a way of its usage by medical specialists.

The chapter entitled ***An Introduction to ECG Signal Processing and Analysis*** by A. Gacek provides a comprehensive overview of the history, developments, and information supporting technology that is efficient and effective methods of processing and analysis of ECG signals with their emphasis on the discovery of essential and novel diagnostic information.

ECG Signal Analysis, Classification, and Interpretation: A Framework of Computational Intelligence authored by A. Gacek and W. Pedrycz is a general introduction to the principles, algorithms, and practice of Computational Intelligence (CI) and elaborates on those facets in relation with the ECG signal analysis. It discusses the main technologies of Computational Intelligence (neural networks, fuzzy sets, and evolutionary and population-based optimization), identifies their focal points, and stresses an overall synergistic character of the discipline, which ultimately gives rise to the highly synergistic CI environment. Furthermore, the main advantages and limitations of the CI technologies are discussed. The design of information granules is elaborated on; their design realized on the basis of numeric data as well as pieces of domain knowledge is considered.

The next chapter, ***A Generic and Patient-Specific Electrocardiogram Signal Classification System*** is authored by T. Ince, S. Kiranyaz, and M. Gabbouj. They report on a generic and patient-specific classification system designed for robust and accurate detection of ECG heartbeat patterns. They exploit the concept of morphological wavelet transform. By invoking its time–frequency localization properties inherent to wavelets, it becomes possible to separate the relevant ECG waveform morphology descriptors from the noise, interference, baseline drift, and amplitude variation of the original signal. The essential technologies of CI explored in this study stress an interesting synergy of neurocomputing where a neural network has been designed with the use of Particle Swarm Optimization (PSO).

P. Carvalho, J. Henriques, R. Couceiro, M. Harris, M. Antunes, and J. Habetha in their contribution entitled ***Model-Based Atrial Fibrillation Detection*** elaborate on the strategy based on a Computational Intelligence approach, combining expert knowledge and neural networks. This makes use of the three principal physiological characteristics being applied by cardiologists in their medical reasoning. Such a knowledge-based approach has an inherent advantage of increasing interpretability of the results, while improving robustness of the detection process. The authors exploit public databases (MIT-BIH Arrhythmia and QT databases from Physionet).

The principles and applicability of Evolutionary Computation (EC) are covered in the chapter entitled ***An Introduction to the Use of Evolutionary Computation Techniques for Dealing with ECG Signals*** and authored by G. Leguizamon and C.A. Coello. They present a comprehensive and carefully structured introduction to the EC fundamentals including a unified perspective of the most representative algorithms present in the area. Some other well-known bio-inspired metaheuristics that have been adopted for dealing with the treatment of ECG signals are also covered.

Diagnostic processes are knowledge-rich and knowledge-driven pursuits. To emphasize and exploit this aspect, M.H. Wang, C.S. Lee, G. Acampora, and V. Loia in their study entitled ***Electrocardiogram Application Based on Heart Rate Variability Ontology and Fuzzy Markup Language*** present a fuzzy markup language (FML)-based HRV ontology applied to the ECG domain knowledge. The ontology technologies are used to construct the personalized HRV ontology, and the FML is used to describe the knowledge base and rule base of the HRV. An experimental platform has been constructed to test the performance of the ontology.

The chapter entitled ***Learning in Artificial Neural Networks*** authored by A. Pâdua Braga offers a general overview of Artificial Neural Networks learning from the perspectives of Statistical Learning Theory and multi-objective optimization. The vital issue of a sound trade-off between the empirical risk obtained from the data set and the model complexity is elaborated on with direct implications on multi-objective learning. Subsequently, the main concepts of multi-objective learning are discussed in the context of ECG classification problems.

Kernel methods have recently enjoyed visible importance. The paper entitled ***A Review of Kernel Methods in ECG Signal Classification*** (J.L. Rojo Álvarez, G. Camps-Valls, A.J. Caamaño-Fernández, and J.F. Guerrero-Martínez) forms a well-rounded view at this recent technology by underlining their consistent and well-founded theoretical framework for developing nonlinear algorithms. It is shown that kernel characteristics are particularly appropriate for biomedical signal processing and analysis, and hence one can witness the widespread use of these techniques in biomedical signal processing in general, and in ECG data analysis, in particular. This chapter provides a survey of applications of kernel methods in this context of ECG signal analysis.

G. Bortolan, I. Christov, and W. Pedrycz in the chapter, ***Hyperellipsoidal Classifier for Beat Classification in ECG Signals,*** stress important interpretability facets of ECG pattern classifiers by presenting so-called hyperbox classifiers. Different techniques based on a combination of fuzzy clustering and genetic algorithms are put together to form an efficient learning environment. The hyperbox classifiers have been investigated for the detection and classification of different types of heartbeats in electrocardiograms (ECGs), which are of major importance in the diagnosis of cardiac dysfunctions. The experiments were reported for the MIT-BIH arrhythmia database. The chapter elaborates on several ways of combining fuzzy clustering and genetic algorithm in identifying the optimal hyperboxes and forming a family of hyperellipsoids.

A.I. Hernandez, J. Dumont, M. Altuve, A. Beuchee, and G. Carrault in their study, ***Evolutionary Optimization of ECG Feature Extraction Methods: Applications to the Monitoring of Adult Myocardial Ischemia and Neonatal Apnea Bradycardia Events,*** propose an automated method, based on evolutionary computing, to optimize parameters used in signal processing methods (filter cut-off frequencies, thresholds, etc.) being applied to ECG signals. This is of particular importance for signal processing applied to the detection and segmentation of individual ECG beats. This optimization method is described and applied to two different monitoring applications, namely the detection of myocardial ischemia episodes on adult patients and the characterization of apnea-bradycardia events in preterm infants.

Given the organization of the material, the volume could serve as a useful reference material for graduate students and senior undergraduate students in courses in biomedical system design expert systems, bioinformatics, and bioengineering, especially those aimed at ECG signal analysis and interpretation. The volume will appeal to the practitioners. The book brings forward a new conceptual and algorithmic framework of Computational Intelligence to the practice of biomedical signal processing.

We would like to take this opportunity to express our sincere thanks to the authors for reporting on their innovative research and sharing insights into the area. The reviewers deserve our thanks for their constructive input. We highly appreciate a continuous support and professionalism of the staff of Springer.

We hope that the readers will find this publication of genuine interest and help in research, educational, and practical endeavors.

Zabrze, Poland *Adam Gacek*
Edmonton, Alberta, Canada *Witold Pedrycz*

Contents

Chapter 1
An Introduction to ECG Interpretation

Jarosław Wasilewski and Lech Poloński

1.1 Introduction

Electrocardiography is a method that registers electrical activity against time. The changes in electrical potential difference (voltage) during depolarization and repolarisation of the myocardial fibers are recorded by electrodes positioned on the surface of the chest and on the limb (limb leads). The sources of the electrical potentials are contractile cardiac muscle cells (cardiomyocytes). The ECG waveform is either printed onto graph paper that runs at a constant speed or shown on a computer screen. The advantages of electrocardiography come with its low cost, immediate availability and easy implementation. The procedure itself is also non-invasive.

The electrocardiogram (ECG) is used to investigate some types of abnormal heart function including arrhythmias and conduction disturbances, as well as heart morphology (e.g., the orientation of the heart in the chest cavity, hypertrophy, and evolving myocardial ischemia or infarction). It is also useful for assessing performance of pacemarkers.

1.2 The Electrical Conduction System of the Heart

Cardiac muscle is composed of two main cell types: cardiomyocytes, which generate electrical potentials during contraction, and cells specialized in the generation and conduction of the action potentials. These specialized electrical cells depolarize spontaneously. At rest, cardiomyocytes are polarized with an electrical membrane

J. Wasilewski (✉) · L. Poloński
Silesian Center for Heart Disease, Zabrze ul. Marii Skłowowskiej-Curie 9, Zabrze, Poland
e-mail: jaroslaw-wasilewski@wp.pl; scchs@slam.katowice.pl

A. Gacek and W. Pedrycz (eds.), *ECG Signal Processing, Classification and Interpretation: A Comprehensive Framework of Computational Intelligence*,
DOI 10.1007/978-0-85729-868-3_1, © Springer-Verlag London Limited 2012

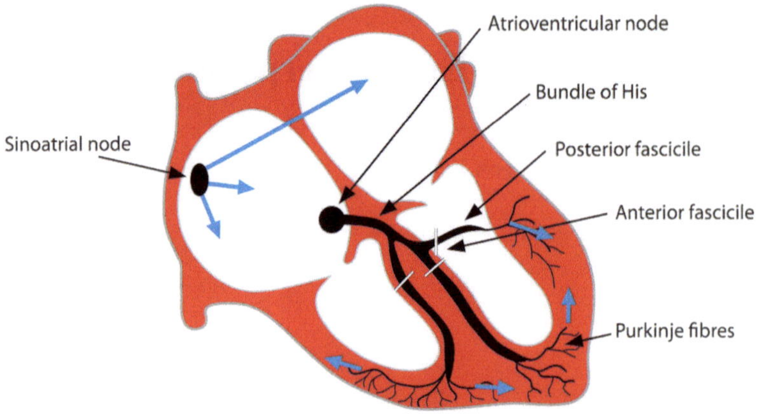

Fig. 1.1 The electrical conduction system of the heart

potential of about −90 mV. Excitation by an external stimulus can trigger a rapid reversal of the electrical potential of working myocardial cells (depolarization). The depolarization is usually due to a sudden increase in permeability of the membrane to sodium, which allows positively charged sodium ions to enter the cell. In some cardiac cells the action potential is carried by calcium ions instead of sodium ions. The downward swing of the action potential, or repolarisation phase, is mainly due to the movement of potassium ions out of the cell. After depolarization, the muscle returns to its original electrical state. During the repolarisation, the cardiac muscle is incapable of being stimulated (i.e., is refractory), which protects it against premature activation.

The conduction system of the heart is shown in Fig. 1.1. The sinoatrial node (S-A) has the highest rate of spontaneous depolarization and acts as the primary pacemaker. At normal condition, the S-A node generates impulses that stimulate the atria to contract. This node is located in the superior wall of the right atrium, close to the opening of the superior vena cava. Other elements of the conduction system include the atrioventricular node (A-V), located between the atria and the ventricles, in the lower atrial septum adjacent to the annulus of the mitral valve, and the bundle of His. The bundle of His divides into a right and left branch at the level of membranous part of the interventricular septum. The left branch is further branched into an anterior and posterior bundle. The Purkinje fibers are the final component of the conduction system, which are intertwined with muscle fibers and the papillary muscles. Their task is to conduct the wavefronts directly to the two ventricles so that they contract simultaneously. The Purkinje fibers have intrinsic automaticity (ventricular escape rhythm) generating approximately 30 bpm (beats per minute). The cells of the A-V node also depolarize spontaneously but at a higher rate (about 40–50 bpm) and this automaticity is called (escape) junctional rhythm. In physiological conditions the automaticity of these rescue pacemakers is suppressed by the activity of the S-A node.

If electrical activity appears on the ECG recording later than expected (i.e., the R-R interval is longer than the R-R interval in sinus rhythm), this means that an action potential originated in one of the lower pacemakers. However, the appearance of activity earlier than expected indicates the presence of a premature ectopic beat.

Extrasystolic beats are usually followed by compensatory pause. A full compensatory pause occurs after ventricular premature beats, see Fig. 1.16, and an incomplete compensatory pause occurs in cases of supraventricular premature beats. This happens because of the depolarization of the A-V node if the activity is supraventricular and its changes firing rate of the S-A node (Fig. 1.4).

The activity of the S-A node is regulated mainly by the autonomic nervous system. An activation of sympathetic fibers causes an increase in the heart rate, while activation of the parasympathetic fibers results in a decrease in this rate. The normal heart rate at rest is approximately 60–70 bpm but is lower at night during sleep. The heart rhythm is normally regular except for minor variations with respiration especially in young individuals.

Using the terminology associated with electrical devices, the conduction system of the heart can be described as a pacemaker (S-A node), a resistor that simultaneously acts like a fuse (the A-V node) and two insulated electrical cables (branches of the bundle of His) (Fig. 1.1). The term "resistor" for the property of the A-V node is appropriate because it slows down the depolarization (conduction velocity through the A-V node is slower than in other parts of the conducting system −0.05 m/s vs. 4 m/s, respectively). This delay enables the transfer of blood from the atria to the ventricles and is responsible for ensuring that the sequence of ventricular contraction follows atrial contraction.

The comparison between the A-V node and a "fuse" is appropriate because the A-V node possesses Wenckebach's point, which is thought to maintain the ratio of maximum conduction of the supraventricular impulses to ventricles at 1:1. Under normal conditions this is about 180 impulses/min. In certain situations, such as in atrial fibrillation, Wenckebach's point provides protection against the propagation of atrial fibrillation to ventricular fibrillation. In the presence of accessory conduction pathways bypassing the atrioventricular A-V node, this mechanism can fail and atrial flutter or fibrillation can therefore progress to ventricular flutter or fibrillation.

A properly functioning conduction system guarantees an appropriate heart rate and sequential contractions of the atria and ventricles. Cardiac electrical dysfunction can be caused by damage to or improper functioning of any of the components of the conduction system separately or in combination with other problems (for example, sinus bradycardia and bundle-branch block). Other causes of cardiac arrhythmias can be a pathological stimulus generation (for example, premature ectopic beats) or pathological conductive loops. Re-entry, which is a recurrence of electrical impulses, is the most common mechanism responsible for the occurrence of paroxysmal and persistent tachycardia. A common arrhythmia that arises in this manner is atrial flutter. For this phenomenon to occur, a re-entry circuit formed by two conduction pathways is necessary. Impulses in the first pathway travel at ahigh velocity (the fast pathway) while impulses in the second pathway travel at a considerably lower velocity (the slow pathway). This means there is a delay between the arrival of the two signals, so that when the second impulse arrives, the cells are no longer refractory.

1.3 Electrical Axis and Orientation of the Heart in the Chest Cavity

Bipolar limb leads (I, II, III) developed by Willem Einthoven (Fig. 1.2) aim to calculate the mean depolarization vector of the heart in the frontal plane (the electrical axis of the heart) (Figs. 1.20a, b). The normal range of the electric axis lies between $+30^\circ$ and -110° in the frontal plane.

The morphology of the ECG recorded depends on the orientation of the heart. The unipolar augmented limb leads of Goldberger (aVR, aVL, and aVF) are used in determining the orientation of the heart. If the position of the heart is vertical as, for example, in asthenic women, the net deflection of the QRS complex in lead aVF is positive and it resembles lead V6 in morphology. Meanwhile, the QRS complex

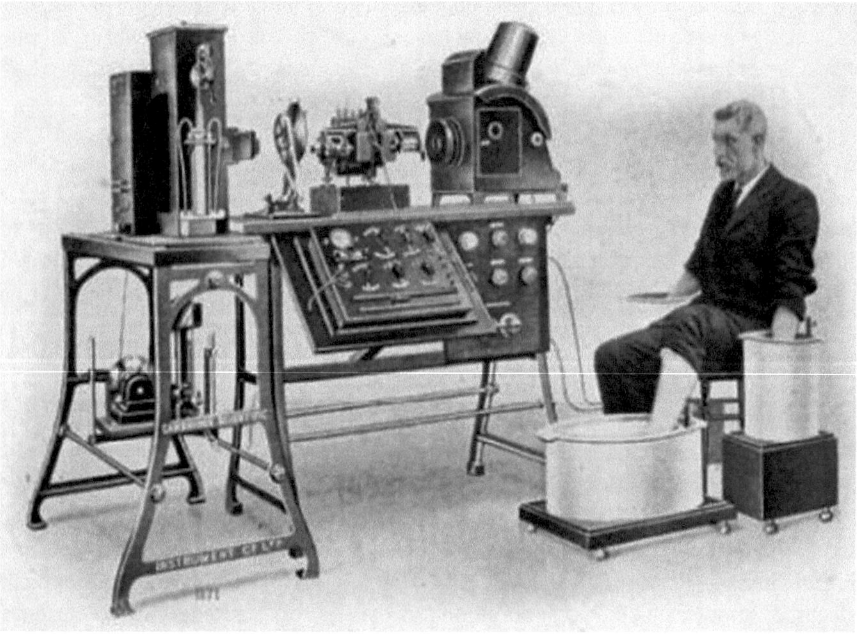

Fig. 1.2 The ECG machine constructed by Willem Eindhoven (1860–1927). The patient is connected to the galvanometer and both hands and one leg are immersed in saline containers. The electrodes connected by cables to the galvanometer are called the limb leads. Eithoven was awarded the Nobel Prize for his discovery of mechanism of electrocardiography

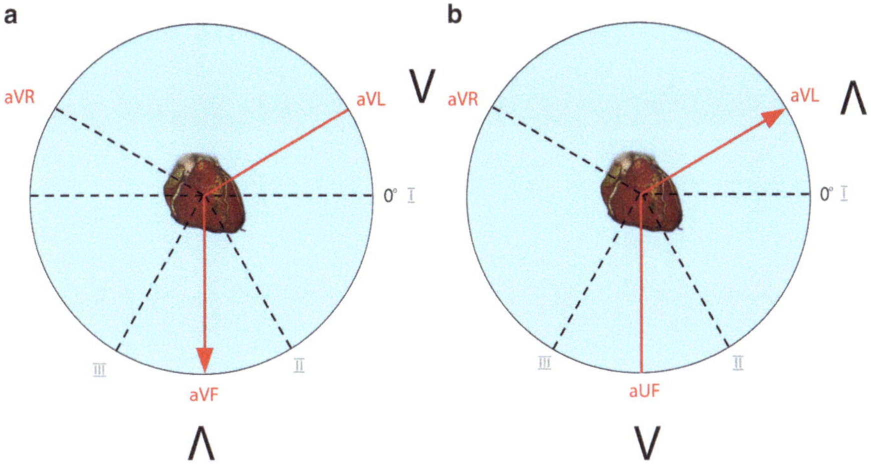

Fig. 1.3 The orientation of the heart in chest cavity. *Panel* (**a**) – vertical position. *Panel* (**b**) – horizontal position of the heart. A fundamental principle of ECG recording is that when the wave of depolarization travels toward a recording lead this results in positive or upward deflection. In contrast, if the wave of depolarization travels away, it results in negative or downward deflection

in lead aVL is negative and resembles lead V1 (Fig. 1.3a). In contrast, when the orientation of the heart is horizontal, for example, in an endomorphic individual or in someone whose diaphragm is in a high position, the QRS complex in lead aVF resembles lead V1 (the net deflection of the QRS complex is negative) and lead aVL resembles lead V6 (Fig. 1.3b).

The placement of Wilson's unipolar precordial leads is as follows:

V1: 4th intercostal space, right of the sternum
V2: 4th intercostal space, left of the sternum
V3: halfway between V2 and V4
V4: 5th intercostal space, left midclavicular line
V5: anterior axillary line, where it is intersected by a perpendicular line from lead V4
V6: midaxillary line, where it is intersected by a perpendicular line from lead V4

The chest leads sense the ECG in the transverse or horizontal plane. Leads V1 and V2 are placed above the anterior wall of the right ventricle. For this reason they are referred to as right ventricular leads. When the heart is normally oriented along the long axis, leads V5 and V6 are placed above the lateral wall of the left ventricle and are therefore known as left ventricular leads. The transitional zone between the left and right ventricles (interventricular septum) is found at the level of lead V3 and V4 (equal amplitudes of the R-wave and S-wave). In cases where the heart is rotated around its long axis the transitional zone is displaced, for example during an acute pulmonary embolism. The right ventricle is enlarged in this situation and the transitional zone is often shifted to the right toward the leads V5 or even V6

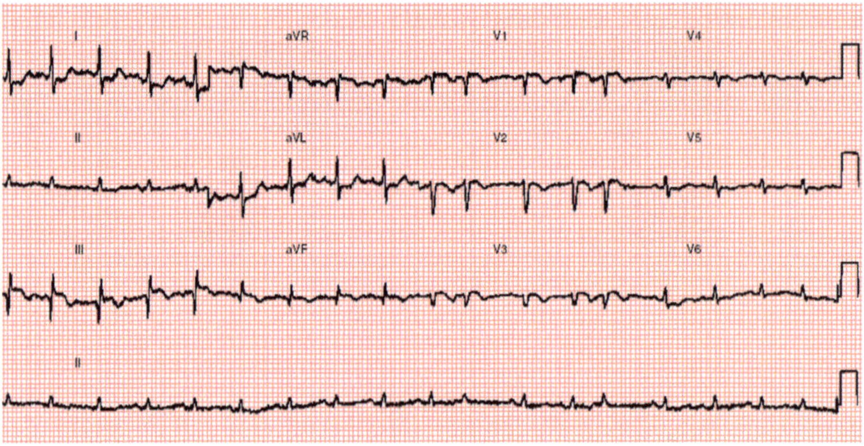

Fig. 1.4 Acute pulmonary embolism. The transitional zone in the chest leads is located near lead V5. In this situation the right ventricular leads are V1–V4. The first left ventricular lead is V6. This ECG shows the ST segment elevation in leads III, aVF, and V1–V3 with negative T-waves in these leads (characteristic pattern of ischaemia of the right ventricle). The eleventh and fourteenth cardiac cycles are premature supraventricular beats. The compensatory pause is incomplete. The RR interval including premature contractions is shorter than double the regular R-R interval of sinus rhythm (This figure was published in Poloński and Wasilewski (2004), p. 8, Fig. 2.4. Copyright Elsevier Urban & Partner Sp. z.o.o, 2006, Wrocław)

(see Fig. 1.4). According to the ECG shown in Fig. 1.4 the right ventricular leads are V1–V4 and the left ventricular lead is V6. For this reason, the right ventricular leads are best defined as lying to the right of the transitional zone, while the left ventricular leads lie to the left of the transitional zone. In patients with cyanotic congenital heart defect with significant hypertrophy and enlargement of the right ventricle, most or even all of the precordial leads can be found overlying the right ventricle. In these situations the displacement of the transitional area is accompanied by a high voltage wave in V1 and V2, which is typical for right ventricular hypertrophy.

1.4 Waves, Segments, and Intervals

There are certain elements in the ECG waveform (Fig. 1.5):

- The isoelectric line: a horizontal line when there is no electrical activity on ECG.
- Segments: the duration of the isoelectric line between waves
- Intervals: the time between the same segments of adjacent waves.

The P-wave is the first deflection of the ECG. It results from depolarization of the atria. Atrial repolarisation occurs during ventricular depolarization and is obscured. The QRS complex corresponds to the ventricular depolarization.

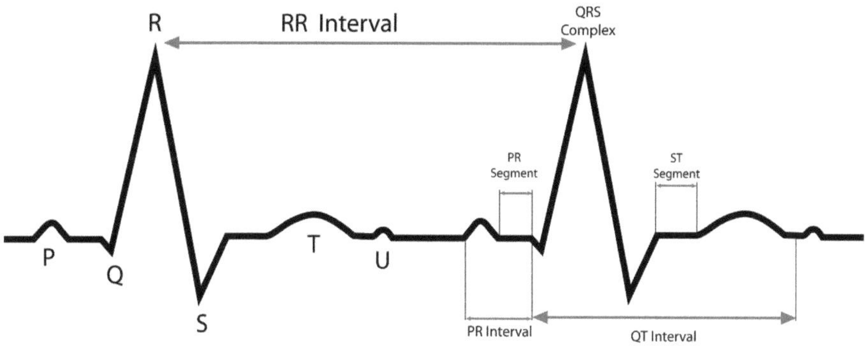

Fig. 1.5 The ECG waves, segments, and intervals

The T-wave represents ventricular repolarisation, i.e., restoration of the resting membrane potential. In about one-quarter of population, a U-wave can be seen after the T-wave. This usually has the same polarity as the preceding T-wave. It has been suggested that the U-wave is caused by after-potentials that are probably generated by mechanical–electric feedback. Inverted U-waves can appear in the presence of left ventricular hypertrophy or ischaemia.

The PQ segment corresponds to electrical impulses transmitted through the S-A node, bundle of His and its branches, and the Purkinje fibers and is usually isoelectric. The PQ interval expresses the time elapsed from atrial depolarization to the onset of ventricular depolarization. The ST-T interval coincides with the slow and rapid repolarisation of ventricular muscle. The QT interval corresponds to the duration of the ventricular action potential and repolarisation. Then TP interval is the period for which the atria and ventricles are in diastole. The RR interval represents one cardiac cycle and is used to calculate the heart rate.

1.5 Interpretation of the ECG

After describing the predominant heart rhythm, the mean electrical axis, and the position of the heart in the chest, the next step of the ECG analysis is to evaluate the shape, amplitude, and duration of the waves, segments, and intervals.

1.6 The P-wave

The P-wave is usually positive in most leads (but it is always negative in aVR) (Fig. 1.18). It can sometimes have a negative deflection in leads III and V1 or be biphasic in these leads and in lead aVL. The normal duration of the P-wave is no longer than 0.12 s, and the voltage in the limb leads should not exceed 0.25 and 0.15 mV in the precordial leads. A P-wave that is notched, and exceeds the values given above (voltage, duration, and polarization in the appropriate leads) is considered abnormal. This can result from atria enlargement and hypertrophy or from atrial depolarization generated in locations other than the S-A node.

1.7 The PQ Interval

The normal range for the PQ interval is 0.12–0.20 s. Longer PQ intervals are seen in cases of first- or second-degree atrioventricular block. The PQ interval can be shortened in pre-excitation syndromes, in which depolarizations from the atria are transmitted to the ventricles via an anomalous accessory conduction pathway that bypasses the A-V node.

1.8 The QRS Complex

This is the largest group of waves on the ECG and represents ventricular depolarization. The first downward deflection is the Q-wave. The first upward deflection is called the R-wave. The S-wave is the last downward deflection of the QRS complex. The Q-wave is not a constant component of the QRS (ventricular) complex.

During physiological conduction through the branches of the bundle of His, the left and right ventricle are depolarized simultaneously and contract along the direction of ventricular outflow tract. Ventricular depolarization propagates from the medial part of the septum downward through the apex of the heart and further along the free wall of the ventricles toward the base of the heart. The normal duration of the QRS complex does not exceed 0.12 s. The voltage usually varies between 1.5 and 2.0 mV. Durations greater than 0.12 s are most likely due to an asynchronous depolarization of both ventricles. This occurs in cases of bundle-branch block, pre-excitation syndromes, or premature ventricular contraction. In these situations, one ventricle is depolarized earlier than the other. In such cases the QRS complex consists of one R-wave followed by an R'-wave. These waves correspond to the depolarization of one and then the other ventricle, respectively. In this situation the QRS complex gets subsequently wider. If the widened and notched QRS complex is most pronounced in the right ventricular leads V1 and V2 (Fig. 1.6) then it could be caused by a right bundle-branch block. Analogously, if a notched QRS complex is recorded in the left ventricular leads V5 and V6, it may result from a left bundle-branch block (Fig. 1.7). If there is a pre-excitation syndrome with an accessory conduction pathway located on the right side, then the QRS complex mimics left bundle-branch block morphology. Similarly, if a premature beat originates in the right ventricle, then the QRS complex can also resemble left bundle-branch block. In both of these situations the right ventricle is

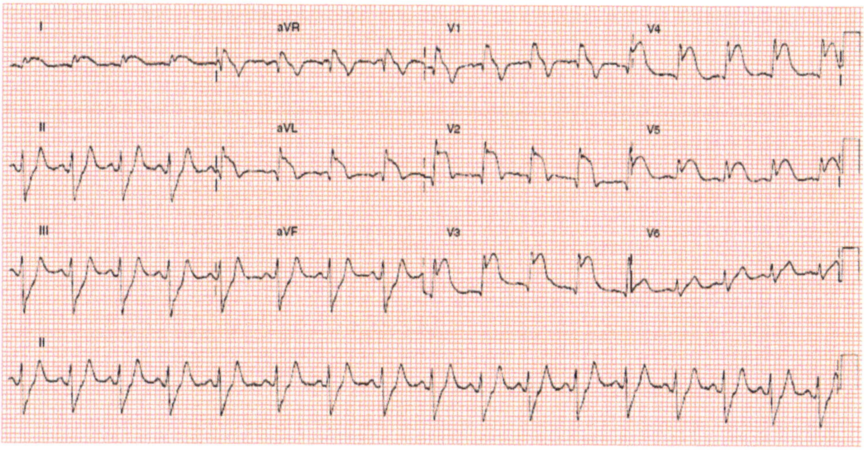

Fig. 1.6 Right bundle-branch block during an anterior wall MI showing ST segment elevation in leads V1–V6 and in leads I and aVL. There is a reciprocal ST segment depression in leads II, III, and aVF (This figure was published in Poloński and Wasilewski (2004), p. 112, Fig. 10.1.2a. Copyright Elsevier Urban & Partner Sp. z.o.o, 2006, Wrocław)

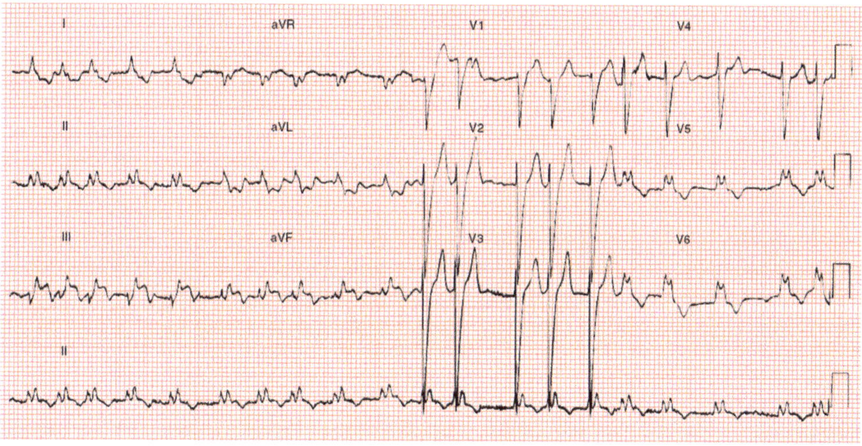

Fig. 1.7 Irregular heart rhythm (atrial fibrillation and left bundle-branch block). Notched and widened QRS complex with secondary changes in the ST segment and T-wave (ST segment depression and T-waves opposite to net deflection of QRS complex). Note the ST segment elevation in leads II, II and aVF (an inferior wall MI) (This figure was published in Poloński and Wasilewski (2004), p. 118, Fig. 10.2.2. Copyright Elsevier Urban & Partner Sp. z.o.o, 2006, Wrocław)

depolarized first, as in left bundle-branch block. In pre-excitation syndromes with an accessory conduction pathway located on the left side of the heart, or when a premature beat originates in the left ventricle, the widened QRS complex occurs in the right ventricular leads. In this case the QRS complex will resemble right

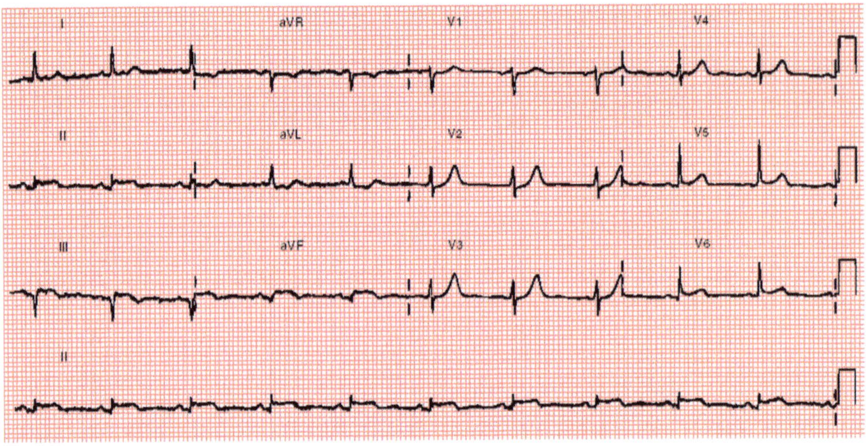

Fig. 1.8 ST segment elevation in lead III equal to the elevation in lead II, with a reciprocal ST segment depression in lead aVL. ST segment in lead I runs in the isoelectric line. The QS complex is present in leads III and aVF. ST segment elevation in leads V5 and V6. High R-wave (R-wave voltage is greater than S) in lead V2 with a positive T-wave. Evolution of inferoposterolateral wall MI (This figure was published in Poloński and Wasilewski (2004), p. 81, Fig. 8.1.5. Copyright Elsevier Urban & Partner Sp. z.o.o, 2006, Wrocław)

bundle-branch block (Fig. 1.16). Widening of the QRS complex is also seen in ventricular hypertrophy although in this situation the voltage criteria for hypertrophy must also be satisfied.

A small Q-wave is present in leads V5 and V6 and comes as a manifestation of depolarization of the septum. Each Q-wave in the precordial leads (except for the QS complex in V1) or widened and deep Q-waves in leads V5 or V6 are considered to be pathological and indicate the presence of necrotic tissue after a myocardial infarction (MI). A Q-wave in leads II, III, and aVF is considered pathological when the duration is longer than 0.03 s and its amplitude greater than 25% of the height of the R-wave and 50% of the voltage of the R-wave in lead aVL. In the case of a myocardial scar of the left ventricle posterior wall the equivalent of a Q-wave in leads V1 and V2 is an R-wave greater than the S-wave in one of these leads. Usually in this situation, the T-wave in leads V1 and V2 is positive (Figs. 1.8 and 1.16).

1.9 The ST Segment

The ST segment is a part of the ECG from the QRS complex (the J point) to the onset of the T-wave. It is normally isoelectric. The most important reason for ST segment elevation is an MI (Fig. 1.9), but it can also occur in the course of other diseases such as pericarditis (Fig. 1.10) and pulmonary embolism (Fig. 1.4) or can be a persistent abnormality in subjects with a post-MI left ventricular aneurysm.

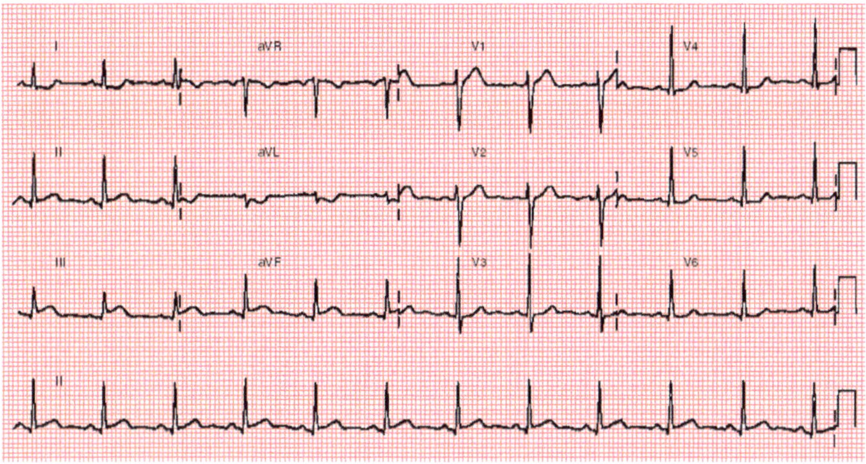

Fig. 1.9 ST segment elevation in leads II, III, and aVF. The ST segment elevation in lead III is higher than in lead II. The ST segment elevation in the right ventricular lead V1 and the lack of a reciprocal ST segment depression in lead V2 indicate that the MI of the inferior wall of the left ventricle is accompanied by a right ventricular MI (This ECG pattern suggests right coronary occlusion above the origin of the right ventricular branch) (This figure was published in Poloński and Wasilewski (2004), p. 94, Fig. 8.2.5a. Copyright Elsevier Urban & Partner Sp. z.o.o, 2006, Wrocław)

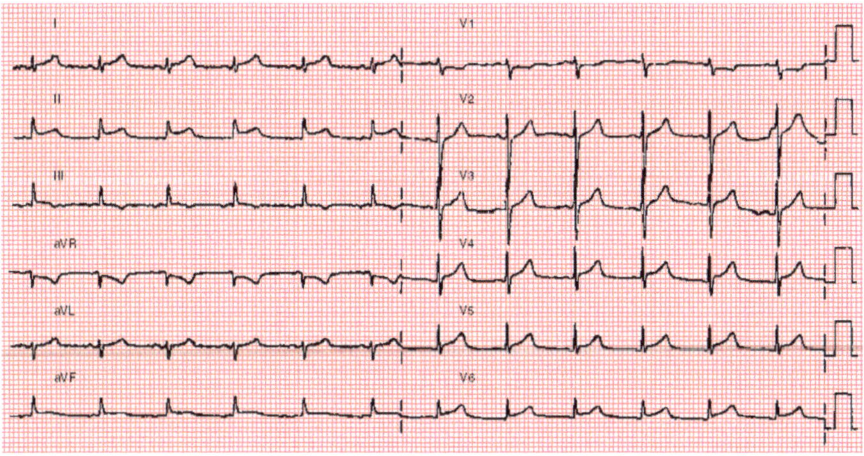

Fig. 1.10 Acute pericarditis. The widespired ST segment elevation. ST segment depression in leads aVR and V1. Note the upward concavity of the ST segment elevation and notching at the J point in leads I, II, III, and V4–V6 (This figure was published in Poloński and Wasilewski (2004), p. 6, Fig. 2.1. Copyright Elsevier Urban & Partner Sp. z.o.o, 2006, Wrocław)

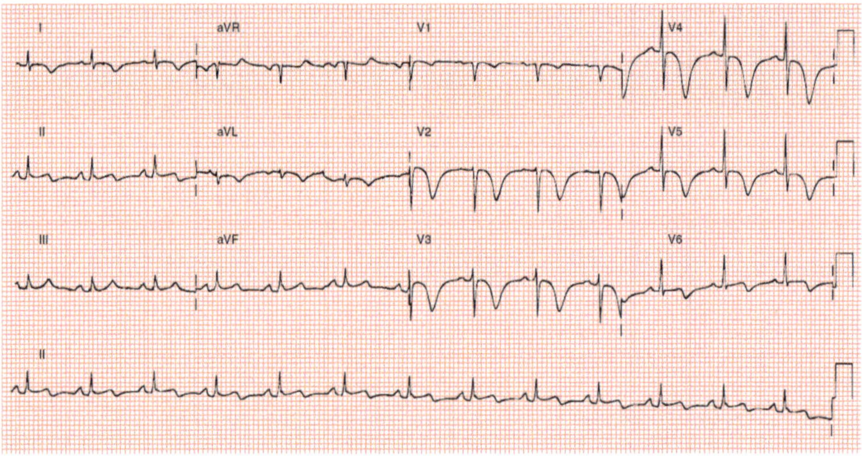

Fig. 1.11 Anterior wall MI during an occlusion of the anterior descending artery (LADT-wave pattern). Note the presence of deep symmetrical negative T-waves in leads V2–V5 and negative T-wave in leads I and aVL, biphasic T-wave in lead V6 and a positive T-wave in lead aVR (This figure was published in Poloński and Wasilewski (2004), p. 11, Fig. 2.6a. Copyright Elsevier Urban & Partner Sp. z.o.o, 2006, Wrocław)

Other situations include a dissecting aortic aneurysm (if the dissection involves the ostium of the coronary arteries), Brugada's syndrome, hyperkalaemia, hypothermia, hypervagotonia, and early repolarisation syndrome. A displacement of the ST segment secondary to the alternation of the sequence of depolarization accompanies bundle-branch block (Figs. 1.7 and 1.16), prexcitation syndromes, and premature ventricular contraction (T-wave polarity opposite to that of the R wave).

An ST segment depression in leads aVR and V6 with an ST elevation in most of the leads is found in exudative pericarditis (Fig. 1.10). A horizontal or oblique downward depression, of the ST segment, especially in patients with chest pain, is the most specific sign of ongoing myocardial ischaemia.

1.10 T-Wave

The T-wave should be positive in most leads except for aVR and sometimes in V1, in which it can be horizontal or negative. Deeply negative T-waves can be a sign of MI, e.g., due to occlusion of the left anterior descending artery (LAD-T-wave pattern) (Fig. 1.11). Other situations include hypertrophic cardiomyopathy and subarachnoid haemorrhage. T-wave inversion sometimes occurs without obvious causes (idiopathic global T-wave inversion).

1.11 The QT Interval

The QT interval is measured from the beginning of the QRS complex to the end of the T-wave. The length of the QT interval is directly affected by the heart rate (the slower the heart rate, the longer the interval). To eliminate this influence, a corrected QT (QTc) should be calculated using either Bazett's formula ($QTc = QT/RR^{0.5}$) or Fridericia's formula ($QTc = QT/RR^{0.33}$). The disadvantage is that these formulas overestimate the QT interval when the heart rate is fast and underestimate it when the heart rate is slow. Prolongation of the QT interval can be caused by many factors, including some medications, and it is also associated with the increased risk of polymorphic tachycardia known as torsades des pointes ("twisting of the points") – sudden cardiac death can result (Dessertenne 1966). The normal range for the QT interval is up to 0.44 s.

1.12 Adjacent and Opposing Leads

When assessing the ECG it is important to be familiar with the adjacent and opposing leads. The placement of the leads in relation to the structure of the heart is shown in Fig. 1.12. The adjacent leads are: lead II and aVF and lead aVF and III. These leads represent the inferior wall of the left ventricle. The adjacent limb leads are also leads I and aVL, and represent the basal segment of the left ventricle. Among precordial leads adjacent leads are for example V5 and V6 placed in front of the lateral wall of the left ventricle. The opposing leads (groups of leads where the displacement of the ST segment in one direction is accompanied by the displacement of the ST segment in the reciprocal direction in the other group of leads) are defined as follows: leads I and aVL are opposing to leads II, III, and aVF; whether the highest ST segment elevation is seen in lead aVL, the deepest ST segment depression is present in lead III (Fig. 1.13). In unipolar leads opposing leads for V1 and V2 are leads V7 and V8 covering the posterior wall. In a plane perpendicular to the front of the limbs, the reciprocal ST segment depression in leads V1–V3 are present, with an ST elevation in the inferior wall leads or as an ST elevation in lead aVR with an ST segment depression in lead V6 and vice versa.

Knowledge about adjacent and opposing leads is necessary for assessing ECG changes seen in an ST elevation MI and helps determine the infarct-related artery, and even the localization of the occlusion. In case of an inferior wall infarct caused by occlusion of the right coronary artery, the displacement of the vector of the ST segment elevation in the limb leads is to the right, while in a myocardial infarction associated with occlusion of the circumflex coronary artery, the displacement of the ST segment elevation vector is to the left. The association between the ECG, the angiographic localization of the infarct, and diagnostic algorithms is discussed in further detail elsewhere (Poloński and Wasilewski 2004).

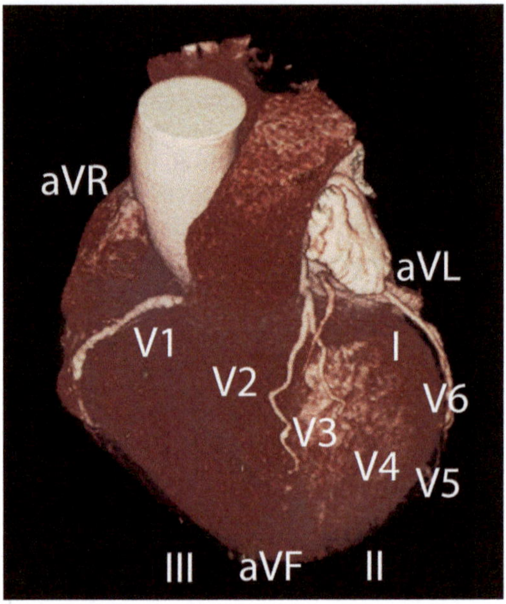

Fig. 1.12 Myocardial infarction due to the right coronary artery, the vector of the ST segment elevation is directed to the right toward lead III (the ST segment elevation in lead III is greater than in lead II and the ST segment depression in lead aVL is greater than in lead I). If the left circumflex artery is responsible for the MI then the ST segment elevation is in lead II ≥ III and there is no ST segment depression in lead I (the ST segment elevation vector is directed to the left toward lead II). In an anterior wall MI the highest ST segment elevation is seen in leads V2 and V3. In a MI with occlusion of the diagonal artery or the marginal artery, ST segment elevation appears in leads I and aVL, which are the leads representing the basal segment of the heart (Fig. 1.13). ST segment elevations are accompanied by ST segment depression in the opposite leads (reciprocal or reflected ST depression)

1.13 Negative or "Inverted" Leads

Negative leads are leads that are not present in the 12-lead ECG but are formed by inversion of the 12 standard leads. The angle between them, in contrast with the opposite leads, is always 180° (opposite orientation). The names of the negative leads are analogous to the 12 standard leads, but are preceded by a minus sign. An ECG in which negative leads are analyzed is called a 24-lead ECG. It offers supplemental clinical information without increasing the number or even altering the position of the 10 standard electrodes (Figs. 1.13 and 1.15).

Even though leads V1 (V2R) and V2 (V1R) are defined as right ventricular leads, this designation is not precise. In the absence of hypertrophy or enlargement of the right ventricle, these leads represent a view of the left ventricle posterior wall as a mirror image (Figs. 1.14–1.17). The action potential of the right ventricle is too small to have any vital influence on the ECG waveform in these leads. Consequently,

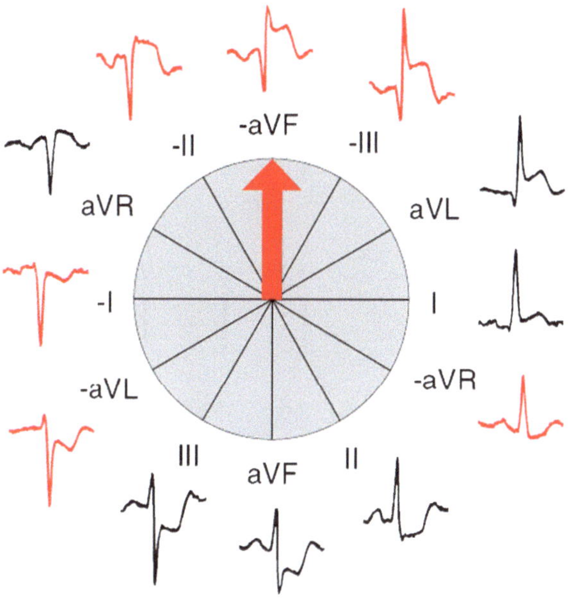

Fig. 1.13 The limb leads and corresponding negative limb leads. ST segment depressions in leads II, aVF, and III represent reciprocal ST segment elevation on the opposing leads I and aVL. Displacement of the ST segment is also seen in the all negative leads. MI of the basal segment of the heart due to occlusion of the diagonal branch (This figure was published in Poloński and Wasilewski (2004), p. 35, Fig. 2.1c. Copyright Elsevier Urban & Partner Sp. z.o.o, 2006, Wrocław)

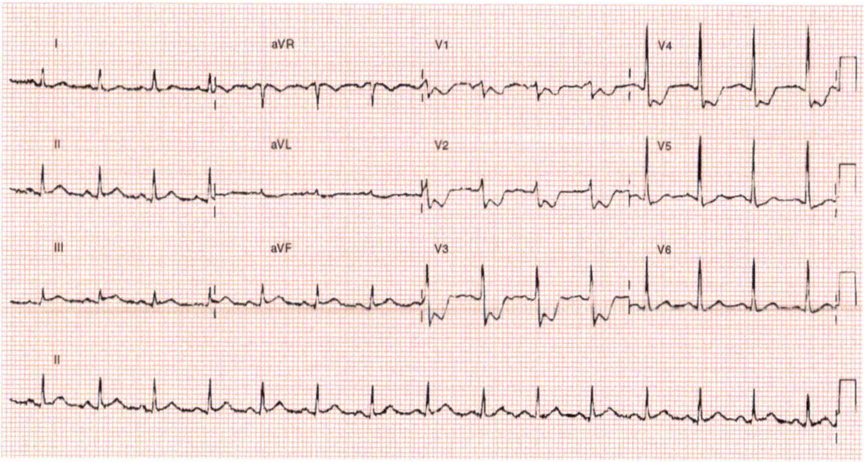

Fig. 1.14 ST segment elevation in leads II, III, and aVF, in which the elevation in lead II is equal to that in lead III. A small reciprocal ST segment depression can be seen in lead aVL. A reverted Pardee wave is present in leads V1–V4 ("up-sidedown injury"). ST segment elevation in lead V6. Inferoposterolateral wall MI. Diagnosis of posterior wall MI was made from reciprocal changes appear in leads V1–V4 (This figure was published in Poloński and Wasilewski (2004), p. 98, Fig. 8.4.3a. Copyright Elsevier Urban & Partner Sp. z.o.o, 2006, Wrocław)

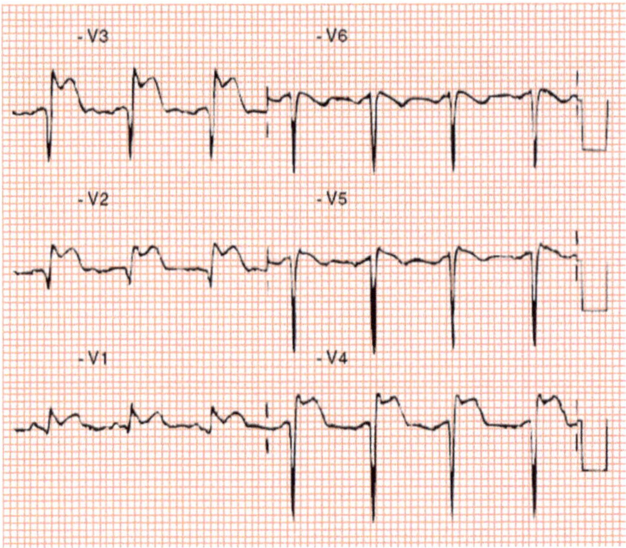

Fig. 1.15 Precordial leads shown in Fig. 1.14 are presented as their negative counterpart. Pardee's wave is clearly seen in leads −V1 to −V4. The maximal information that could be gained without the placement of additional electrodes but adding inverted leads for evaluation of ST-segment displacement (This figure was published in Poloński and Wasilewski (2004), p. 99, Fig. 8.4.3c. Copyright Elsevier Urban & Partner Sp. z.o.o, 2006, Wrocław)

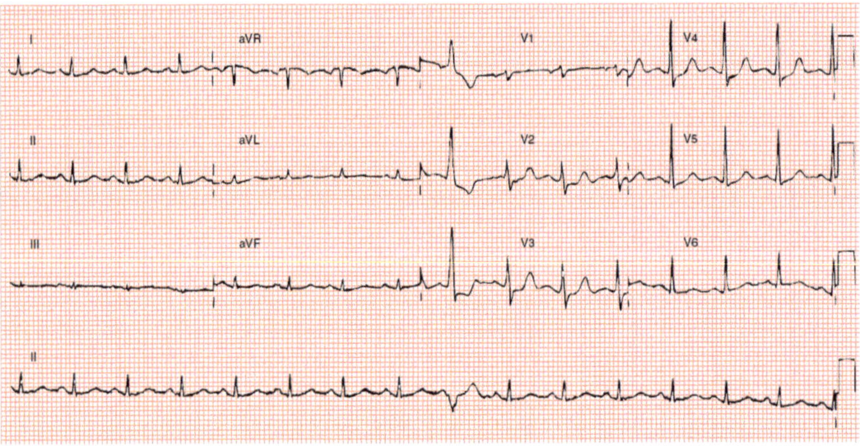

Fig. 1.16 The same patient as in Fig. 1.14, but the ECG is recorded 1 h after the patency of the artery has been restored. Note the high voltage R-wave in lead V2 (the amplitude of R-wave is greater than S) and a positive T-wave. The ninth cardiac cycle is a premature ventricular beat. The RR interval that contains the extrasystole is twice as long as the RR interval in sinus rhythm. A full compensatory pause is present. The premature ventricular contraction has morphology that resembles a right bundle-branch block and indicates that the premature ventricular contraction originates in the left ventricle (This figure was published in Poloński and Wasilewski (2004), p. 99, Fig. 8.4.3b. Copyright Elsevier Urban & Partner Sp. z.o.o, 2006, Wrocław)

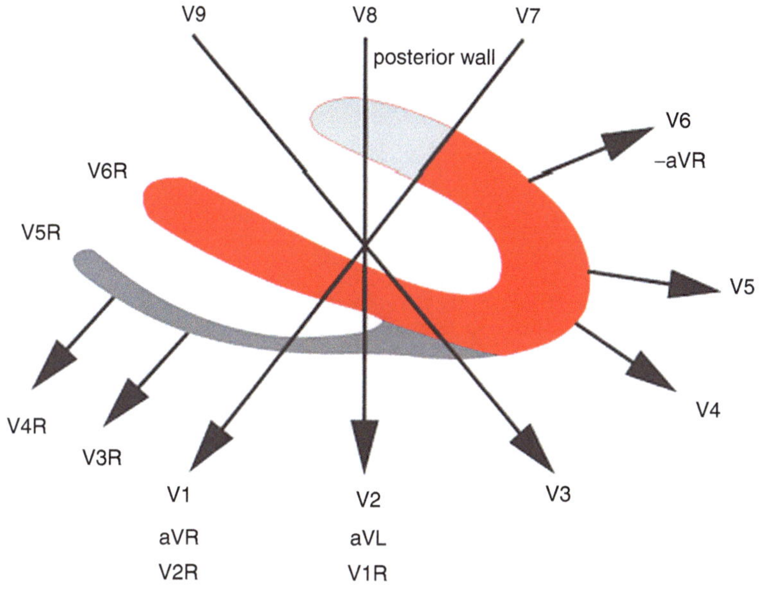

Fig. 1.17 The schematic diagram shows the placement of the precordial leads and their position in relation to leads aVL and aVR. The opposite leads related to leads V1 and V2 are leads V7 and V8 (This figure was published in Połoński and Wasilewski (2004), p. 29, Fig. 5.1. Copyright Elsevier Urban & Partner Sp. z.o.o, 2006, Wrocław)

the right ventricle is said to be "invisible" in the ECG. Under this assumption, the equivalent of the small Q-wave in V6 is a small R-wave in lead V1. The equivalence of a high R-wave in V6 is a deep negative S-wave in lead V1. The theory of opposite leads helps explain why, in case of left ventricular hypertrophy, there is an increase in the R-wave voltage in lead V6, which is accompanied by further S-wave voltage increase in lead V1. According to the Sokolow-Lyon index, left ventricular hypertrophy can be diagnosed when the sum of the voltages of the R-wave in V6 and the S-wave in V1 is greater than 35 mV (Sokolow and Lyon 1949).

Knowledge of adjacent and opposite leads not only helps to identify the orientation of the heart axis but also explains why, in lead aVR, the P-waves and T-waves and QRS complex are negative (Fig. 1.18). It also explains why in left axis deviation the QRS complex is positive in lead I and negative in lead III. If the average of depolarization vector in frontal plane is moving toward an electrode, this electrode records a positive deflection (lead I). At the same time, a wave of depolarization is moving away from lead III and this lead records a negative deflection (Figs. 1.19 and 1.20a). This effect is reversed if the electrical axis deviates to the right. Then the depolarization vector approaches lead III (the positive QRS complex in lead III), and distances itself from lead I (the negative QRS complex in lead I) (Figs. 1.19 and 1.20b).

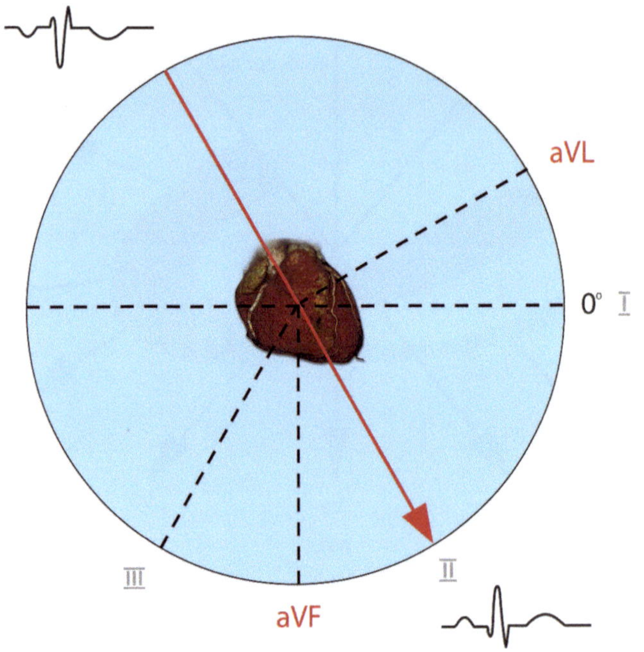

Fig. 1.18 The morphology of the ECG in leads aVR and II. Positive electrical impulses in the ECG directed toward the electrode (lead II) are registered as upward deflections, while the same impulses moving away from the electrode (aVR) are registered as downward deflections. In sinus rhythm when the depolarization is spread normally in the cardiac muscle the P-wave in lead II, the QRS complex, and the T-wave are positive

A detailed discussion of issues associated with arrhythmias and conduction problems are beyond the scope of this chapter. Hundreds of books, monographs, studies, and ECG articles have been dedicated to these topics; this is an old diagnostic procedure despite which a continuous progress is still being made (Fig. 1.21).

1.14 Conclusions

Applying digital methods to the ECG increases the resolution of the signal, thus enhancing its diagnostic capabilities. At the same time sophisticated methods also make it possible to apply algorithms that automatically interpret the ECG both in terms of morphology (the evaluation of multiple leads) and arrhythmias and conduction disorders (usually monitoring of a single lead is sufficient). Careful assessment of the ECG helps determine the mechanism and origin of the electrical impulse and propagation of electrical wave in the cardiac muscle and provides a wealth of useful information about the orientation of the heart, hypertrophy and

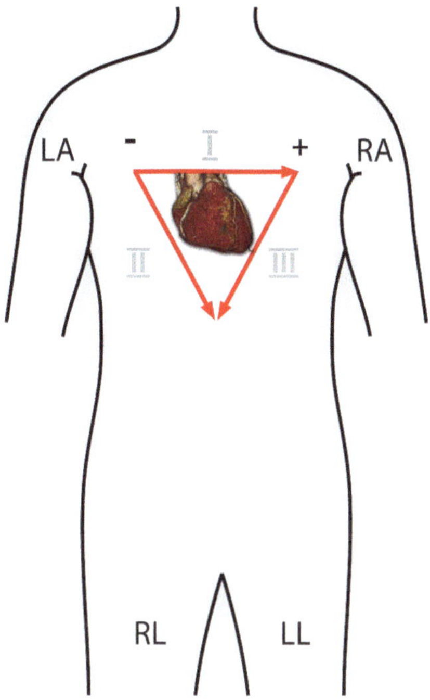

Fig. 1.19 The orientation of the bipolar leads. Lead I is placed horizontally and directed from the right to the left shoulder. The direction of lead II is from the right shoulder toward the lower left limb, while the third lead is directed from the left shoulder toward the lower right limb. In the Einthoven triangle, the angle created by lead II is 60° while the angle created by lead III is 120°. The deflection in a lead is highest when the electromotor vector is approaching the electrode

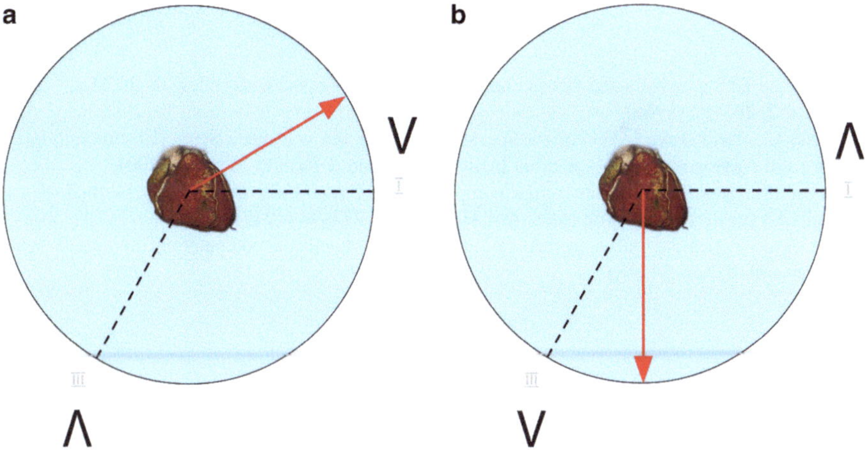

Fig. 1.20 (**a**) Sinistrogram. (**b**) Dextrogram

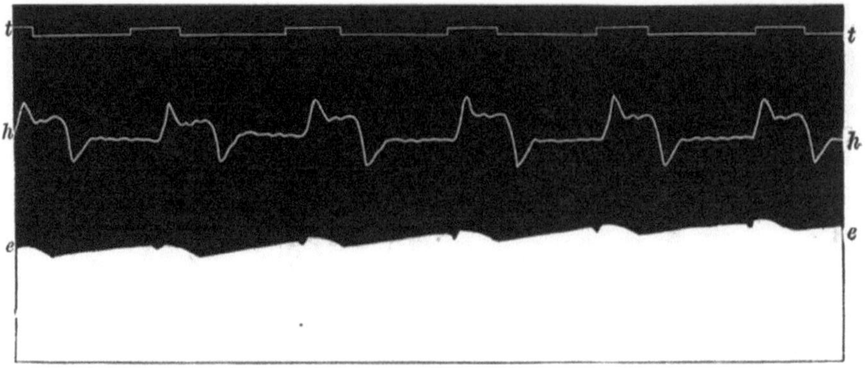

Fig. 1.21 The first human ECG recorded in 1887 by August Desire Walter (1856–1922) (Waller 1887). Walter presented his work in 1889 at the First International Congress of Physiologists, while Einthoven, the father of modern electrocardiography, watched

ischaemia, injury, or necrosis. Although simple to implement, the ECG can be very difficult to interpret. While computer programs and protocols to assess the ECG are helpful in establishing a preliminary diagnosis, an overall patient's clinical status should be taken into consideration when interpreting the ECG.

References

Dessertenne F.: La tachycardie ventriculaire a deux foyers opposes variables. Arch. Mal. Coeur. Vaiss. **2**, 263–72 (1966)

Poloński L., Wasilewski J.: Elektrokardiografia i Angiografia w Zawale Serca (Electrocardiography and Angiography in Myocardial Infarction). Urban & Partner, Wrocaw (2004)

Sokolow M., Lyon T.P.: The ventricular complex in right ventricular hypertrophy as obtained by unipolar precordial and limb leads. Am. Heart. J. **38**, 273–94 (1949)

Waller A.G.: A demonstration in man of electromotive changes accompanying the heart's beat. J. Physiol. **8**, 229–34 (1887)

Chapter 2
An Introduction to ECG Signal Processing and Analysis

Adam Gacek

2.1 Introduction

ECG signals are reflective of electric activities of a heart muscle. They are related to a variety of intertwined and complex chemical, electrical, and mechanical processes present in heart. They convey a great deal to valuable diagnostic information not only describing functioning of heart but also other systems such as circulation or nervous systems.

The ECG signal has been a subject of studies for over 100 years. The first recording of electrical activities of heart was realized in 1887 by an English physiologist August Waller who used surface electrodes placed on a skin and connected to the capillary electrometer. He was the first to call the registered signal electrocardiogram. Nevertheless W. Einthoven is regarded to be the father of electrocardiography who in 1902 recorded the first electrocardiogram with the use of a string galvanometer. In 1906 M. Cremer realized a recording of the first esophageal electrocardiogram with the help of a special esophageal probe (electrode) (Cremer 1906). This type of electrocardiography has been intensively developed in the 1970s of the last century to be used as a technique helpful in the differentiation of atria rhythm irregularity. Cremer recorded also the first fetal electrocardiogram. In 1924 W. Einthoven received the Nobel Prize for the invention of electrocardiography and its development. Since then there has been a substantial research in the area of electrocardiography. Since the 1940s, electrocardiography has become a routine method in heart diagnostics. There has been a significant development of diagnostic techniques based on ECG analysis (say, exercise test EKG, monitoring of patients in intensive care, high resolution electrocardiography, heart rhythm variability HRV, heart mapping).

A. Gacek (✉)
Institute of Medical Technology and Equipment, Zabrze, Poland
e-mail: adamg@itam.zabrze.pl

A. Gacek and W. Pedrycz (eds.), *ECG Signal Processing, Classification and Interpretation: A Comprehensive Framework of Computational Intelligence*,
DOI 10.1007/978-0-85729-868-3_2, © Springer-Verlag London Limited 2012

ECG signal is one of the best-recognized biomedical signals. Its high diagnostic capabilities have been demonstrated. In the last decades there has been a significant growth of interest in the development of efficient methods of processing and analysis of ECG signals with intent of the formation of useful diagnostic information. Those pursuits have been realized in parallel with information technologies, especially in the realm of digital signal processing realized both in hardware and software.

In virtue of the essence of ECG signals, they often have been a source of imprecise information. In the design of diagnostic systems, it becomes of interest to make them user-friendly. These factors have triggered interest in the exploitation of the technology of Computational Intelligence (CI). In this context, it is worth recalling that the first studies in the area of intelligent systems go back to the use of techniques of Artificial Intelligence (AI) with a wealth of its symbolic processing. The description of ECG signals in terms of sequences of symbols has resulted in techniques of syntactic pattern description and classification. In essence, a continuous ECG signal is represented in the form of sequences of symbols, which are analyzed and classified based on the machinery of formal grammars. We can refer here to syntactic methods used to detect the characteristic waves of ECG signals (Horowitz 1975), detection of arrhythmias (Udupa and Murphy 1980) signal filtering (Papakonstantinou and Gritazali 1981), and ECG signal analysis (Papakonstantinou and Gritazali 1981; Skordolakis 1986; Papakonstantinou et al. 1986; Trahanias and Skordolakis 1990). There are also studies devoted to the analysis and classification of ECG signals by using combinations of syntactic and probabilistic methods.

One of the first approaches, which fully exploits techniques of AI, comes in the form of semantic nets applied to the analysis of ECG signals (Stockman and Kanal 1983). In this method the signal is represented in the form of a OR/AND graph while the classification process is concerned with a graph search. Another important collection of techniques stems from the concept of rule-based systems where an ECG signal is described in the form of "if-ten" rules (Kundu et al. 1993). The reasoning mechanism relies on the use of the so-called modus ponens. The reliance on this concept, though, requires that a knowledge base is complete meaning that for any signal there is a set of rules to be used in the inference process. The reduction of the size of the rule base along with an enhancement of reasoning processes realized in presence of uncertainty becomes possible when invoking a so-called *generalized* modus ponens (Kundu et al. 1998). For the detailed discussion the reader may refer to (Kundu et al. 2000); one of the conclusions coming from this study and the references reported therein is that the AI methods are more often used to ECG signal interpretation and quite seldom are involved in the description of the features of the signal used in its description.

Considering a certain historical framework, it is worth noting that the technology of neural networks being an integral component of Computational Intelligence has been applied to ECG signal analysis and classification. One of the first applications of neurocomputing was in ECG signal compression applied to signals collected in

Holter ECG systems (Iwata et al. 1990) and in the detection of QRS complexes (Xue et al. 1992; Xue and Reddy 1997). In the second half of the 1990s, we have witnessed a rapidly growing number of applications of neural networks to ECG signal analysis and classification. With this regard, it is worth recalling other applications such a detection of ventricular late potentials VLPs (Xue and Reddy 1997) and ECG signal analysis (Silipo and Marchesi 1998; Barro et al. 1998). For instance, radial basis function (RBF) neural networks were used in ECG signal classification (Silipo et al. 1999). Neural networks were used to arrhythmia analysis (Wang et al. 2001), determination of P waves (Botter et al. 2001), and classification of heart evolution with the use of second order cumulants (Osowski and Linh 2001). The concept of neural networks in the form of a collection of subnetworks (experts) was presented in (Hu et al. 1997). Neural networks in conjunction with the methods of frequency-temporal signal analysis were used to detect ventricular late potentials (VLPs) (Wu et al. 2001) and classification of heart evolution in an on-line mode in which case neural networks were used in conjunction with Hermite functions (Linh et al. 2003).

In the literature, we can also note a stream of studies exploiting the technology of fuzzy systems (Czogała and Łęski 2000b). For instance, fuzzy systems were used in the analysis of ECG and EEG signals in (Moon et al. 2002). Fuzzy rule-based systems were used in the detection of arrhythmias (Chowdhury and Ludeman 1994) as well as a construction of ECG signals (Wang et al. 1991). Some other applications of fuzzy sets to ECG signal analysis include a detection and classification of QRS segments (Czogała and Łęski 1998, 2000a). In this case a fuzzy signal is formed through a transformation of the numeric (standard) ECG signal into a series of membership functions. In (Łęski and Henzel 1999a, b) a fuzzy signal was used to feature extraction. In (Pedrycz and Gacek 2001a) presented was a concept of fuzzy automata (Moore and Mealy) applied to ECG signal classification. An interesting development was reported in (Pedrycz et al. 2000; Pedrycz and Gacek 2001b) where shadowed sets were used to signal granulation (quantization). Examples of information granulation to ECG signal modeling and classification were presented in (Pedrycz and Gacek 2002; Gacek and Pedrycz 2005, 2006; Bortolan and Pedrycz 2002a, b). More recently, ideas of information granulation were used to ECG signal compression and classification. With this regard used were ideas of data clustering (Gacek and Jeżewski 2003a, b) and Genetic Algorithms (GAs) (Gacek and Pedrycz 2003).

This brief analysis points at a growing role and interest of CI to ECG signal analysis, processing, and classification. It has to be noted though that the CI methods are still in the research phase and only a few medical devices commercially available use some components of CI. The limitations come from the fact that these methods quite commonly come with a considerable computing overhead, which requires the use of hardware system resources. Over time this limitation becomes less essential given the progress of information technologies. It supports a conclusion that the technology of CI will become more readily available and implemented in ECG systems including those operating in the on-line mode.

ECG signal processing and analysis comprises a sequence of steps among which the most essential include

- Amplification of signal and its A/C conversion
- Noise elimination
- Feature selection

The quality and effectiveness of the methods used at these steps imply the quality of the overall process of classification and interpretation of ECG signals. Both signal amplification and A/C conversion are realized in hardware while all filtering and noise elimination are realized through the use of advanced technologies of information processing; here we witness a growing role being played by Computational Intelligence.

2.2 A Nature of ECG Signals

ECG signals are reflective of an electric activity of heart. The ECG signal is some kind of an electric provocation spread in the heart muscle cells. Under the influence of this provocation, the heart muscle cells shrink, which as a result, causes a mechanical effect in the form of cyclic shrinking of heart atria and ventricles. As an effect of heart muscle shrinking, the blood circulates in the human organs. The propagation electric provocation in the heart muscle forms a depolarization wave of the bioelectric potentials of the neighboring heart cells. The propagation of the depolarization wave, see Fig. 2.1, is caused due to a quick movement of positive ions of sodium (Na+). After moving of the depolarization wave, the heart muscle cells return to their rest state recovering before starting resting negative potential. This state is called a repolarization phase. The depolarization and

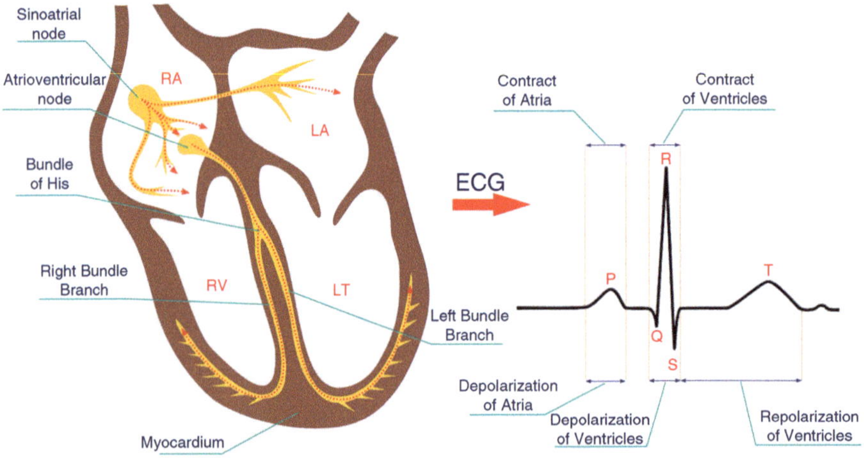

Fig. 2.1 Propagation of the depolarization wave in the heart muscle

repolarization phenomena of the heart muscle cells are caused by the movement of ions. This is the essence of the heart electric activity. Movement of ions in the heart muscle cells is the electric current, which generates the electromagnetic field around the heart. There is possibility to measure the electric potential at each point of the electromagnetic field.

The potential difference recorded at the two points of the electromagnetic field reflects the ECG signal. The shape of the ECG signal and a cyclic repetition of its characteristic parts including P-QRS-T complex, constitute essential information about operation of the electrical conduction system of the heart. By analyzing the ECG signals recorded simultaneously at different points of the human body, we can obtain essential diagnostic information related to heart functioning. It is concerned not only with the electrophysiological parameters of the heart, but it is also connected with its anatomical and mechanical properties. In essence, the ECG signal is an electric signal generated directly by the heart muscle cells. The information included in the ECG signal is directly related to the source of the signal, that is, the heart itself. As opposed to other biomedical signals, ECG signals are received directly at the recording points as electrical signal. Recorded ECG signals do not require conversion. ECG signals are recorded as a difference of electric potentials at the two points inside of the heart, on its surface or on a surface of the human body. The potential difference corresponds to the voltage recorded between two points where the measurements were taken. This voltage is the amplitude of the ECG signal recorded in the two-pole (two electrode) system. Such a two-electrode system applied to the recording of the ECG signal is referred to as an ECG lead. In this two-pole ECG recording system, one electrode is an active measurement electrode while the second electrode is the reference one. The changes during time, of voltage variation between the ECG recording electrodes, depict a course of ECG signal during time. The ECG signal recorded on paper or electronic data carrier is called an electrocardiogram.

2.3 The Main Properties of ECG Signals

ECG signals are one of the best-known biomedical signals. Given their nature, they, bring forward a number of challenges during their registration, processing, and analysis. Characteristic properties of biomedical signals include their nonstationarity, noise susceptibility, and variability among individuals. ECG signals exhibit all these properties. In particular, a highly undesirable aspect of these signals is their high susceptibility to various types of noise. The registered ECG signals are always affected by noise. The main sources of noise include:

Changes of the body-electrode impedance resulting from physic-chemical processes present in this region as well as the movement of the patient. These phenomena cause a so-called effect of a baseline wandering. These distortions are slow-varying distortions (Wiese et al. 2005; Pawar et al. 2007b).

Changes of a mutual position of heart and the electrodes caused by respiratory movements of a patient. This results in some slow-changing disturbances.

Contraction of skeletal muscles caused by the movement of the patient or inappropriate temperature of the environment. This causes so-called muscle disturbances. They are very difficult to deal with because of the broad spectrum of frequency of these disturbances, whose frequency overlaps with the frequency of the ECG signal itself (Fernandez-Chimeno et al. 2006).

Interference of electromagnetic nature (Bruce 2000). These disturbances are referred to as power interferences.

Interferences caused by high power devices such as e.g., diathermy. These disturbances are of impulse nature (Santopietro 1977; Fernandez-Chimeno et al. 2006).

By taking into consideration all causes of disturbances affecting ECG signals, their list includes the following categories:

Low frequency (slow-changing) interferences
Muscle interferences
Power-induced electromagnetic interferences
Electromagnetic interferences of impulse character

As already noted, the most difficult to deal with are interferences of low frequency and those of muscle origin. They are difficult to filter without affecting important diagnostic information contained in the original ECG signal. Depending upon the nature of the ECG test, the signals could be affected to some extent, which also depends on the location of the points of registration of the ECG signals. The ECG signals registered from various points could have a very much diversified amplitude and quite often exhibit a very low signal-to-noise ratio (SNR). Typically, the amplitudes of ECG signals collected on the body surface have amplitude of several mV. Higher signal amplitudes are those coming from heart ventricles. Whereas ECG fetal signals exhibit amplitudes in the range of μV. Similar amplitudes of ECG signals are encountered when dealing with an analysis of heart micropotentials. In these two cases we encounter a highly undesirable SNR, which could be as bad as −20 dB (Jesus and Rix 1986). For some segments of the ECG signal, this detrimental SNR values are quite natural. We observe this situation in the initial region of the P, Q, and T waves when detecting delayed potentials of the ECG signal. In case of non-standard rest ECG test, such as an analysis of heart micropotentials (Ahmed and Milne 1975; Berbari et al. 2005) the amplitudes of the registered signals are in the range of μV. In spite of the fact that the patient is not moving, the muscle noise as well as noise of electronic interface itself give rise to disturbances whose amplitudes exceed many times the amplitude of the useful signal. The fetal ECG signals, registered on mother abdomen surface, have particularly unfavorable values of SNR. It is caused by the effect that the ECG signal is the joint signal coming from the mother and the fetus. In this case, the signal coming from the mother treated as a noise has amplitude in the range of mV while the fetal signal has amplitude of μV so that the useful signal is affected by noise whose amplitude is 1,000 times higher than the original source of diagnostic information. For instance, if we consider that the micropotentials have amplitude of 5 μV and visually the signal in the rest state is regarded to be noise-free when the amplitude of disturbances is no larger than 50 μV, then the amplitude of disturbances is ten times higher than the useful signal. We are faced with similar problems when dealing with some specialized testing such as those involving analysis of high frequency electrocardiograms (Maniewski 2000; Mroczka et al. 2000; Narayanaswamy 2002), where in order to detect ischemic heart disease (IHD), the signals in the range of 80–150 Hz are analyzed. In this case the recorded signal is of the amplitude of a few μV. Important features of ECG concern their variability across individuals (patients) and across time. This means that the shape of the signal as well as its repeatability to the characteristic regions change over time and are dependent on each individual. If we consider a shape of the ECG signal present in a certain lead within the population of healthy individuals, there will be differences among these signals. A similar situation will be encountered in case of patients with some heart problems. This implies that in the analysis of ECG signals we cannot rely on some templates – prototypes as such do not exist. The limitation associated with this is quite substantial, as we cannot consider typical methods of signal processing and classification where we often rely on the use of such templates. For instance, in exercise tests we realize muscle noise suppression via averaging parts of the ECG signals including QRS complexes. From the averaging process we have to exclude those complexes that are of a different shape than the one which has been acknowledged to be dominant for a given patient. The algorithm has to exhibit some abilities of unsupervised learning given the fact that such a dominant shape cannot be determined in advance.

The ECG signal is reflective of interrelated processes of chemical, electrical, and mechanical nature that are present in the heart. They depend upon the features specific to a given individual, say a form of ventricles as well as the properties of the electrical conduction system of the heart (ECSH).

The mathematical description of these phenomena is still incomplete. In spite of this, cardiologists are considering the shape of the ECG signal and its key features, and are capable to assess the functioning of the heart and detect changes occurring in the heart muscle. The assessment is realized in a heuristic manner based on the existing knowledge and acquired experience.

For the purposes of ECG diagnostics defined was a typical ECG signal (viewed as normal) that reflects the electrical activity of the heart muscle place during a single heart evolution. As shown in Fig. 2.2, defined are some characteristic segments, points, and parameters used to capture the essence of the signal.

In medical diagnostics, the relationships between the shape and parameters of the signal and the functioning of the heart are often expressed in terms of linguistic statements resulting in some logic expressions. For instance, we have the terms such as "extended R wave," "shortened QT interval," "unclear Q wave," elevated ST segment," "low T wave," etc. In all these examples we encounter some linguistic terms (which can be formalized in the language of fuzzy sets). In books about cardiological diagnostics we usually do not encounter detailed numeric relationships or formulas but instead rather verbal descriptions characterizing the relationships between the signals and functioning of the heart.

The expert cardiologist forms his/her own model of the process, which is described in a linguistic fashion. It is noted that the model is formed on a basis of acquired knowledge and experience.

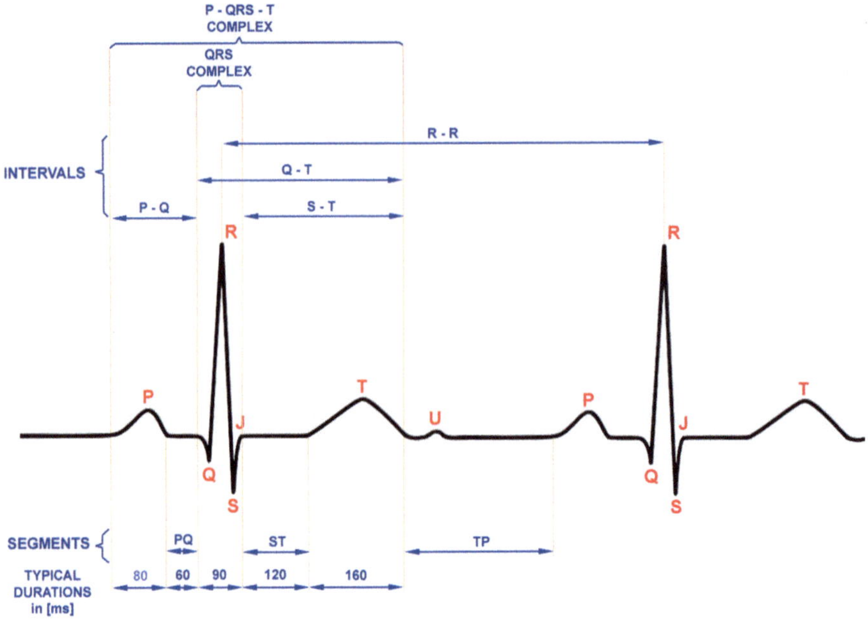

Fig. 2.2 Typical shape of ECG signal and its essential waves and characteristic points

2.4 Processing and Analysis of ECG Signals

As noted, ECG signals form a source of important diagnostic information in cardiology. In order to take advantage of it, the signals have to be properly registered and processed in such a way that we can proceed with their effective analysis and interpretation (Sornmo and Laguna 2005; Acharya et al. 2007). ECG signals are quasi-periodic of relatively low amplitude of several mV. They are often affected by noise. The registration of the signal requires their amplification and further processing in order to suppress noise to highest extent. Further ECG signal analysis is realized based on these recordings for which the noise has been suppressed. The first step of the overall processing is an analog-to-digital (A/D) conversion. In the sequel the digital ECG signal is filtered to eliminate noise and further processed to enhance effectiveness of methods of feature selection, classification, and interpretation applied to the signal. Information granulation has been regarded as one of the interesting and promising alternatives with this regard; in essence the methods arising there could be sought as a certain way of realization of data compression.

An overall process of ECG signal processing and analysis comprises the following phases, refer to Fig. 2.3

Signal amplification
A/C conversion

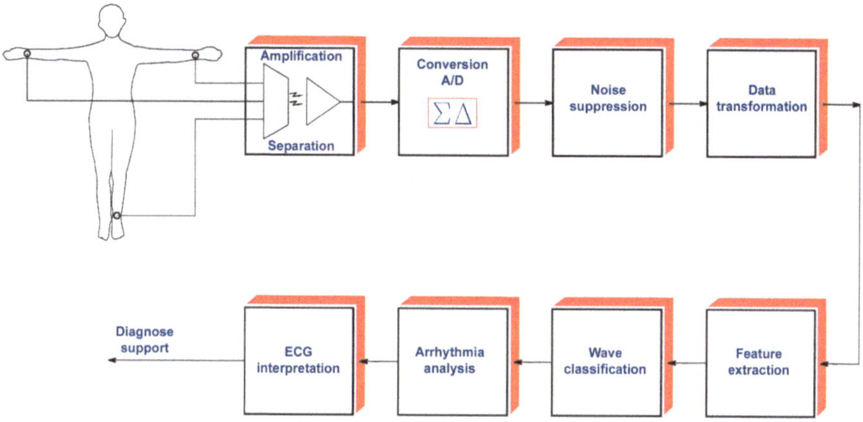

Fig. 2.3 Main phases of ECG signal processing and analysis

Noise suppression (reduction)
Data compression
Feature selection
Signal classification
Interpretation

2.4.1 Amplification of ECG Signals

Depending upon the needs, ECG signals can be registered from various parts of the body. Most commonly, the registration is realized from the skin of chest and limbs. For the needs of electrophysiological diagnostics, the signals are registered directly from the inside of atria and heart ventricles or from esophagus. Depending on the registration area, the amplitude of the signal is in the range of several μV to mV. The first step of signal processing is concerned with signal amplification under conditions of galvanic separation implied by safety requirements. In modern electrocardiographic systems, one uses signal amplifiers with galvanic separation, see (von Maltzahn and Nagel 2006). In these systems, the signal is amplified several times, typically 3–10 times. In particular applications, the ECG signal can be significantly amplified up to few hundred times. The amplifiers offer galvanic separation up to 5 kV.

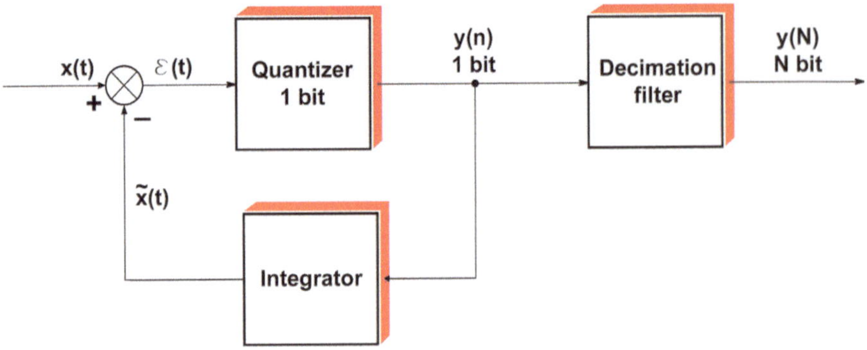

Fig. 2.4 A schematic view of the simplified 1 bit ΣΔ A/D converter

2.4.2 A/C Conversion

Once amplified, the signals are converted into its digital form. For this purpose commonly used are A/C converters of sigma-delta (ΣΔ) type of high resolution (22 bits) and a low-noise level (Stranneby 2001). These converters operate in the oversampling mode that is with the sampling frequency that significantly exceeds the one resulting from the Shannon-Nyquist sampling theorem.

Figure 2.4 illustrates a simplified scheme of a 1-bit ΣΔ A/D converter.

As shown there, the converter consists of a ΣΔ modulator combined with a decimation filter The essence of these converters comprises a rough approximation of the input signal $x(t)$, denoted here by $x^{\sim}(t)$, computation of the approximation error and its quantization. In the sequel this quantized error becomes integrated providing a new value of the approximation of the original signal.

A digital decimation filter present at the output of the A/C converter realizes three functions. It reduces a sampling frequency, increases the length of word from one to M bits, and reduces noise generated by the 1 bit ΣΔ modulator. The sampling frequency of ECG signals when the ΣΔ converters are being used is in the range of 4,000 Hz.

2.4.3 Noise Suppression

As noted earlier, ECG signals are always affected by noise. Among different types of noise, low frequency and muscle noises are the most difficult to handle.

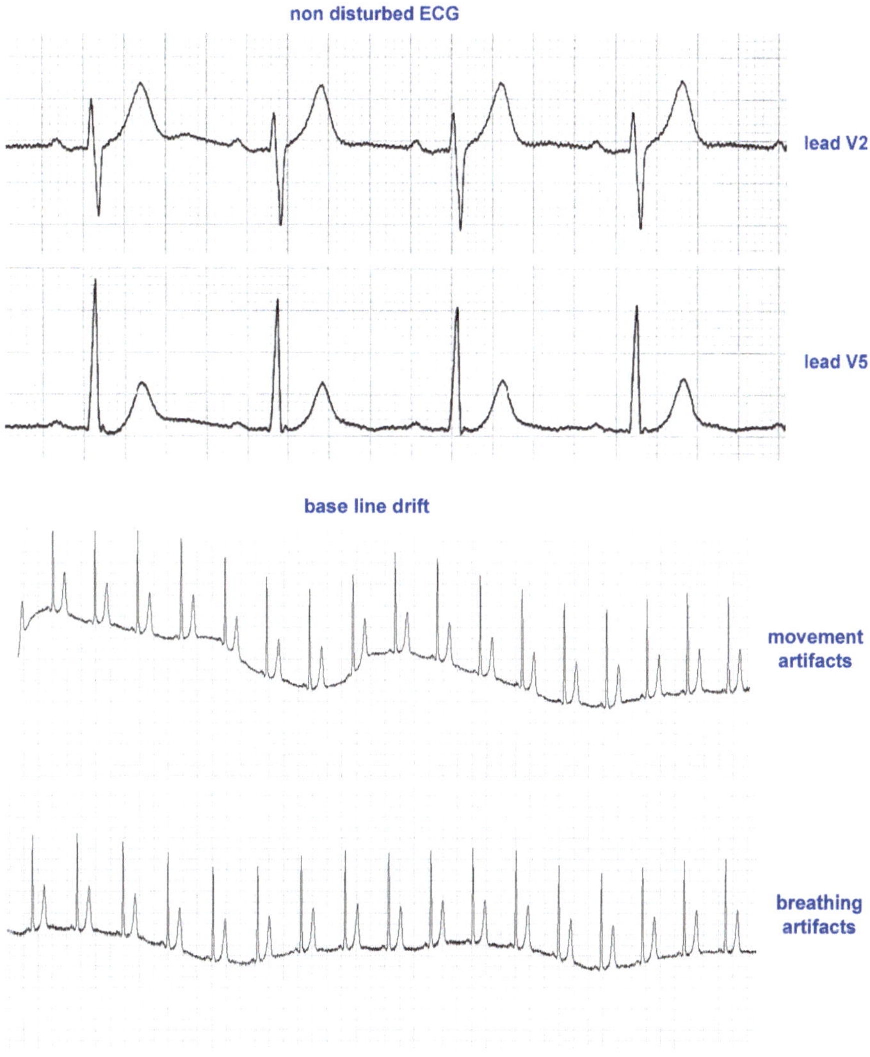

Fig. 2.5 Low frequency noise present in ECG signal

2.4.3.1 Low Frequency Noise

This noise is a result of changes of impedance between the electrode and a body of the patient. The impedance changes as a result of changes of distances between the source of signal (heart) and the electrode caused by the movement of the patient including breathing and changes of contact between the body and the electrode, which to a significant extent is caused by the movement of the body of the patient, Fig. 2.5.

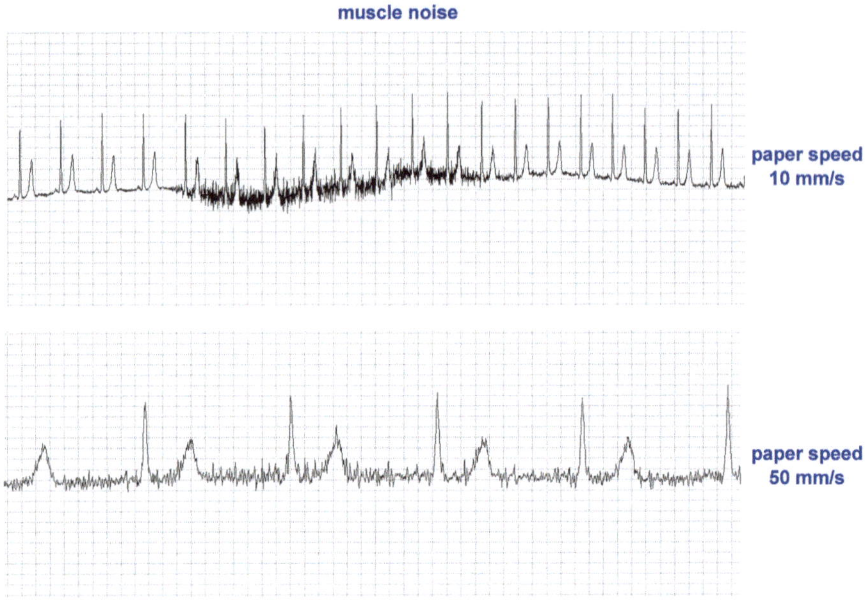

Fig. 2.6 Example of muscle noise of ECG signals

The low frequency noise is located in the frequency below 1 Hz. However, in some types of examinations, say exercise examination of ECG (Santopietro 1977; Su et al. 2007; Bailon et al. 2006), this range of frequencies is far higher and can reach the frequency of several Hz. In exercise test of ECG, the amplitude of low frequency noise becomes higher which calls for the use of more effective means of noise suppression. A similar situation appears in systems of long-term registration and monitoring of ECG signals (Holter systems).

2.4.3.2 Muscle Noise

The noise of this nature is caused by the contraction of skeletal muscles, which appear because of the movement of the patient (related with the movement or inappropriate ambient temperature in which the ECG examination is being carried out).

Muscle signals, Fig. 2.6, are always associated with ECG signals. The highest level of noise is present in stress tests. In these conditions, the noise is caused by intensive muscle contractions during running on a treadmill or the load of the patient caused by cycloergometer.

The movement of the patient is present during a long-term recording of ECG signals under normal conditions (which is present in Holter testing). In this case, the level of muscle noise depends quite significantly on a level of activity (movement) of the patient, which could vary within the testing.

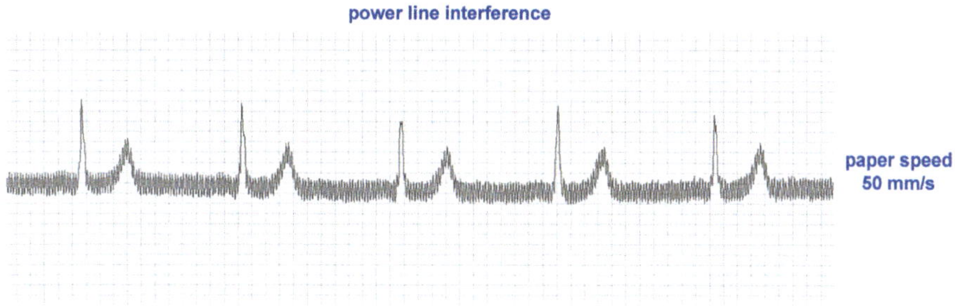

Fig. 2.7 Power line interference in ECG signal

Muscle noise becomes present in rest tests caused by involuntary contractions of skeletal muscle resulting from the ambient temperature, which could be too low or too high. This phenomenon is particularly undesirable in case of registering microvolt heart potentials, that is micropotentials recorded on the surface of the body, in the esophagus or in the heart ventricles. The main problem arises here because of the overlap of the spectrum of the signal and noise to a significant extent. The spectrum of the signal forms a range of 0.005–150 Hz whereas the noise spectrum covers the range of frequencies from 20 to 80 Hz. The attempts to filter muscle noise lead to significant distortions of the ECG signal. With the increase of the effectiveness of the muscle noise, the resulting distortions of the signal may result in incorrect classification results produced by medical doctors as well as computerized systems.

2.4.3.3 Electromagnetic Noise

The noise of this type becomes present as a result of influence of the electromagnetic field generated by power supplied to the measurement system (Fig. 2.7) or generated by other medical devices (Bruce 2000; Lin and Hu 2008).

The frequency spectrum of the power line interferences is relatively narrow and centered around the frequency of AC power supply. This noise is relatively easy to filter. For this purpose the band prohibitive filters are used with narrow frequency characteristics; the filters could be analog but most predominantly digital. An efficient way to suppress power noise is to construct registration devices in such a way so that proper shielding and noise elimination is provided.

Electromagnetic noise is also relatively easy to eliminate through band prohibitive filtering. The spectrum of this noise overlaps to a limited extent of the ECG frequencies, meaning that the required methods of noise filtering do not distort the original signal.

Among the electromagnetic noise we can distinguish noise caused by the power supplies where the amplitude of voltage and current changes with frequency of 50 or 60 Hz. In this case, we are talking about typical power supply type of noise.

The power supply could be a source of sporadic impulse-like noise. It is often caused by turning on high-power devices such as diathermy equipment, Roentgen machines, and tomography devices.

2.4.4 Data Transformation

Another important phase of the overall processing of ECG signals concerns a transformation of data (samples of signals) to some other format in order to enhance effectiveness of processing and further interpretation. In general, we can say that the transformation forms a sort of compression process. On the one hand, we reduce an amount of information to be processed and analyzed. On the other, we extract a limited number of features, which exhibit high discriminatory properties (which is of relevance in case of signal classification).

As a result of the signal transformation, the original signal can be represented in a digital format or as a series of linguistic information granules described in terms of some parameters or described in a linguistic fashion. The transformation viewed in this way is applied to on-line ECG systems, say telemedicine systems, systems for exercise test of ECG, or Holter systems.

The development of ideas and algorithms supporting the transformation of ECG signals started in the 1960s of the past century. In this period, a transformation method called AZTEC was quite popular. Following some rules, the method is aimed at the approximation of the ECG signal by a series of linear segments that are either horizontal or elevated. Since then we witness a rapid development of other methods including orthogonal transformation (Ahmed and Milne 1975), entropy coding (Ruttimann and Pibperger 1979), long-term prediction (Nave and Cohen 1993), wavelet transformations (Hilton 1997; Tai et al. 2005), SVD analysis (Kanjilal et al. 1997; Wei et al. 2001), and information granulation (Gacek and Pedrycz 2006).

2.4.5 A Detection of P-QRS-T Complex – A Region of Interest

A characteristic feature of ECG signal comes with a cyclic occurrence of its components consisting of the P-QRS-T complex. The ECG signal in this region is reflective of performance of the conduction system of the heart that pertains to a single heart evolution involving contraction of atria and ventricles. This part of the ECG signal forms a region of interest (ROI) as it contains the most essential diagnostic information. During ECG signal processing and analysis, an important task is to detect each section containing the P-QRS-T complex, refer to Fig. 2.2, and a determination ofso-called fiducial points (Sayadi and Shamsollahi 2008). These points determine the beginning and the end of location of P and T, Q, R, S, I and a location of the center of the ST interval. The most essential is the determination of the R point.

A detection of the part of the signal containing the O-QRS-T complex is realized through a detection of the most characteristic basis point of the region called FR (referred to as a centering point) that corresponds to the location of the R point in time. The time intervals between successive R points are used to determine a frequency of heart activity being one of the diagnostic indicators used in cardiology. The overall P-QRS-T complex is taken as the part of the ECG signal present in some time interval that is formed by taking n_b samples and n_f samples of the signal located before and after the location of the R point. The analysis of ECG signal in the temporal window (ROI) deals with the determination of the remaining basis points of the P-QRS-T complex.

The simplest methods of detection of the R point involve finding a sample of the signal of the highest amplitude at the point where the first derivative crosses zero or the signal exceeds a certain predetermined threshold level. Such methods, although computationally simple, are based on a single sample of the signal, which makes the method sensitive to noise. Given this, these methods are used only when dealing with noise-free signals such as those coming from rest of the examinations. Some other simple methods based on the use of three points are known as a double-level method (Rompelman et al. 1986). In this method, the centering point of $x(t)$ in the region of interest is computed as an average of two time moments t_1 and t_2 that correspond to the crossing points of the rising and falling slope of the signal determined for some level L (Rompelman et al. 1986) We obtain

$$FP = \frac{t_1 + t_2}{2},$$

where $x(t_1) = x(t_2) = L$ while the predetermined threshold level is described in the form

$$L = a \cdot \max |x(t)|.$$

Typically, the value of a is set to 0.6 (Jane et al. 1991). As presented above, the method is aimed at processing continuous signals. The discrete time version of the signal is formed by looking at the samples for which the difference between their amplitudes and the threshold L attains a minimal value. The double-level method determines the basis points FR with accuracy that is higher than the one arising from the sampling period of the signal. However, as the method is simple and lacks robustness, the result is rounded off to the closest sample.

In the literature, we encounter a number of important methods, which were proposed to detect basis points of the ECG signal, especially those present in the QRS complex. Among others, we encounter wavelet analysis (Kadambe et al. 1999; Li and Zheng 1995) and banks of filters (Afonso et al. 1999). One can also point at the methods based on slope analysis (Ahmed and Milne 1975) or the derivative analysis (Haque et al. 2002).

By a thorough analysis of the methods of the determination of the basis points, we note that there is a tendency of moving from simple methods, in which the determination of the FR point uses one or several samples of the signal to the algorithms that are more complex and where the determination of the FR point relies on the entire collection of the samples of the signal. This tendency is motivated by intent of constructing methods that are more robust to noise. Obviously, this comes with a higher computing overhead associated with the determination of the basis points. In some sense it relates with the increasing computing capabilities available today. On the other hand, we can envision that too high computing overhead might become an obstacle of using some methods. For instance, in the Holter system, when we decide to proceed with some initial preprocessing during signal acquisition in a portable registration device, the simple methods are only applicable (say, the double point method). On the other hand, if we realize the entire ECG signal analysis on a stationary Holter analyzer, we can considering using more complex methods of the determination of the centering points. Evidently, it leads to a longer analysis time or necessitates the use of computers of higher processing power.

2.4.6 Feature Extraction

The successive step of ECG signal analysis is a formation of a feature space that is a collection of descriptors that fully capture the essence of the signal. More precisely, we are interested in the features that exhibit high discriminatory power, which is of importance to any classification of ECG signals and their interpretation. Those features are mostly present in a time domain; however they could be defined in the frequency domain. It is also possible to extract features of a different nature, which relate with some unconventional features such as those exploiting methods of data approximation, data segmentation, and information granulation.

Of paramount importance are the features exhibiting some diagnostic properties. As examples, we can recall here, see Fig. 2.2,

Time intervals between consecutive R points
Distance PQ, PR, QT
Amplitudes of P, Q, R, S, T
Duration of P, R, and T waves
A location of the center of the ST interval
A slope of the ST interval.

These features, being so-called primitive features are determined directly from the ECG signal.

For diagnostic purposes extracted are also some other features, called derivative features which are constructed based on the primitive ones. For instance, we can recall here

Shift of the QRS complex versus baseline – known as offset
Areas of waves of P, R, and T
Position of the heart axis

Corrected distance Qt denoted also as Qt_c, which is determined following the Bazett equation

$$Qt_c = \frac{QT}{\sqrt{RR}}$$

where RR stands for a distance between successive R waves.

A ratio of successive intervals RR_i described as $\partial_R = \frac{RR_i}{RR_{i+1}}$.

The features of the ECG signal constructed on a basis of a shape of the signal, segments of the signal that repeat in a cyclic fashion that cover a single heart evolution, namely a P-QRS-T complex. Once classified, these complexes along with other parameters of the ECG signal form a basis for further analysis and interpretation.

2.4.7 Classification of ECG Signals

The classification of ECG signals boils down to the discrimination of P-QRS-T complexes as belonging to one of the existing classes (de Chazal et al. 2004; Evans et al. 1994; Hu et al. 1997; Osowski and Linh 2001; de Chazal and Reilly 2006). The discrimination is mostly based on an analysis of the shape of the QRS complex itself. At the same time considered is also a location of the waves P and T relative to the QRS complex and a location of the successive QRS complexes. In classification, the following features come with significant discriminatory properties.

Shape of the QRS complex expressed in terms of its width, shape, and a slope of the R wave

Lengths of intervals within the P-QRS-T complex

Length of the RR interval

At this level, we distinguish between the following main classes of P-QRS-T complexes

- Ventricular complexes VC,
- Supraventricular complexes SVC,
- Premature ventricular complexes PVC,
- Premature supraventricular complexes PSVC,
- Myocardial infarct complexes MIC, wide QRS complexes with the elevation of the ST segment, and upside down T wave,
- WPW complexes, characteristic of Wolf Parkinson White syndrome – wide QRS complex with the characteristic deviation from the increasing slope – so-called delta wave.

The P-QRS-T identified in the classification of ECG signals form a basis for analysis of the heart rhythm disturbances, which is the next phase of ECG signal processing.

2.4.8 *An Analysis of Rhythm Disturbances*

The objective of the ECG testing is an identification of heart dysfunctions and an identification of their causes. The essence of these testing relies on the assessment of the functioning of the heart. During such testing carried out is an analysis of the changes of some essential cardiac parameters of diagnostic nature. The most generic is the analysis of the heart rhythm disturbances. The rhythm disturbances are associated with abnormalities of action of the stimuli generation system of the heart or with abnormal conduction of these stimuli. In the first case, there are the heart rhythm disturbances, and in the second one we are concerned with the heart conduction disturbances. (Dubin 2000; Hampton 2003).

These abnormalities can be classified as follows:

- Irregular rhythms,
- Substitute rhythms,
- Premature stimulations,
- Tachyarhytmies.

These deviations in the conductance of electrical impulses in the heart muscle manifest in so-called heart blocks (Hampton 2003) which block conductance of a depolarization wave. These blocks could concern sinus node, atrioventricular, or main branches of the electrical conduction system of the ventricles. Here we distinguish the following main categories of conduction disturbance (Dubin 2000):

- Sinus blocks,
- Atrio blocks,
- His bundle branch blocks,
- Hemiblocks (infarct blocks).

In this analysis, an important role is played by the changes in the Heart Rate Variability (HRV) (Acharya et al. 2007; Almeida et al. 2006). Here one analyzes the changes of the time intervals between successive R waves (RR interval). During normal human activities, the length of distances RR varies. The rhythm frequency and the variability of changes in successive heart evolution to a significant extent is reflective of the influence of the autonomic system on electrical activity of the sinus node. The quantitative assessment of the heart rhythm variability is an indirect indicator of the activity of the autonomic system (T.F. of the ESC/ASPE 1996).

In recent years one can note an increasing interest in the development of methods of analysis of heart rhythm disturbances (Almeida et al. 2006; Mateo and Laguna 2000).

2.4.9 *Interpretation of ECG Signals*

Interpretation constitutes a final stage of the overall process of signal processing of ECG signals realized in electrocardiographic systems. The objective is to understand the results of the ECG testing and offer an interpretation in order to provide diagnosis and consider further testing. The final interpretation is always realized by the specialist so the computer system provides a decision-support environment. The currently available systems embrace this phase of the overall analysis by focusing on data understanding (Boudreau Conover 2002; Gertsch 2003; Kowalak and Turkington 2007; Lippincott Williams & Wilkins 2005), quite often exploiting the technology of Computational Intelligence. In this phase of interpretation (Alesanco and García 2008; Skillmasters 2006; Lippincott Williams & Wilkins 2005) not only the results of ECG tests are considered but they are augmented by results of other tests as well as personal data of the patient.

Processing of ECG data associated with the interpretation process is often realized in the setting of expert systems. In this case, formulated is a certain diagnostic hypothesis concerning a heart status. This hypothesis must be verified by a cardiologist. In spite of this, to a significant extent the automatic interpretation of ECG signals can support medical diagnosis. The level of the improvement associated with this depends upon the effectiveness of the processing methods applied to ECG signals.

2.5 Categories of ECG Tests

ECG tests are the generic tests used to assess functioning of the heart muscle reflected by the ECG signal measured at different points of the body. Depending on the location area, we distinguish among the main ECG tests:

- Invasive – recording of ECG inside or on heart surface,
- Semi-invasive – recording of ECG in oesophagus,
- Nonivasive – recording of ECG on the body, mainly on the chest.

Likewise, ECG tests can be also classified as routine ones and those of specialized nature. The routine ECG tests could be further classified depending upon a way in which the tests were administered. We have the following categories:

- Rest ECG examination – multi-lead ECG recording in rest state,
- Exercise ECG examination – multi-lead ECG recording in exercise state (patient is loaded by means of cycloergometer or treadmill),
- Holter ECG recording and monitoring – several-lead ECG recording in normal life conditions,
- Spatial ECG recording – vectocardiography – orthogonal-lead ECG recording,
- Mapping of heart – multi-channel ECG recording on the heart muscle or on the Chest.

Similarly, in case of the specialized ECG tests we can offer a classification depending upon a leading electrocardiographic parameter, which is subject to analysis in order to detect some irregularities in heart functioning. In this case we identify the following categories of tests:

- Heart micropotentials analysis – high resolution electrocardiography,
- Sinus rhythm variability analysis – HRV analysis,
- Heart rhythm disturbances analysis – arrhythmia analysis,
- Baroreflex examination –.BRS (Baroreflex Sensitivity),
- Repolarization analysis – analysis of QT segment duration and dispersion,
- Microvolt T wave variability analysis – alternation of T wave (T-wave afternans TWA).

The specialized ECG tests come with their own specificity which means that the diagnostic information is conveyed in quite limited changes of parameters, either specified in time or frequency domain. The detection of changes in these parameters in a noisy ECG signal becomes a difficult task. Practically, its direct identification realized by a cardiologist is impossible; it can be done based on the registered ECG signal.

The required diagnostic information in case of such specialized ECG tests is obtained through running advanced algorithms. In particular, this concerns problems dealing with noise suppression and a precise determination of the basis points.

In what follows, we discuss some specific tests in detail.

2.5.1 Analysis of Heart Micropotentials LVP

This is a high-resolution analysis of ECG signals. This test is aimed at the assessment of potential threat of occurrence of ventricle frequent contraction. In this case, of particular interest are late heart potentials LVP (Narayanaswamy 2002). By LVP one means irregular (up to 25 mV) meshed waves of the extended QRS complex obtained as a result of averaging hundreds of correlated QRS complexes. These complexes are registered at high sampling frequency (2,000–4,000) Hz and at high amplification (5,000–40,000). The occurrence of late potentials in patients after heart attack forms an independent indicator of a danger of permanent frequent ventricle contraction, which leads to the sudden heart arrest. In this case, an analysis of an average QRS complex can be realized in a time domain (Simpson method), frequency domain (Fourier analysis), or in time–frequency domain (say, through autoregressive time series modeling or through a generalized Wigner transformation).

In the analysis of the late ventricle potentials, the Simpson method is the standard one. It is based on the analysis of a vector S formed on a basis of the three orthogonal leads X, Y, Z.

$$S = \sqrt{X^2 + Y^2 + Z^2}$$

referred to as a filtered QRS complex or a Simpson vector (Simson 1981).

2.5.2 *Microvolt Variability of T Wave (T-Wave Alternans TWA)*

The analysis of the microvolt variability of the T wave (Monasterio et al. 2009) is a non-invasive diagnostic test done to detect threats of the sudden heart arrest. These tests are realized for patients after heart attack and other serious damages of heart muscle or for which there is a danger of serious disturbances of heart rhythm. The testing of the microvolt variability of the T wave (repolarization variability) is based on the testing of the changes of the vector and amplitude of the T wave present in the ECG signal. The changes alternate and its magnitude is low (expressed in mV). This test is of high resolution and like the analysis of heart microptentials it calls for highly specialized methods of signal analysis.

2.5.3 *Analysis of Variability of Sinus Rhythm HRV*

This testing is concerned about an analysis of the changes of heart rhythm. This analysis helps us evaluate the quality of the autonomic heart control system. The autonomic nervous system controlling functioning of the heart consists of sympathetic and parasympathetic systems. These two systems work in two opposite directions with regard to the frequency of heart action, controlling it depending upon the existing situation. The heart rhythm is increased when there is an increasing activity of the sympathetic system. When the activity of the parasympathetic system increases, the heart rhythm decreases. In a healthy individual, there exist some fluctuations of the rhythm within the bounds of the adaptation. However under certain stimulus (say, alcohol, nicotine, some medications) and as a consequence of some diseases (for instance, infarct of myocardium, diabetes second type, failure of kidneys), the adjustment of the heart rhythm is made difficult and the variability is significantly reduced (Acharya et al. 2006; Almeida et al. 2004; T.F. of the ESC/ASPE 1996).

The analysis of the variability of heart rhythm reduces to the analysis of changes of the length of RR distances for QRS complexes of sinus origin. An essential component of the analysis is a precise localization of the peaks of the R waves.

The analysis of RR distances (RR periods) is done in a time domain, frequency domain by utilizing methods of time–frequency analysis or other nonlinear methods (Acharya et al. 2006; Sornmo and Laguna 2005; T.F. of the ESC/ASPE 1996).

2.6 Conclusions

ECG signals are electrical signals generated and conducted by cells of the heart muscle. They offer valuable diagnostic information about the functioning of the heart and, indirectly, other organs. The nature and properties of ECG signals have been a subject of intensive study for over 100 years. The ECG signals, even though they are the most recognized biomedical signals, are still a subject of intensive research both in the realm of cardiology as well as biomedical engineering. Cardiologists are interested in the diagnostic properties of ECG signal while at the engineering end the interest lies in the processing and analysis of such signals. As a result, there is an emergence of new medical technology exploiting ECG signals. The specific properties of these signals, as discussed in the chapter, give rise to a number of challenges in the signal acquisition, processing, analysis, which definitely exacerbate a way in which the diagnostic information becomes obtained.

ECG signals are nonstationary, susceptible to noise, and exhibit a high variability. They are a source of imprecise information. All of these imply that the processing and analysis of ECG signals calls for the use of effective methods of signal processing that can function given all the limitations outlined above. In particular, this concerns techniques of noise suppression, efficient signal representation, and feature extraction.

There is no doubt that in this area in the recent years the technology of Computational Intelligence has played a visible role. We can envision that it will be even more instrumental in the future.

References

Aaronson, P.I., Ward, J.P., Wiener C.M.: The Cardiovascular System at a Glance, Blackwell Publishing Ltd. (2004)

Acharya, U.R., Joseph, K.P., Kannathal, N., Lim, C.M., Suri, J.S.: Heart rate variability: a review. Med. Biol. Eng. Comput. **44**, 1031–1051 (2006)

Acharya, U.R., Suri, J.S., Spaan, J.A.E., Krishan,S.M.: Advances in Cardiac Signal Processing. Springer, Berlin (2007)

Afonso, V.X., Tompkins, W.J., Nguyen, T.Q., Luo, S.: ECG beat detection using filter banks. IEEE Trans. Biomed. Eng. **46**(2), 192–202 (1999)

Ahmed, N., Milne, P.I.: Electrocardiographic data compression via orthogonal transforms. IEEE Trans. Biomed. Eng. **BME-22**, 484–487 (1975)

Alesanco, A., García, J.: Automatic real-time ECG coding methodology guaranteeing signal interpretation quality. IEEE Trans. Biomed. Eng. **55**(11), 2519–2527 (2008)

Almeida, R., Pueyo, E., Martínez, J.P., Rocha, A.P., Laguna, P.: Quantification of the QT variability related to HRV: robustness study facing automatic delineation and noise on the ECG. Comput. Cardiol. **31**, 769–772 (2004)

Almeida, R., Gouveia, S., Rocha, A.P., Pueyo, E., Martínez, J.P., Laguna, P.: QT variability and HRV interactions in ECG: quantification and reliability. IEEE Trans. Biomed. Eng. **53**(7), 1317–1329 (2006)

Bailon, R., Sornmo, L., Laguna, P.: A robust method for ECG-based estimation of the respiratory frequency during stress testing. IEEE Trans. Biomed. Eng. **53**(7), 1273–1285 (2006)

Barro, S., Fernandez-Delgado, M., Regueiro, J.A., Sanchez, E.: Classifying multichannel ECG patterns with an adaptive neural network. IEEE Eng. Med. Biol. Mag. **17**(1), 45–55 (1998)

Berbari, E.J., Bock, E.A., Cházaro, A.C., Sun, X., Sörnmo, L.: High-resolution analysis of ambulatory electrocardiograms to detect possible mechanism of premature ventircular beats. IEEE Trans. Biomed. Eng. **52**(4), 593–599 (2005)

Bortolan, G., Pedrycz, W.: Fuzzy descriptive models: an interactive framework of information granulation. IEEE Trans. Fuzzy Syst. **10**(6), 743–755 (2002a)
Bortolan, G., Pedrycz,W.: An interactive framework for an analysis of ECG signals. Artif. Intell. Med. **24**, 109–132 (2002b)
Botter,E., Nascimento, C.L., Yoneyama, T.: A neural network with asymmetric basis function for feature extraction of ECG P waves. IEEE Trans. Neural Netw. **12**(5), 1252–1255 (2001)
Boudreau Conover, M.: Understanding Electrocardiography. Elsevier Health Sciences, St. Louis (2002)
Bruce, E.N.: Biomedical Signal Processing and Signal Modeling. Wiley, New York (2000)
de Chazal, P., Reilly, R.B.: A patient-adapting heartbeat classifier using ECG morphology and heartbeat interval features. IEEE Trans. Biomed. Eng. **53**(12), 2535–2543 (2006)
de Chazal, P., O'Dwyer, M., Reilly, R.: Automatic classification of heartbeats using ECG morphology and heartbeat interval features. IEEE Trans. Biomed. Eng. **51**(7), 1196–1206 (2004)
Chowdhury, E., Ludeman, L.C.: Discrimination of cardiac arrhythmias using a fuzzy rule-based method. In: The Proceedings of the Conference Computers in Cardiology, 25–28 September, pp. 549–552. Bethesda, USA (1994)
Cox, J.R., Nolle, F.N., Fozzard, H.A., Oliver, G.C.: AZTEC preprocessing program for real-time ECG rhythm analysis. IEEE Trans. Biomed. Eng. **BME-15**, 128–129 (1968)
Cremer,M.: Üeber die Direkte Ableitung der Aktionsstrome des Menslichen Herzensvom Oesophagus uber das Elecktrokardiogram des Fotus. Munch, Med. Wochr. **53**, 811 (1906)
Czogala, E., Leski, J.: Application of entropy and energy measure of fuzziness to processing of ECG signal. Fuzzy Sets Syst. **97**(1), 9–18 (1998)
Czogala, E., Leski, J.: Entropy and energy measures of fuzziness in ECG signal processing. W monografii. In: Szczepaniak, P.S., Lisboa, P.J.G., Kacprzyk, J. (eds.) Fuzzy Systems in Medicine, pp. 227–245. Physica-Verlag, Springer-Verlag Com., Heidelberg, New York (2000).
Czogala, E., Leski, J.: Fuzzy and Neuro-Fuzzy Intelligent Systems. Physica-Verlag, Springer-Verlag Com., Heidelberg, New York (2000)
Dubin, D.: Rapid interpretation of EKG's, 6th ed. Cover Inc., Tampa (2000)
Evans, S., Hastings, H., Bodenheimer, M.: Differentiation of beats of ventricular and sinus origin using a self-training neural network. PACE **17**, 611–626 (1994)
Fernandez-Chimeno, M., Quilez, M., Silva, F.: Understanding electrosurgical unit perturbations in order to address hospital operating room electromagnetic compatibility. IEEE Trans. Biomed. Eng. **53**(6), 1205–1207 (2006)
Gacek, A., Pedrycz, W.: A genetic segmentation of ECG signals. IEEE Trans. Biomed. Eng. **50**(10), 1203–1208 (2003)
Gacek, A., Jeżewski, J.: Representation of ECG signals using the segmentation technique. Biocybern. Biomed. Eng. **23**(4), 33–43 (2003a)
Gacek, A., Jeżewski, J.: w-FCM: clustering with weights and its application to ECG signal analysis. Polish J. Med. Phys. Eng. **9**(2), 931–941 (2003b)
Gacek,A., Pedrycz, W.: Logic characterization and classification of ECG signals. In: Leonides, C.T. (ed.) Medical Imaging Systems Technology. Methods in Cardiovascular and Brain Systems, pp. 183–206. World Scientific, Hackensack/London (2005)
Gacek, A., Pedrycz, W.: A granular description of ECG signals. IEEE Trans. Biomed. Eng. **53**(10), 1972–1982 (2006)
Gertsch, M.: The ECG: A Two-Step Approach to Diagnosis. Springer, New York (2003)
Hampton, J.R.: The ECG in Practice, 4th edn. Elsevier Science Limited, Oxford, United Kingdom (2003)
Haque, M.A., Rahman, M.E., Sayeed, C.A.A., Uddin, B.M.Z.: A fast algorithm in detecting ECG characteristic points. Proceedings of the ICECE, Dhaka, pp. 160–163 (2002)
Hilton, M.L.: Wavelet and wavelet packet compression of electrocardiograms. IEEE Trans. Biomed. Eng. **394**(May), 402–444 (1997)
Horowitz, S.: A syntactic algorithm for peak detection in waveforms with applications to cardiography. CACM **18**(5), 281–285 (1975)

Hu, Y., Palreddy, S., Tompkins, W.J.: A patient-adaptable ECG beat classifier using a mixture of experts approach. IEEE Trans. Biomed. Eng. **44**(9), 891–900 (1997)

Huang, B., Wang, Y., Chen, J.: 2-D compression of ECG signals using ROI mask and conditional entropy coding. IEEE Trans. Biomed. Eng. **56**(4), 1261–1263 (2009)

Iwata, A., Y. Nagasaka, Suzumura, N.: Data compression of the ECG using neural network for digital Holter monitor. IEEE Eng. Med. Biol. Mag. **9**(3), 53–57 (1990)

Jane, R., Rix, H., Caminal, P., Laguna, P.: Alignment methods for averaging of high-resolution cardiac signals: a comparative study of performance. IEEE Trans. Biomed. Eng. **38**(6), 571–579 (1991)

Jesus, S., Rix, H.: High resolution ECG analysis by an improved signal averaging method and comparison with a beat-to-beat approach. J. Biomed. Eng. **10**, 25–32 (1986)

Kadambe, S., Murray, R., Boudreaux-Bartels, G.: Wavelet transform-based QRS complex detector. IEEE Trans. Biomed. Eng. **46**(7), 838–848 (1999)

Kanjilal, P.P., Palit, S., Saha, G.: Fetal ECG extraction from single-channel maternal ECG using singular value decomposition. IEEE Trans. Biomed. Eng. **44**(1), 51–59 (1997)

Kowalak, J.L., Turkington, C.: Lippincott Manual of Nursing Practice series: ECG Interpretation. Lippincott Williams & Wilkins, Ambler (2007)

Köhler, B.U., Hennig, C., Orglmeister, R.: The principles of software QRS detection. IEEE Eng. Med. Biol. Mag. **21**(Jan.–Feb.), 42–57 (2002)

Kundu, M., Nasipuri, M., Basu, D.K.: A reasoning system for on-line interpretation of ECG signal. TENCON'93, Beijing, pp. 827–838 (1993)

Kundu, M., Nasipuri, M., Basu, D.K.: A knowledge based approach to ECG interpretation using fuzzy logic. IEEE Trans. Syst. Man Cybern. – Part B Cybern. **28**(2), 237–243 (1998)

Kundu, M., Nasipuri, M., Basu, D.K.: Knowledge-based ECG interpretation: a critical review. Pattern Recognit. **33**, 351–373 (2000)

Lee, R.G., Chol, I.C., Lai, C.C., Liu, M.H., Chiu, M.J.: A novel QRS detection algorithm applied to the analysis for heart rate variability of patients with sleep apnea. J. Biomed. Eng. Appl. Basis & Commun. **17**(Oct.), 258–262 (2005)

Lewandowski, P., Meste, O., Maniewski, R., Mroczka, T., Steinbach, K., Rix, H.: Risk evaluation of ventricular tachycardia using wavelet transform irregularity of the high-resolution electrocardiogram. Med. Biol. Eng. Comput. **38**, 666–673 (2000)

Li, C., Zheng, C.: Tai: detection of ECG characteristic points using wavelet transforms. IEEE Trans. Biomed. Eng. **42**(1), 21–28 (1995)

Lin, Y.-D., Hu, Y.H.: Power-line interference detection and suppression in ECG signal processing. IEEE Trans. Biomed. Eng. **55**(1), 354–357 (2008)

Linh,T.H., Osowski, S., Stodolski, M.: On-line heart beat recognition using Hermite polynomials and neuro-fuzzy network. IEEE Trans. Instrum. Meas. **52**(4), 1224–1231 (2003)

Lippincott Williams & Wilkins: Interpreting Difficult ECGs: A Rapid Reference. Lippincott Williams & Wilkins, Philadelphia (2005)

Leski, J., Henzel, N.: A new fuzzy method for high-resolution localization of ECG waves. Proceedings of the FUZZ-IEEE, Seoul, pp 154–157 (1999a)

Leski, J., Henzel, N.: Biomedical signal averaging with highly-quantized weights. Proceeding of the IEEE-EMBS, Atlanta, p. 428 (1999b)

von Maltzahn, W.W., Nagel, J.H.: Chapter 52: Biopotential amplifiers. In: Bronzino, J.D. (ed.) Medical Devices and Systems. CRC Press, Hartford (2006)

Maniewski, R.: High resolution electrocardiography measurement and analysis. Biocybern. Biomed. Eng. **20**(1), 5–17 (2000)

Mateo, J., Laguna, P.: Improved heart rate variability signal analysis from the beat occurrence times according to the IPFM model. IEEE Trans. Biomed. Eng. **47**(8), 985–996 (2000)

Monasterio, V., Laguna, P., Martínez, J.P.: Multilead analysis of T-wave alternans in the ECG using principal component analysis. IEEE Trans. Biomed. Eng. **56**(7), 1880–1890 (2009)

Moon, B.S., Lee, H.C., Lee, Y.H., Park, J.C., Oh, I.S., Lee, J.W.: Fuzzy systems to process ECG and EEG signals for quantification of mental workload. Inform. Sci. **142**(1–4), 23–35 (2002)

Mroczka, T., Lewandowski, P., Maniewski, R., Liebert, A., Spioch, M., Steinbach, K.: Effectiveness of high resolution ECG spectral analysis in discrimination of patients prone to ventricular tachycardia and fibrillation. Med. Sci. Monit. **6**(5), 1018–1026 (2000)

Narayanaswamy, S.: High resolution electrocardiography. Indian Pacing Electrocardiography J. **2**, 50–56 (2002)

Nave, G., Cohen, A.: ECG compression using long-term prediction. IEEE Trans. Biomed. Eng. **40**(9), 877–885 (1993)

Osowski, S., Linh, T.: ECG beat recognition using fuzzy hybrid neural network. IEEE Trans. Biomed. Eng. **48**(11), 1265–1271 (2001)

Papakonstantinou, G., Skordolakis, E., Gritazali, F.: A attribute grammar for QRS detection. Pattern Recognit. **19**, 297–303 (1986)

Papakonstantinou, G., Gritazali, F.: Syntactic filtering of ECG waveforms. Comput. Biomed. Res. **14**, 158–167 (1981)

Pawar, T., Anantakrishnan, N.S., Chaudhuri, S., Duttagupta, S.P.: Transition detection in body movement activities for wearable ECG. IEEE Trans. Biomed. Eng. **54**(6), 1149–1153 (2007a)

Pawar, T., Chaudhuri, S., Duttagupta, S.P.: Body movement activity recognition for ambulatory cardiac monitoring. IEEE Trans. Biomed. Eng. **54**(5), 874–883 (2007b)

Pedrycz, W., Gacek, A.: Learning of fuzzy automata. Int. J. Comput. Intell. Appl. **1**(1), 19–33 (2001a)

Pedrycz, W., Gacek, A.: Information granulation and signal quantization. Kybernetes **30**(2), 179–192 (2001b)

Pedrycz, W., Gacek, A.: Temporal granulation and its application to signal analysis. Inform. Sci. **143**, 47–71 (2002)

Pedrycz, W., Vasilakos, A.V., Gacek, A.: Information granulation for concept formation. Proceedings of ACM Symposium on Applied Computing, vol. 1, 19–21 March 2000, Villa Como, pp. 484–489 (2000)

Piętka E.: Feature extraction in computerized approach to the ECG analysis. Pattern Recognit. **24**, 139–146 (1991)

Rangayyan, R.M.: Biomedical Signal Analysis. A Case-Study Approach. IEEE Press, Wiley-Interscience, John Wiley & Sons, Inc. (2002)

Rompelman, O., Janssen, R.J., Koeleman, A.S.M., Van Der Akker, T.J., Ros, H.H.: Practical limitations for the estimation of P-wave and QRS-complex occurrence times. Automedica **6**, 269–284 (1986)

Ruttimann, U.E., Pibperger, H.V.: Compression of the ECG by prediction or interpolation and entropy encoding. IEEE Trans. Biomed. Eng. **BME-26**(11), 613–623 (1979)

Santopietro, R.F.: The origin and characterization of the primary signal, noise, and interference sources in the high frequency electrocardiogram. Proc. IEEE **65**(5), 707–713 (1977)

Sayadi, O., Shamsollahi, M.B.: Model-based fiducial points extraction for baseline wandered electrocardiograms. IEEE Trans. Biomed. Eng. **55**(1), 347–351 (2008)

Silipo, R., Marchesi, C.: Artificial neural networks for automatic ECG analysis. IEEE Trans. Acoustics Speech Signal Process. **46**(5), 1417–1425 (1998)

Silipo, R., Bortolan, G., Marchesi, C.: Design of hybrid architectures based on neural classifier and RBF pre-processing for ECG analysis. Int. J. Approx. Reason. **21**(2), 177–196 (1999)

Simson, M.B.: Use of signals in the terminal QRS complex to identify patients with ventricular tachycardia after myocardial infarction. Circulation **64**, 235–242 (1981)

Skillmasters: Expert ECG Interpretation. Skillmasters Series. Lippincott Williams & Wilkins, Philadelphia (2006)

Skordolakis, E.: Syntactic ECG pattern processing: a review. Pattern Recognit. **19**(4), 305–313 (1986)

Sornmo, L., Laguna, P. Biomedical Signal Processing in Cardiac and Neurological Applications, Biomedical Engineering. Academic Press, New York (2005)

Stockman, G.C., Kanal, L.N.: Problem reduction representation for the linguistic analysis of waveforms. IEEE Trans. Pattern Anal. Mach. Intell. **5**(3), 287–298 (1983)

Stranneby, D.: Digital Signal Processing: DSP and Applications. Elsevier Inc., Burlington (2001)

Su, S.W., Wang, L., Celler, B.G., Savkin, A.V., Guo, Y.: Identification and control for heart rate regulation during treadmill exercise. IEEE Trans. Biomed. Eng. **54**(7), 1238–1246 (2007)

Suzuki, Y.: Self-organizing QRS-wave recognition in ECG using neural networks. IEEE Trans. Neural Netw. **6**(6), 1469–1477 (1995)

Tai, S.C., Sun, C.C., Tan, W.C.: 2-D ECG compression method based on wavelet transform and modified SPIHT. IEEE Trans. Biomed. Eng. **52**(6), 999–1008 (2005)

T.F. of the ESC/ASPE: Heart rate variability: standards of measurement, physiological interpretation, and clinical use. Eur. Heart J. **17**, 354–381 (1996)

Trahanias, P., Skordolakis, E.: Syntactic pattern recognition of the ECG. IEEE Trans. Pattern Anal. Mach. Intell. **12**(7), 648–657 (1990)

Udupa, K., Murphy, I.S.N.: Syntactic approach to ECG rhythm analysis. IEEE Trans. Biomed. Eng. **27**(7), 425–430 (1980)

Wang, J.T., Sehmi, A.S., Jones, N.B., Bono, D.P.: A knowledge-based systems for qualitative ECG simulation and ECG analysis. In: The Proceedings of the Conference Computers in Cardiology, 25–28 September 1994, pp. 733–736. Bethesda, USA (1991)

Wang, Y., Zhu, Y., Thakor, N.V., Xu, Y.: A short-time multifractal approach for arrhythmia detection based on fuzzy neural network. IEEE Trans. Biomed. Eng. **48**(9), 989–995 (2001)

Wei, J.J., Chang, C.J., Chou, N.K., Jan,G.J.: ECG data compression using truncated singular value decomposition. IEEE Trans. Biomed. Eng. **290**(Dec.), 299–295 (2001)

Wiese, S.R., Anheier, P., Connemara, R.D., Mollner, A.T., Neils, T.F., Khan, J.A., Webster, J.G.: Electrocardiographic motion artifact versus electrode impedance. IEEE Trans. Biomed. Eng. **52**(1), 136–139 (2005)

Wu, S., Qian, Y., Gao, Z., Lin, J.: A novel method for beat-to-beat detection of ventricular late potentials. IEEE Trans. Biomed. Eng. **48**(8), 931–935 (2001)

Xue, Q., Hu, Y.H., Tompkins, W.J.: Neural-network-based adaptive matched filtering for QRS detection. IEEE Trans. Biomed. Eng. **39**(4), 317–329 (1992)

Xue, Q., Reddy, B.R.: Late potentials recognition by artificial neural networks. IEEE Trans. Biomed. Eng. **44**(2), 132–143 (1997)

Chapter 3
ECG Signal Analysis, Classification, and Interpretation: A Framework of Computational Intelligence

Adam Gacek and Witold Pedrycz

3.1 Introduction

There has been a significant number of various information technologies applied to ECG signal analysis, interpretation, and classification. Along with the steady progress of hardware, new more advanced algorithmic developments have been reported upon. There are several compelling reasons behind this progress, which mainly results from the exposure to the challenges inherently associated with the domain of ECG signal processing, analysis, and interpretation:

- ECG signals are one of the most important sources of diagnostic information. Their proper acquisition and processing provide an indispensible vehicle to support medical diagnosis. Acquired signals are affected by noise and call for advanced filtering techniques.
- A description and classification of ECG signals call for nonlinear mechanisms producing a suitable set of features (descriptors) of the signal so that the ensuing classifiers come with significant discriminatory capabilities. We witness a great deal of various ways used to describe ECG signals followed by a numerous classifiers.
- It is expected that any computerized interpretation of ECG signals has to be user-friendly, meaning that the results of classification/interpretation could be easily comprehended by a human user. This requirement calls for an effective way of dealing with knowledge acquisition and knowledge manipulation when working with numeric signals.

A. Gacek (✉)
Institute of Medical Technology and Equipment, Zabrze, Poland
e-mail: adamg@itam.zabrze.pl

W. Pedrycz
Department of Electrical & Computer Engineering, University of Alberta, Edmonton, Canada and Systems Research Institute Polish Academy of Sciences, Warsaw, Poland
e-mail: pedrycz@ece.ualberta.ca

A. Gacek and W. Pedrycz (eds.), *ECG Signal Processing, Classification and Interpretation: A Comprehensive Framework of Computational Intelligence*,
DOI 10.1007/978-0-85729-868-3_3, © Springer-Verlag London Limited 2012

Quite often these problems are intertwined and need to be dealt with in a holistic manner. We notice that some of them (preprocessing, filtering) require advanced nonlinear processing techniques while the others (interpretation) call for knowledge-oriented techniques. Altogether, a comprehensive methodological and algorithmic environment, which is offered by Computational Intelligence, comes as a viable alternative.

In this study, we discuss the main conceptual, methodological, and algorithmic pillars of Computational Intelligence (CI), identify their main features and elaborate on their role in signal processing.

To a significant extent, the content of this study is self-contained and the most essential ideas are elaborated on from scratch. The reader can benefit from some introductory knowledge of the subject matter on neural networks, fuzzy sets, and evolutionary computing; see, for instance Pedrycz (1997), Pedrycz and Gomide (2007). The presentation is delivered in a top-down approach. We start with some methodological aspects of the individual technologies of Computational Intelligence, highlighting their main features and stressing the essential advantages and limitations. Furthermore we show that the three main technologies of CI are naturally inclined to form useful synergistic linkages. Practical insights identifying advantages and possible limitations of these technologies are carefully addressed. Information granularity and processing information granules arise as an important component of CI by forming the front- and back-ends of its constructs. We elaborate on these important analysis and design aspects in Sect. 3.4 including a study on information granularity used in signal representation. The design of information granules regarded as semantically sound abstractions is discussed as well. Here we discuss ways where not only numeric data – experimental evidence is taken into account but various tidbits of domain knowledge are also used in the formation of information granules.

As far as the notation is concerned, we follow the symbols being in common usage. Patterns (data) $\boldsymbol{x}_1, \boldsymbol{x}_2, \ldots, \boldsymbol{x}_N$ are treated as vectors located in n-dimensional space $\boldsymbol{R}^n$, $||.||$ is used to denote a distance (Euclidean, Mahalanobis, Hamming, Tchebyshev, etc.). Fuzzy sets will be described by capital letters; the same notation is being used for their membership functions. Class labels will be denoted by $\omega_1, \omega_2, \ldots$, etc. while the corresponding sets of integers will be described as $\boldsymbol{K} = \{1,2,\ldots,K\}, \boldsymbol{N} = \{1,2,\ldots,N\}$, etc.

3.2 Neural Networks and Neurocomputing

There exists an immensely vast body of literature on neural networks. Neural networks are viewed as highly versatile distributed architectures realizing a concept of universal approximation (Wassermann 1989; Haykin 1999), which offer a very much attractive feature of approximating nonlinear (continuous) mappings to any desired level of accuracy and in this way supporting various classification tasks.

The two main taxonomies encountered in neurocomputing concern: (a) topologies of networks and (b) a variety of ways of their development (training) schemes.

Table 3.1 Neurocomputing: advantages and limitations along with some design guidelines

Advantages	Universal approximation capabilities
	Significant learning abilities, a large repository of algorithms, well-developed and validated training methods
	Distributed processing
	Potential for significant fault tolerance
	Efficient realizations of networks
Limitations	Black-box architectures (require effort to interpret constructed networks)
	Mostly gradient-based learning with all limitations associated with this type of learning
	Non-repetitive results of learning of the networks (depending upon initial learning condition, parameters of the learning algorithm, etc.)
	Slow, inefficient learning in presence of high-dimensional and large data sets

With regard to the first coordinate of the taxonomy, one looks at a way in which individual neurons are arranged together into successive layers and a way in which processing is realized by the network, namely being of feedforward or feedback format. Typically, within the spectrum of learning scenarios one distinguishes between supervised learning and unsupervised learning; however there are a number of interesting learning schemes, which fall in-between these two extreme positions (say, learning with partial supervision, proximity-based learning, etc.).

One needs to be aware of some limitations of neural networks that start manifesting in practical scenarios (those drawbacks might be alleviated to some extent but it is unlikely they will vanish completely). From the perspective of practice of neural networks, we compiled a list of advantages and shortcomings of neurocomputing; refer to Table 3.1.

From the perspective of applications, we should be aware that neural networks could offer a highly competitive solution; however, one has to proceed very prudently with the learning process. Most importantly, the learning results might not be repetitive: running the same method while starting from a slightly different initial configuration (say, a different random initialization of the connections of the neurons) may result in quite substantial differences in the performance of the constructed network. Likewise setting different numeric values of the learning environment (say, a learning rate) could lead to a different solution. A formation of the input space, which becomes of a genuine challenge, when dealing with highly dimensional data and a large number of data themselves, requires attention. Ignoring this problem may result in a highly inefficient learning producing quite poor, non-competitive results lacking generalization abilities.

We should stress that by no means neural networks can be sought as a plug-and-play technology. To the contrary, its successful usage does require careful planning, data organization and data preprocessing, a prudent validation, and a careful accommodation of any prior domain knowledge being available. The black box nature of neural networks can bring some hesitation and reluctance to use the neural network solution and one has to be prepared for further critical evaluation of the obtained results.

3.3 Evolutionary and Biologically Inspired Computing: Toward a Holistic View at Global Optimization

The attractiveness of this paradigm of computing stems from the fact that all pursuits are realized by a population of individual – potential solutions so that this offers a very much appealing opportunity of exploring or exploiting a search space in a holistic manner (Goldberg 1989). The search is realized by a population – a collection of individuals, which at each iteration (generation) carry out search on their own and then are subject to some processes of interaction.

In case of genetic algorithms, evolutionary methods, and population-based methods (say, genetic algorithms, evolutionary strategies, particle swarm optimization), in general, a population undergoes evolution; the best individuals are retained, they form a new population through recombination. They are subject to mutation. Each operator present in the search process realizes some mechanism of exploration or exploitation of the search space. A general processing scheme can be outlined as follows

{evaluate population (individuals)
select mating individuals (selection process)
recombination
mutation}

The above basic sequence scheme is repeated (iterated).

In contrast to evolutionary methods, in the swarm-based methods (Engelbrecht 2005), we encounter an interesting way of sharing experience. Each particle relies on its own experience accumulated so far but it is also affected by the cognitive component where one looks at the performance of other members of the population as well as an overall behavior of the population.

The essential phase of any evolutionary and population-based method (directly affecting its performance) is a representation problem. It is concerned about a way how to represent the problem in the language of the search strategy so that (a) the resulting search space is made compact enough (to make the search less time consuming), and (b) is well reflective of the properties of the fitness function to be optimized. By forming a suitable search space we avoid forming extended regions of the search space where the fitness function does not change its values.

The *forte* of the methods falling under the rubric of these population-based optimization techniques is the genuine flexibility of the fitness function – there is a great deal of possibilities on how it can be formulated to capture the essence of the optimization problem. This translates into an ability to arrive at a suitable solution to the real-world task.

The inevitable challenges come with the need to assess how good the obtained solution really is and a formation of the feature space itself.

The advantages and limitations of this paradigm of computing and optimization are collected in Table 3.2.

Table 3.2 Evolutionary and biologically inspired computing: advantages and limitations along with some design guidelines

Advantages	Mechanisms of global search General form of fitness function Abilities to deal with a wide range of structural and parametric optimization
Limitations	Construction of search space (encoding and decoding mechanisms) Selection/adjustments of control parameters (e.g., crossover rate, mutation rate, recombination parameters) Assurance of optimality of solutions

3.4 Information Granularity and Granular Computing

Information granules permeate numerous human endeavors (Bargiela and Pedrycz 2002, 2003; Zadeh 1997; Pedrycz and Bargiela 2002). No matter what problem is taken into consideration, we usually express it in a certain conceptual framework of basic entities, which we regard to be of relevance to the problem formulation and problem solving. This becomes a framework in which we formulate generic concepts adhering to some level of abstraction, carry out processing, and communicate the results to the external environment. Consider, for instance, image processing. In spite of the continuous progress in the area, a human being assumes a dominant and very much uncontested position when it comes to understanding and interpreting images. Surely, we do not focus our attention on individual pixels and process them as such but group them together into semantically meaningful constructs – familiar objects we deal with in everyday life. Such objects involve regions that consist of pixels or categories of pixels drawn together because of their proximity in the image, similar texture, color, etc. This remarkable and unchallenged ability of humans dwells on our effortless ability to construct information granules, manipulate them, and arrive at sound conclusions. As another example, consider a collection of time series. From our perspective we can describe them in a semi-qualitative manner by pointing at specific regions of such signals. Specialists can effortlessly interpret various diagnostic signals including ECG recordings. They distinguish some segments of such signals and interpret their combinations. Experts can interpret temporal readings of sensors and assess the status of the monitored system. Again, in all these situations, the individual samples of the signals are not the focal point of the analysis and the ensuing signal interpretation. We always granulate all phenomena (no matter if they are originally discrete or analog in their nature). Time is another important variable that is subjected to granulation. We use seconds, minutes, days, months, and years. Depending upon a specific problem we have in mind and who the user is, the size of information granules (time intervals) could vary quite dramatically. To the high-level management time intervals of quarters of year or a few years could be meaningful temporal information granules on basis of which one develops any predictive model. For those in charge of everyday operation of a dispatching plant, minutes and hours could form a viable scale of time granulation. For the designer of high-speed integrated circuits and digital systems, the temporal information granules concern nanoseconds, microseconds, and perhaps microseconds. Even such commonly encountered and simple examples are convincing enough to lead us to ascertain that (a) information granules are the key components of knowledge representation and processing, (b) the level of granularity of information granules (their size, to be more descriptive) becomes crucial to the problem description and an overall strategy of problem solving, and (c) there is no universal level of granularity of information; the size of granules is problem-oriented and user-dependent.

What has been said so far touched a qualitative aspect of the problem. The challenge is to develop a computing framework within which all these representation and processing endeavors could be formally realized. The common platform emerging within this context comes under the name of Granular Computing. In essence, it is an emerging paradigm of information processing. While we have already noticed a number of important conceptual and computational constructs built in the domain of system modeling, machine learning, image processing, pattern recognition, and data compression in which various abstractions (and ensuing information granules) came into existence, Granular Computing becomes innovative and intellectually proactive in several fundamental ways

- It identifies the essential commonalities between the surprisingly diversified problems and technologies used there, which could be cast into a unified framework known as a granular world. This is a fully operational processing entity that interacts with the external world (that could be another granular or numeric world) by collecting necessary granular information and returning the outcomes of granular computing.
- With the emergence of the unified framework of granular processing, we achieve a better grasp as to the role of interaction between various formalisms and visualize a way in which they communicate.
- It brings together the existing formalisms of set theory (interval analysis) (Moore 1966), fuzzy sets (Zadeh 1965, 2005), rough sets (Pawlak 1982, 1991; Pawlak and Skowron 2007) under the same roof by clearly visualizing that in spite of their visibly distinct underpinnings (and ensuing processing), they exhibit some fundamental commonalities. In this sense, Granular Computing establishes a stimulating environment of synergy between the individual approaches.
- By building upon the commonalities of the existing formal approaches, Granular Computing helps build heterogeneous and multifaceted models of processing of information granules by clearly recognizing the orthogonal nature of some of the existing and well-established frameworks (say, probability theory coming with its probability density functions and fuzzy sets with their membership functions).
- Granular Computing fully acknowledges a notion of variable granularity whose range could cover detailed numeric entities and very abstract and general information granules. It looks at the aspects of compatibility of such information granules and ensuing communication mechanisms of the granular worlds.

Table 3.3 Granular computing: advantages and limitations along with some design guidelines

Advantages	Efficient knowledge representation in the form of information granules and granular models
	Transparency and high interpretability of resulting constructs
	Diversity of formal schemes of representation of information granules
Limitations	Lack of effective learning abilities
	Prescriptive nature of granular constructs
	Scalability issues

- Interestingly, the inception of information granules is highly motivated. We do not form information granules without reason. Information granules arise as an evident realization of the fundamental paradigm of abstraction.

Granular Computing forms a unified conceptual and computing platform. Yet, it directly benefits from the already existing and well-established concepts of information granules formed in the setting of set theory, fuzzy sets, rough sets, and others. While Granular Computing offers a unique ability to conveniently express the problem in the language of information granules, it also exhibits some limitations, refer to Table 3.3.

While all the three classes of technologies discussed so far offer tangible benefits and help address various central problems of intelligent systems, it becomes apparent that they are very much complementary. The strength of one technology is a quite visible limitation of some other. It is not surprising that there have been various ways of forming hybrid approaches dwelling upon the complementarity of neurocomputing, fuzzy sets (Granular Computing), and evolutionary methods, out of which a concept of Computational Intelligence (CI) has emerged.

3.5 Computational Intelligence: An Agenda of Synergy of Learning, Optimization, and Knowledge Representation

Computational Intelligence can be defined in many different ways. Let us start by recalling two definitions or descriptions, which are commonly encountered in the literature

> A system is computationally intelligent when it: deals with only numerical (low-level) data, has pattern recognition components, does not use knowledge in the AI sense; and additionally when it (begins to) exhibit (1) computational adaptivity; (2) computational fault tolerance, (3) speed approaching human-like turnaround, and (4) error rates that approximate human performance (Bezdek 1992, 1994)

The description provided by W. Karplus comes as follows

> CI substitutes intensive computation for insight how the system works. Neural networks, fuzzy systems, and evolutionary Computation were all shunned by classical system and control theorists. CI umbrellas and unifies these and other revolutionary methods

The first description captures the essence of the area. Perhaps today such a definition becomes slightly extended by allowing for some new trends and technologies, which are visible in the design of intelligent systems. Nevertheless the essence of CI is well-captured.

The comprehensive monograph on CI (Pedrycz 1997) emphasizes the importance of synergy of the contributing and very much complementary technologies of fuzzy sets, neurocomputing and evolutionary optimization. In a nutshell, CI is about effective and omnipresent mechanisms of synergy exploited in a variety of tasks of analysis and design of intelligent systems. The reader may refer to Fulcher and Jain (2008) and Mumford and Jain (2009), which serve as comprehensive sources of updated material on Computational Intelligence.

The emergence of CI is justifiable and in some sense, unavoidable. Over time, being faced with more advanced problems, increased dimensionality, and complexity of systems one has to deal with, neural networks, fuzzy sets, and evolutionary computing started to exhibit some clear limitations. This is not startling at all as their research agendas are very much distinct and they focus on different aspects of the design of intelligent systems. The synergistic environment, in which knowledge representation, learning, and global optimization go hand in hand, becomes highly desirable.

Let us elaborate in more detail on knowledge representation as being captured by fuzzy sets. Fuzzy sets offer a unique and general opportunity to look at information granules as semantically meaningful entities endowed with detailed numeric description. For instance, consider an information granule termed *high* amplitude of signal. On the one hand, *high* is just a single symbol and as such could be processed at the level of symbolic processing encountered in Artificial Intelligence (AI). For instance, it could be one of the symbols used in syntactic pattern classifier captured by a collection of syntactic production rules or automata. On the other hand, the same granular entity *high* is associated with the detailed numeric description, which calibrates the concept in presence of available numeric evidence. A suitable level of abstraction helps us establish the most promising tradeoff between detailed and abstract view at the problem/data. Of course, the choice of the tradeoff is problem-driven and depends upon the task and the main objectives specified therein. Likewise, the same information granule *high* can be looked at in less detail and through the use of some partially specified numeric content (that is in the form of higher type information granules, say fuzzy sets of type-2) could be processed in a semi-numeric fashion. In this way, the granularity of information and a formal mechanism used in granulation itself offers a way to position anywhere in-between symbolic view and numeric view of the reality, see Fig. 3.1.

One may emphasize an important and enlightening linkage between Computational Intelligence and Artificial Intelligence (AI). To a significant extent, AI is a synonym of symbol-driven processing faculty. CI effectively exploits numeric data however owing to the technology of Granular Computing, it may invoke computing based on information described at various levels of granularity by inherently associating such granules with their underlying semantics described in a numeric

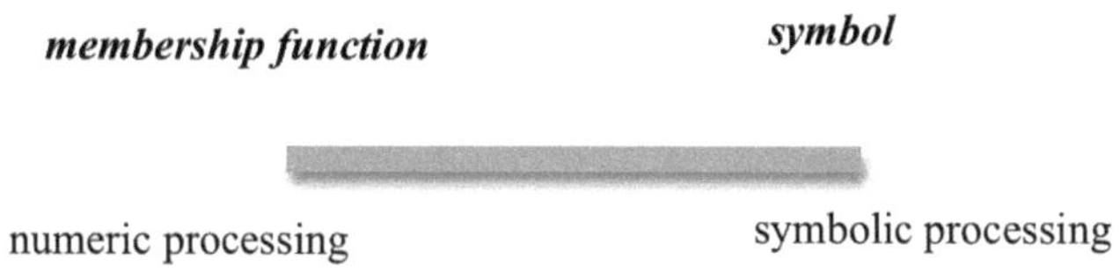

Fig. 3.1 Information granules and their interpretation depending upon the nature of granulation: a spectrum of in-between symbolic and numeric processing

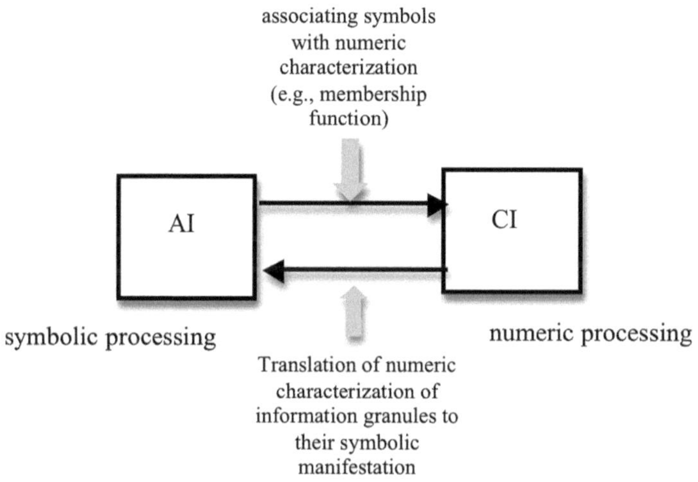

Fig. 3.2 CI and AI constructs: forming linkages between numeric and symbolic processing through information granulation

or semi-numeric fashion (e.g., membership functions, characteristic functions, or interval-valued mappings). The granularity of results supports the user-friendly nature of CI models. They can also form an important construct to be further used in facilitating an interaction with the user as well as forming linkages with symbolic processing of AI constructs as illustrated in Fig. 3.2.

The three fundamental components of CI along with an emphasis on their synergy of the main function can be portrayed as illustrated in Fig. 3.3.

The three axes present there correspond to knowledge representation, highlighting the component of information granularity (along with its abstraction facet), learning (adaptive) abilities (second axis), and global structural optimization (evolutionary methods). Each point positioned in the cube is reflective of the involvement of the corresponding technologies in the construction of the CI system. For instance, neuro-fuzzy systems (classifiers) are located on a plane with no involvement of evolutionary optimization. Evolutionary neurofuzzy systems occupy an interior of the CI hypercube.

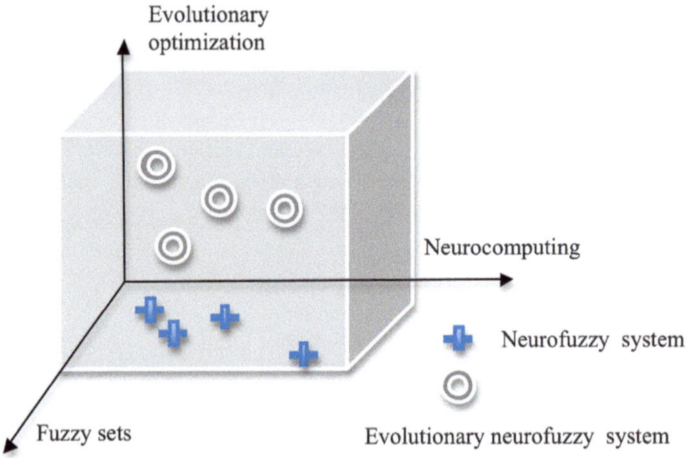

Fig. 3.3 A cube of constructs of Computational Intelligence; shown are several selected design scenarios illustrating a level of involvement of the individual technologies

The results of the queries on Computational Intelligence and ECG (done on Google Scholar – accessed on January 20th, 2011) clearly indicate a substantial interest in the area:

ECG & fuzzy sets 4,470
ECG & neural networks 14,600
ECG & particle swarm optimization 1,320
ECG & genetic algorithms 7,360

3.6 Formal Platforms of Information Granularity

There exists a plethora of formal platforms in which information granules are defined and processed.

Sets (intervals) realize a concept of abstraction by introducing a notion of dichotomy: we admit element to belong to a given information granule or to be excluded from it. Sets are described by characteristic functions taking on values in $\{0,1\}$. A family of sets defined in a universe of discourse $\boldsymbol{X}$ is denoted by $\boldsymbol{P}(\mathbf{X})$.

Fuzzy sets (Zadeh 1965, 2005) offer an important generalization of sets. By admitting partial membership to a given information granule we bring an important feature which makes the concept to be in rapport with reality. The description of fuzzy sets is realized in terms of membership functions taking on values in the unit interval. A family of fuzzy sets defined in $\boldsymbol{X}$ is denoted by $\boldsymbol{F}(\mathbf{X})$.

Probability-based information granules are expressed in the form of some probability density functions or probability functions. They capture a collection of elements resulting from some experiment. In virtue of the concept of probability, the granularity of information becomes a manifestation of occurrence of some elements.

Rough sets (Pawlak 1982, 1991; Pawlak and Skowron 2007) emphasize a roughness of description of a given concept X when being realized in terms of the indiscernibility relation provided in advance. The roughness of the description of X is manifested in terms of its lower and upper approximations of a certain rough set. A family of fuzzy sets defined in $\boldsymbol{X}$ is denoted by $\boldsymbol{R}(\mathbf{X})$.

Shadowed sets (Pedrycz 1998) offer a description of information granules by distinguishing among elements, which fully belong to the concept, are excluded from it and whose belongingness is completely unknown. Formally, these information granules are described as a mapping $X\colon \boldsymbol{X} \rightarrow \{1, 0, [0, 1]\}$ where the elements with the membership quantified as the entire [0,1] interval are used to describe a shadow of the construct. Given the nature of the mapping here, shadowed sets can be sought as a granular description of fuzzy sets where the shadow is used to localize partial membership values, which in fuzzy sets are distributed over the entire universe of discourse. A family of fuzzy sets defined in $\boldsymbol{X}$ is denoted by $\boldsymbol{S}(\boldsymbol{X})$.

Probability-grounded sets are defined over a certain universe where the membership grades are represented as some probabilistic constructs. For instance, each element of a set comes with a truncated to [0,1] probability density function, which quantifies a degree of membership to the information granule. There are a number of variations of these constructs with proabilistic sets (Hirota 1981) being one of them.

Other formal models of information granules involve axiomatic sets, soft sets, and intuitionistic sets.

3.6.1 Information Granules of Higher Type and Higher Order

In general, we distinguish between information granules of higher type and higher order.

Higher type information granules. The quantification of levels of belongingness to a given information granule is granular itself rather than numeric as encountered in sets or fuzzy sets. This type of quantification is of interest in situations it is not quite justifiable or technically meaningful to quantify the membership in terms of a single numeric value. These situations give rise to ideas of type-2 fuzzy sets or interval-valued fuzzy sets. In the first case the membership is quantified by a certain fuzzy set taking on values in the unit interval. In the second case we have a subinterval of [0,1] representing membership values. One can discuss fuzzy sets of higher type in which the granular quantification is moved to the higher levels of

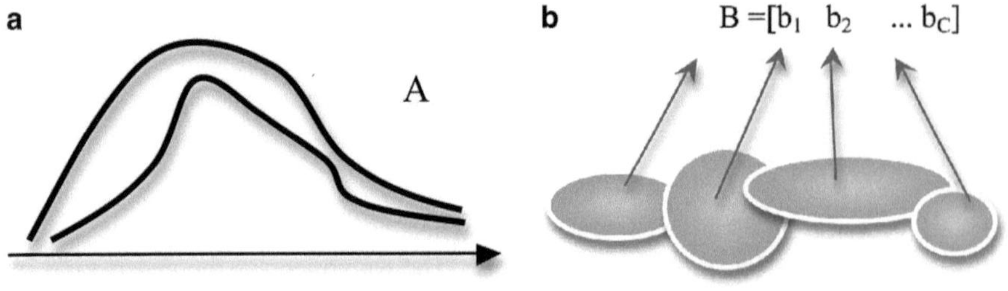

Fig. 3.4 Examples of information granules of type-2 (type-2 fuzzy set A) (**a**) and order 2 fuzzy set B (defined over a collection of fuzzy sets) (**b**)

the construct. For instance, one can talk about type-3, type-4, ... fuzzy sets. Albeit conceptually sound, one should be aware that the computing overhead associated with further processing of such information granules becomes more significant. In light of the essence of these constructs, we can view probabilistic granules to be treated as higher type information granules as we admit membership values to be granulated in a probabilistic manner.

Higher order information granules. The notion of higher order of information granules points at a space in which an information granule is defined. Here the universe of discourse is composed of a family of information granules. For instance, a fuzzy set of order 2 is constructed in the space of a family of so-called reference fuzzy sets. This stands in a sharp contrast with fuzzy sets of order 1, which are defined in individual elements of the universe of discourse. One could remark that fuzzy modeling quite often involve order 2 fuzzy sets.

The illustration of these concepts is included in Fig. 3.4.

These types of construct could be generalized by invoking a number of consecutive levels of the structure. In all situations, we could assess whether moving to the higher level or order constructs is legitimate from the perspective of the problem at hand.

3.6.2 *Hybrid Models of Information Granules*

Information granules can embrace several granulation formalisms at the same time forming some hybrid models. This constructs become of particular interest when information granules have to capture a multifaceted nature of the problem. There are a large number of interesting options here. Some of them, which have been found convincing concern

(a) Fuzzy probabilities. Probability and fuzzy sets are orthogonal concepts and as such they could be considered together as a single entity. The concepts of a fuzzy event and fuzzy probabilities (viz. probabilities whose values are quantified in terms of fuzzy sets, say high probability, very low probability) are of interest here.

(b) Fuzzy rough and rough fuzzy information granules. Here the indiscernibility relation can be formed on a basis of fuzzy sets. Fuzzy sets, rather than sets are also the entities that are described in terms of the elements of the indiscernibility relation. The original object X for which a rough set is formed might be a fuzzy set itself rather than a set used in the original definition of rough sets.

3.7 Information Granularity in Signal Representation

In signal characterization, before proceeding with its detailed processing, a careful, prudently thought out representation is an essential prerequisite directly impacting the effectiveness of all ensuing algorithms, in particular influencing classification quality of pattern classifiers built on the basis of such information granules.

Granularity of information plays a primordial role in all these characterization pursuits. Numeric data are represented in the form of information granules and the manifestation of such granules (e.g., as the values of membership functions) is used afterward in a more detailed system design.

Let us highlight the main role information granules play in the constructs of CI such as e.g., neural networks. This role is visible in the formation of data interfaces. The essence of the underlying construct and its role vis-à-vis processing realized by the neural network is profoundly visible in the realization of a new feature space based on information granules. Consider a general scheme portrayed in Fig. 3.5.

Formally speaking, the original data space, typically, n-dimensional space of real number vectors, $\boldsymbol{R}^n$, is transformed via a finite collection of information granules, say, $A_1, A_2, \ldots, A_c$. We say that the input space has been granulated. Each input $\boldsymbol{x}$ is perceived by the following classifier/analyzer through the "eyes" of the information granules, meaning that the following relationship holds, see also Fig. 3.5,

$$\mathcal{G} : R^n \rightarrow [0,1]^c \tag{3.1}$$

Where the result of the mapping is a c-dimensional vector positioned in the [0,1] hypercube.

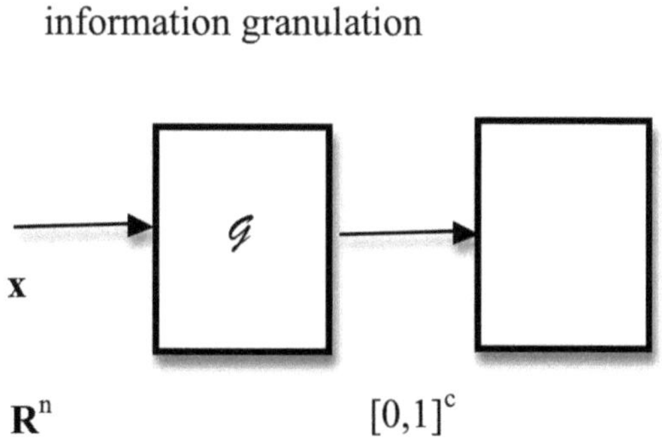

Fig. 3.5 Formation of a new feature space through a collection of information granules

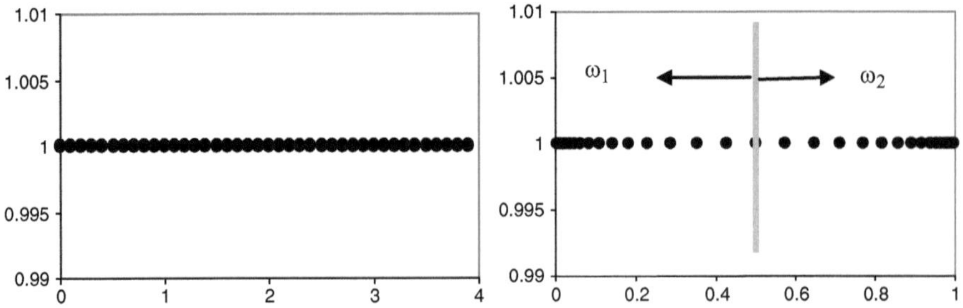

Fig. 3.6 Nonlinear transformation realized by a sigmoid membership function: original patterns distributed uniformly in the feature space are then localized into quite distantly positioned groups

There are at least three important and practically advantageous aspects of the mapping realized by information granules:

Nonlinear mapping of the data space with an intent of forming information granules in such a way that the transformed data $\mathcal{G}(\boldsymbol{x}_1)$, $\mathcal{G}(\boldsymbol{x}_2)$, ..., $\mathcal{G}(\boldsymbol{x}_\mathrm{N})$ are more suitable to construct an effective classifier. We rely on the nonlinearity effect that can be carefully exploited.

The tangible advantage results from the nonlinear character of membership functions. A properly adjusted nonlinearity could move apart patterns belonging to different classes and bring closer those regions in which the patterns belong to the same category. For instance, patterns belonging to two classes and distributed uniformly in a one-dimensional space, see Fig. 3.6, become well separated when transformed through a sigmoid membership function A, $A(x) = 1/(1+\exp(-(x-2)))$ and described in terms of the corresponding membership grades. In essence, fuzzy sets play a role of a nonlinear transformation of the feature space. We note that while the patterns are distributed uniformly, Fig. 3.6a, their distribution in the space of membership degrees $[0,1]$ $u = A(x)$ shows two groups of patterns which are located at the opposite ends of the unit interval with a large separation gap in-between.

Reduction of the dimensionality of the feature space. While the original feature space could be quite high (which is common in many classification problems), the dimensionality of the space of information granules is far lower, $c \ll n$. This supports the developments of the classifiers, especially neural networks and reduces a risk of memorization and poor generalization capabilities. We often witness this role of information granules in the construction of neuro-fuzzy systems.

Information granules as essential constructs supporting the development of interpretable models. For instance, in rule-based systems (classifiers, analyzers), the condition parts (as well as conclusions) comprise information granules – interpretable entities, which make rules meaningful.

3.8 The Concept of Information Granulation–Degranulation

When it comes to numeric information **x** forming a vector in a certain multidimensional space, we can develop an interesting granulation–degranulation scheme (Pedrycz and Gomide 2007). We assume that the information granules forming a collection (codebook) $\boldsymbol{A}$ are described by their prototypes $\boldsymbol{v}_1, \boldsymbol{v}_2, \ldots, \boldsymbol{v}_c$. Such prototypes can be formed as a result of fuzzy clustering (Bezdek 1981; Pedrycz 2005; Hoppner et al. 1999) The granulation–degranulation task is formulated as a certain optimization problem. In what follows, we assume that the distance used in the solutions is the Euclidean one. The granulation of $\boldsymbol{x}$ returns its representation in terms of the collection of available information granules expressed in terms of their prototypes. More specifically, $\boldsymbol{x}$ is expressed in the form of the membership grades u_i of $\boldsymbol{x}$ to the individual granules A_i, which form a solution to the following optimization problem

$$\text{Min} \sum_{i=1}^{c} u_i^m(x)||x - v_i||^2 \tag{3.2}$$

subject to the following constraints imposed on the degrees of membership

$$\sum_{i=1}^{c} u_i(x) = 1 \quad u_i(x) \in [0, 1] \tag{3.3}$$

where "m" stands for the so-called fuzzification coefficient, $m > 1$ [6]. The derived solution to the problem above reads as follows

$$u_i(x) = \frac{1}{\sum\limits_{j=1}^{c} \left(\frac{||x - v_i||}{||x - v_j||} \right)^{2/(m-1)}} \tag{3.4}$$

For the degranulation phase, given $u_i(\boldsymbol{x})$ and the prototypes $\boldsymbol{v}_i$, the vector $\hat{\mathbf{x}}$ is considered as a solution to the minimization problem in which we reconstruct (degranulate) original $\boldsymbol{x}$ when using the prototypes and the membership grades

$$\sum_{i=1}^{c} u_i^m(x)||\hat{x} - v_i||^2 \tag{3.5}$$

Because of the use of the Euclidean distance in the above performance index, the calculations here are straightforward yielding the result

$$\hat{x} = \frac{\sum\limits_{i=1}^{c} u_i^m(x) v_i}{\sum\limits_{i=1}^{c} u_i^m(x)} \tag{3.6}$$

It is important to note that the description of $\boldsymbol{x}$ in more abstract fashion realized by means of A_i and being followed by the consecutive degranulation brings about a certain granulation error (which is inevitable given a fact that we move back and forth between different levels of abstraction). While the above formulas pertain to the granulation realized by fuzzy sets, the granulation–degranulation error is also present when dealing with sets (intervals). In this case we are faced with a quantization error, which becomes inevitable when working with A/D (granulation) and D/A (degranulation) conversion mechanisms.

3.9 The Principle of Justifiable Granularity

The principle of justifiable granularity (Pedrycz and Gomide 2007) is concerned with a formation of a meaningful representation of a collection of numeric values (real numbers), say $\{x_1, x_2, \ldots, x_N\}$. Such a representation comes in the form of a certain information granule rather than a single numeric entity, no matter how such a single individual has been selected. What is being done in statistics is an example of this principle realized in the language of probabilistic information granules. A sample of numeric data is represented not only by its mean or median (which by itself is a very rough description) but also by the standard deviation. Both the mean and the standard deviation imply a realization of a certain probabilistic information granule, such as e.g., a Gaussian one. The probabilistic information granules are just one of the possibilities to build an information granule to represent a collection of numeric data. Some other formal approaches that could be engaged here involve sets, fuzzy sets, rough sets, and others. Formally, we can view the process of granulation as a transformation $\mathcal{G}$ operating on $\{x_1, x_2, \ldots, x_N\}$ resulting in some information granule

$$\mathcal{G} : R \rightarrow G(R) \tag{3.7}$$

where $\boldsymbol{G}(\mathbf{R})$ is a granular construct, for instance interval, $\boldsymbol{G}(\mathbf{R}) = \boldsymbol{P}(\mathbf{R})$ or fuzzy set, $\boldsymbol{G}(\mathbf{R}) = \boldsymbol{F}(\mathbf{R})$, etc.

In case of other formalisms of information granulation, the development of the corresponding granules is guided by a certain optimization criterion, which becomes a crux of the principle of justifiable granularity. In general, in such criteria, we manage two conflicting requirements. The one is about forming an information granule of sufficiently high level of experimental evidence that is accumulated behind it and in this way supports its existence (usage). The second one is about maintaining high specificity of the resulting information granule. In what follows, we show a construction of interval-based information granules in presence of some numeric evidence, see Fig. 3.7.

We span the numeric interval $\Omega(=[a,b])$ in such a way that (1) the numeric evidence accumulated within the bounds of Ω is as high as possible. We quantify this requirement by counting the number of data falling within the bounds of Ω, that is one determines the value of card $\{x_k \in \Omega\}$. This count has to be maximized. At the same time, we require that (2) the support of Ω is as low as possible, which

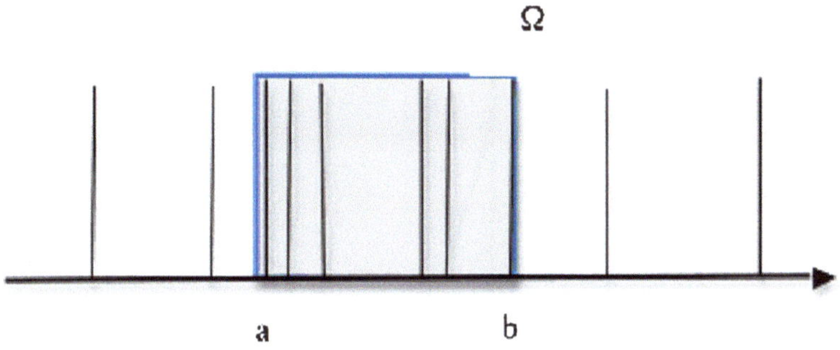

Fig. 3.7 Realization of the principle of justifiable granularity for numeric data and an interval type of information granules

makes Ω specific (detailed) enough. These two requirements are in conflict. To come up with a single performance index Q taken as a product of two functionals f_1 and f_2, $V = f_1 * f_2$ where f_1 is an increasing function of the cardinality of the elements falling within the bounds of the information granule Ω and f_2 is a decreasing function of the support (length) of $|b-a|$. To address the requirements formulated above, our intent is to maximize Q with respect to the boundaries of the interval.

One of the interesting alternatives is to consider the following two expressions:

$$f_1(u) = u \tag{3.8}$$

and

$$f_2(u) = \exp(-\alpha u) \tag{3.9}$$

where $u = |b-a|$ and α is a positive parameter controlling the changes of the function and subsequently offering some flexibility in the produced information granule A. The plots of these two requirements are provided in Fig. 3.8 where it is shown how they are affected by the position of the cutoff point contributing to the realization of the interval information granule.

In the optimization problem, it is helpful to consider a two-step process. First, a numeric representative of the data is determined (say, a mean value, mode or median) and the formation of information granules is realized separately for the lower bound (taking all data that are lower than this numeric representative) and the upper bound (where we consider the data positioned to the right from the numeric representative). The maximization of the expression

$$V(a) = \text{card}(\Omega) * \exp(-a|m-a|) \tag{3.10}$$

is carried out with respect to the unknown lower bound "a." Here "m" stands for the numeric representative of the numeric data we discussed above. Likewise, we proceed with the maximization of the expression (objective function)

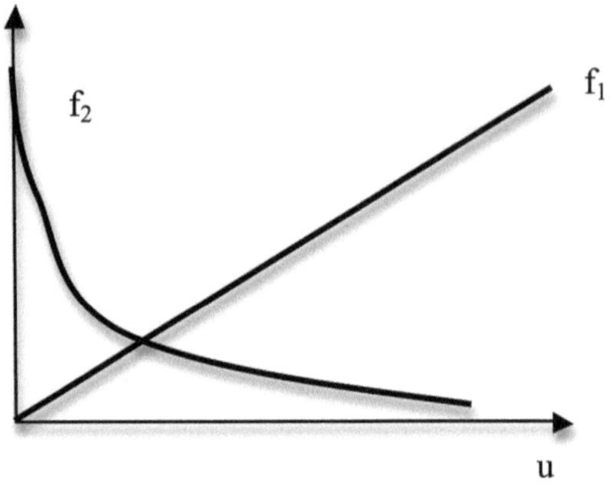

Fig. 3.8 Two functions f_1 and f_2 regarded as functions of the cutoff point (b) of the interval information granule; note a point where a certain balance is noted

$V(b) = \text{card}(\Omega) * \exp(-a|m-b|)$ with "b" being the upper bound of the information granule. It is worth noting that (10) comes with some parameter (α), which is essential to its further usage in granular constructs.

With regard to the above maximization (3.10) one can note an interesting and intuitively appealing relationship between "b" and the values of the parameter α. Consider that the data larger than the numeric representative are $x_1, x_2, \ldots, x_N$ with "m" being a certain numeric representative. In spite of the values of α, the location of optimal "b" is in-between min x_i and max x_i. Given the form of (10) if "b" falls below the lower bound, min x_i, then the performance index is equal to zero. If b moves beyond max x_i, the performance index decreases monotonically. Indeed, take b_1 and b_2 where $b_1 < b_2$. In this case, the performance index $V(b_1)$ is higher than $V(b_2)$, which indicates that moving toward higher values of "b" after exceeding max x_i leads only to the reduced values of the performance index.

In a similar way we can develop an information granule in the form of a certain fuzzy set. Here the only difference is that the cardinality of the set of data in (10) contained within the interval has to be replaced by the sum of membership degrees of the data belonging to the fuzzy set. In this sense, this part of the performance index is a σ-count of the fuzzy set spanned over the data.

The algorithm realizing the principle of justifiable granularity produces an information granule (either an interval or a fuzzy set) based on a collection of numeric data. The nature of the numeric data themselves can be quite different. Two situations are worth highlighting here:

(a) The numeric data could result from measuring some variables present in the system. In this case, information granules are treated as non-numeric data, which can be then used in the design of the model and highlight the structure of a large number of numeric data.
(b) The numeric data are just membership values of some fuzzy sets reported for a certain point of the universe of discourse. The granular representation resulting from the discussed construct gives rise to the information granule of higher type, fuzzy set of type-2, to be more specific. Depending on the nature of the

information granule formed here, we construct interval-valued type-2 fuzzy sets or type-2 fuzzy sets. It is worth stressing that in this manner, we have arrived at a constructive way of designing of type-2 fuzzy sets – the area that has been very much left neglected in the existing studies.

The algorithms supporting the design of information granules presented so far have been concerned with one-dimensional data. In situation of multivariable data, the developed method is applied separately to the individual variables and then the Cartesian products of the information granules are constructed.

3.10 Clustering as a Means of Design of Information Granules

Clustering is a commonly encountered way of forming information granules. The essence of the process is underlined by (3.7). In objective function-based clustering there is usually a certain constraint imposed on the relationship between the resulting information granules. For instance, one requires that the union of information granules "covers" the entire data set, that is $\bigcup_{i=1}^{c} A_c = D$. Obviously the union operation has to be specified in accordance to the formalism of information granules used there. There are a large number of clustering methods, and depending on the formalism being used, we end up with the granules expressed in the language of sets, ***P*(X)**, fuzzy sets ***F*(X)**, rough sets ***R*(X)**, shadowed sets ***S*(X)**, and others. The form of the granules depends on the clustering algorithm and the formulation of the objective function (and partition matrix, in particular). The number of information granules has been another point of comprehensive study as this pertains to the problem of cluster validity.

By having a quick look at the plethora of clustering methods one can conclude that they predominantly realize the concept of closeness between elements: data, which are close to each other form the same information granule. There is another aspect of functional resemblance and this facet is captured through so-called knowledge-based clustering, cf. (Pedrycz 2005).

3.10.1 Unsupervised Learning with Fuzzy Sets

Unsupervised learning, quite commonly treated as an equivalent of clustering is aimed at the discovery of structure in data and its representation in the form of clusters – groups of data.

In reality, clusters, in virtue of their nature, are inherently *fuzzy*. Fuzzy sets constitute a natural vehicle to quantify strength of membership of patterns to a certain group. An example shown in Fig. 3.9 clearly demonstrates this need. The pattern positioned in-between the two well-structured and compact groups exhibits some level of resemblance (membership) to each of the clusters. Surely enough, one

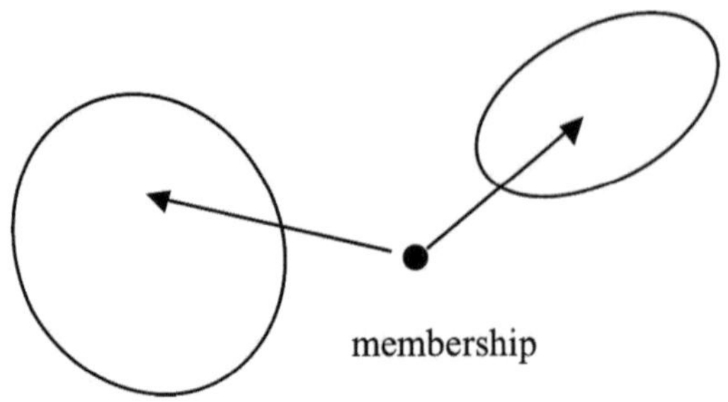

Fig. 3.9 Example of two-dimensional data with patterns of varying membership degrees to the two highly visible and compact clusters

could be hesitant to allocate it fully to either of the clusters. The membership values, e.g., 0.55 and 0.45, are not only reflective of the structure in the data but they also flag the distinct nature of this data – and may trigger some further inspection of this pattern. In this way we remark a user-centric character of fuzzy sets, which make interaction with users more effective and transparent.

3.10.2 Fuzzy C-Means as an Algorithmic Vehicle of Data Reduction Through Fuzzy Clusters

Fuzzy sets can be formed on a basis of numeric data through their clustering (groupings) (Duda et al. 2001; Fukunaga 1990). The groups of data give rise to membership functions that convey a global more abstract and general view at the available data. With this regard Fuzzy C-Means (FCM, for brief) is one of the commonly used mechanisms of fuzzy clustering (Bezdek 1982; Pedrycz 2005).

Let us review its formulation, develop the algorithm and highlight the main properties of the fuzzy clusters. Given a collection of n-dimensional data set $\{\boldsymbol{x}_k\}$, $k = 1, 2, \ldots, N$, the task of determining its structure – a collection of "c" clusters, is expressed as a minimization of the following objective function (performance index) Q being regarded as a sum of the squared distances between data and their representatives (prototypes)

$$Q = \sum_{i=1}^{c} \sum_{k=1}^{N} u_{ik}^{m} ||x_k - v_i||^2 \quad (3.11)$$

Here $\mathbf{v}_i$ s are n-dimensional prototypes of the clusters, $i = 1, 2, \ldots, c$ and $U = [u_{ik}]$ stands for a partition matrix expressing a way of allocation of the data to the corresponding clusters; u_{ik} is the membership degree of data $\boldsymbol{x}_k$ in the i-th cluster. The distance between the data z_k and prototype v_i is denoted by $||.||$. The fuzzification coefficient $m(>1.0)$ expresses the impact of the membership grades on the individual clusters. It implies as certain geometry of fuzzy sets. A partition matrix satisfies two important and intuitively appealing properties

$$(a)\ 0 < \sum_{k=1}^{N} u_{ik} < N, \quad i = 1, 2, \ldots, c$$

$$(b)\ \sum_{i=1}^{c} u_{ik} = 1, \quad k = 1, 2, \ldots, N \tag{3.12}$$

Let us denote by $\boldsymbol{U}$ a family of matrices satisfying (a)–(b). The first requirement states that each cluster has to be nonempty and different from the entire set. The second requirement states that the sum of the membership grades should be confined to 1.

The minimization of Q completed with respect to $U \in \boldsymbol{U}$ and the prototypes $\boldsymbol{v}_i$ of $V = \{\boldsymbol{v}_1, \boldsymbol{v}_2, \ldots, \boldsymbol{v}_c\}$ of the clusters. More explicitly, we write it down as follows

$$\min Q \text{ with respect to } U \in \boldsymbol{U}, \boldsymbol{v}_1, \boldsymbol{v}_2, \ldots, \boldsymbol{v}_c \in \boldsymbol{R}^n \tag{3.13}$$

The successive entries of the partition matrix are expressed as follows

$$u_{st} = \frac{1}{\sum_{j=1}^{c} \left(\frac{\|x_t - v_s\|}{\|x_t - v_j\|} \right)^{2/(m-1)}} \tag{3.14}$$

Assuming the Euclidean form of distance, the prototypes $\boldsymbol{v}_1, \boldsymbol{v}_2, \ldots, \boldsymbol{v}_c$ come in the form

$$v_s = \frac{\sum_{k=1}^{N} u_{ik}^m x_k}{\sum_{k=1}^{N} u_{ik}^m} \tag{3.15}$$

Overall, the FCM clustering is completed through a sequence of iterations where we start from some random allocation of data (a certain randomly initialized partition matrix) and carry out the following updates by adjusting the values of the partition matrix and the prototypes. The iterative process is continued until a certain termination criterion has been satisfied. Typically, the termination condition is quantified by looking at the changes in the membership values of the successive partition matrices. Denote by $U(t)$ and $U(t+1)$ the two partition matrices produced in the two consecutive iterations of the algorithm. If the distance $\|U(t+1) - U(\mathrm{i})\|$ is less than a small predefined threshold ε say $\varepsilon = 10^{-5}$ or 10^{-6}, then we terminate the algorithm. Typically, one considers the Tchebyschev distance between the partition matrices meaning that the termination criterion reads as follows

$$\max_{i,k} |u_{ik}(t+1) - u_{ik}(t)| \leq \varepsilon \tag{3.16}$$

3.10.3 Knowledge-Based Clustering

Clustering and classification are positioned at the two opposite poles of the learning paradigm. In reality, there is no "pure" unsupervised learning as usually there is some limited amount of domain knowledge. There is no fully supervised learning as some labels might not be completely reliable (as those encountered in case of learning with probabilistic teacher).

There is some domain knowledge and it has to be carefully incorporated into the generic clustering procedure. Knowledge hints can be conveniently captured and formalized in terms of fuzzy sets. Altogether with the underlying clustering algorithms, they give rise to the concept of knowledge-based clustering – a unified framework in which data and knowledge are processed together in a uniform fashion.

We can distinguish several interesting and practically viable ways in which domain knowledge is taken into consideration:

A subset of labeled patterns. The knowledge hints are provided in the form of a small subset of labeled patterns $\boldsymbol{K} \subset \boldsymbol{N}$ (Pedrycz and Waletzky 1997a, b). For each of them, we have a vector of membership grades f_{k}, $k \in \boldsymbol{K}$, which consists of degrees of membership the pattern is assigned to the corresponding clusters. As usual, we have $f_{ik} \in [0,1]$ and $\sum_{i=1}^{c} f_{ik} = 1$.

Proximity-based clustering. Here we are provided with a collection of pairs of patterns (Loia et al. 2003) with specified levels of closeness (resemblance) which are quantified in terms of proximity, prox(k,l) expressed for $\boldsymbol{x}_k$ and $\boldsymbol{x}_l$. The proximity offers a very general quantification scheme of resemblance: we require reflexivity and symmetry, that is prox $(k,k) = 1$ and prox $(k,l) =$ prox (l,k); however no transitivity is needed.

"belong" and "not-belong" Boolean relationships between patterns These two Boolean relationships stress that two patterns should belong to the same clusters, $R(\boldsymbol{x}_{\mathrm{k}}, \boldsymbol{x}_{\mathrm{l}}) = 1$ or they should be placed apart in two different clusters, $R(\boldsymbol{x}_{\mathrm{k}}, \boldsymbol{x}_{\mathrm{l}}) = 0$. These two requirements could be relaxed by requiring that these two relationships return values close to one or zero.

Uncertainty of labeling/allocation of patterns. We may consider that some patterns are "easy" to assign to clusters while some others are inherently difficult to deal with meaning that their cluster allocation is associated with a significant level of uncertainty. Let $F(\boldsymbol{x}_{\mathrm{k}})$ stand for the uncertainty measure (e.g., entropy) for $\boldsymbol{x}_{\mathrm{k}}$ (as a matter of fact, F is computed for the membership degrees of $\boldsymbol{x}_{\mathrm{k}}$ that is $F(\boldsymbol{u}_{\mathrm{k}})$ with $\boldsymbol{u}_{\mathrm{k}}$ being the k-th column of the partition matrix). The uncertainty hint is quantified by values close to 0 or 1 depending upon what uncertainty level a given pattern is coming from.

Depending on the character of the knowledge hints, the original clustering algorithm needs to be properly refined. In particular the underlying objective function has to be augmented to capture the knowledge-based requirements. Below shown are several examples of the extended objective functions dealing with the knowledge hints introduced above.

When dealing with some labeled patterns we consider the following augmented objective function

$$Q = \sum_{i=1}^{c} \sum_{k=1}^{N} u_{ik}^{m} ||x_k - v_i||^2 + \alpha \sum_{i=1}^{c} \sum_{k=1}^{N} (u_{ik} - f_{ik} b_k)^2 ||x_k - v_i||^2 \tag{3.17}$$

where the second term quantifies distances between the class membership of the labeled patterns and the values of the partition matrix. The positive weight factor (a) helps set up a suitable balance between the knowledge about classes already available and the structure revealed by the clustering algorithm. The Boolean variable b_k assumes values equal to 1 when the corresponding pattern has been labeled.

The proximity constraints are accommodated as a part of the optimization problem where we minimize the distances between proximity values being provided and those generated by the partition matrix $P(k_1, k_2)$

$$Q = \sum_{i=1}^{c} \sum_{k=1}^{N} u_{ik}^{m} ||x_k - v_i||^2$$

$$||\mathrm{prox}(k_1, k_2) - P(k_1, k_2)|| \rightarrow \mathrm{Min}\ k_1, k_2 \in K \tag{3.18}$$

with $\boldsymbol{K}$ being a pair of patterns for which the proximity level has been provided. It can be shown that given the partition matrix the expression $\sum_{i=1}^{c} \min(u_{ik1}, u_{ik2})$ generates the corresponding proximity value.

For the uncertainty constraints, the minimization problem can be expressed as follows

$$Q = \sum_{i=1}^{c} \sum_{k=1}^{N} u_{ik}^{m} ||x_k - v_i||^2$$

$$||F(u_k) - g_k|| \rightarrow \mathrm{Min}\ k \in K \tag{3.19}$$

where $\boldsymbol{K}$ stands for the set of patterns for which we are provided with the uncertainty values g_k.

Undoubtedly the extended objective functions call for the optimization scheme that is more demanding as far as the calculations are concerned. In several cases we cannot modify the standard technique of Lagrange multipliers, which leads to an iterative scheme of successive updates of the partition matrix and the prototypes. In general, though, the knowledge hints give rise to a more complex objective function in which the iterative scheme cannot be useful in the determination of the partition matrix and the prototypes. Alluding to the generic FCM scheme, we observe that the calculations of the prototypes in the iterative loop are doable in case of the Euclidean distance. Even the Hamming or Tchebyshev distance brings a great deal of complexity. Likewise, the knowledge hints lead to the increased complexity: the prototypes cannot be computed in a straightforward way and one has to resort himself to more advanced optimization techniques. Evolutionary computing arises here as an appealing alternative. We may consider any of the options available there including genetic algorithms, particle swarm optimization, ant colonies, to name some of them. The general scheme can be schematically structured as follows:

– repeat {EC (prototypes); compute partition matrix U;}

3.11 Fuzzy Logic-Oriented Classifiers

Fuzzy sets and information granules, in general, offer a structural backbone of fuzzy classifiers. The crux of the concept is displayed in Fig. 3.10. Information granules are formed in the feature space. They are *logically* associated with classes in the sense that for each class its degree of class membership is a logic expression of the activation levels (matching degrees) of the individual information granules. The flexibility of the logic mapping is offered through the use of the collection of logic neurons (fuzzy neurons) whose connections are optimized during the design of the classifier.

3.11.1 Main Categories of Fuzzy Neurons

There are two main types of logic neurons: aggregative and referential neurons. Each of them comes with a clearly defined semantics of its underlying logic expression and is equipped with significant parametric flexibility necessary to facilitate substantial learning abilities.

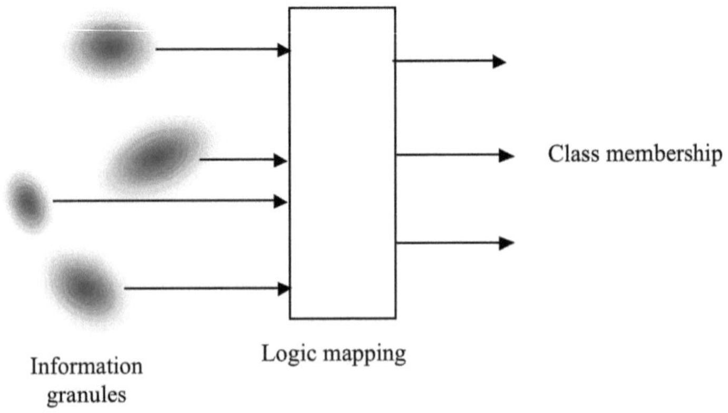

Fig. 3.10 An overall scheme of logic mapping between information granules – fuzzy sets formed in the feature space and the class membership degrees

3.11.1.1 Aggregative Neurons

Formally, these neurons realize a logic mapping from $[0,1]^n$ to [0,1]. Two main classes of the processing units exist in this category (Pedrycz and Rocha 1993; Hirota and Pedrycz 1993).

OR neuron: This realizes an *and* logic aggregation of inputs $\boldsymbol{x} = [x_1 x_2 \ldots x_n]$ with the corresponding connections (weights) $\boldsymbol{w} = [w_1 w_2 \ldots w_n]$ and then summarizes the partial results in an *or*-wise manner (hence the name of the neuron). The concise notation underlines this flow of computing, $y = OR(\boldsymbol{x}; \boldsymbol{w})$ while the realization of the logic operations gives rise to the expression (commonly referring to it as an s-t combination or s-t aggregation)

$$y = \mathop{S}_{i=1}^{n} (x_i t w_i) \tag{3.20}$$

Bearing in mind the interpretation of the logic connectives (t-norms and t-conorms) (Klement et al. 2000), the OR neuron realizes the following logic expression being viewed as an underlying logic description of the processing of the input signals

$$(x_1 \ and \ w_1) \, or \, (x_2 \ and \ w_2) \, or \ldots or \, (x_n \ and \ w_n) \tag{3.21}$$

Apparently the inputs are logically "weighted" by the values of the connections before producing the final result. In other words we can treat "y" as a truth value of the above statement where the truth values of the inputs are affected by the corresponding weights. Noticeably, lower values of w_i discount the impact of the corresponding inputs; higher values of the connections (especially those being positioned close to 1) do not affect the original truth values of the inputs resulting in the logic formula. In limit, if all connections w_i, $i = 1, 2, \ldots, n$ are set to 1 then the neuron produces a plain *or*-combination of the inputs, $y = x_1 \, or x_2 \, or \ldots or \ x_n$. The values of the connections set to zero eliminate the corresponding inputs. Computationally, the OR neuron exhibits nonlinear characteristics (that is inherently implied by the use of the t- and t-conorms (that are evidently nonlinear mappings). The connections of the neuron contribute to its adaptive character; the changes in their values form the crux of the parametric learning.

AND neuron: the neurons in the category, described as $y = \text{AND}(\boldsymbol{x}; \boldsymbol{w})$ with $\boldsymbol{x}$ and $\boldsymbol{w}$ being defined as in case of the OR neuron, are governed by the expression

$$y = \mathop{T}_{i=1}^{n} (x_i s w_i) \tag{3.22}$$

Here the *or* and *and* connectives are used in a reversed order: first the inputs are combined with the use of the t-conorm and the partial results produced in this way are aggregated *and*-wise. Higher values of the connections reduce impact of the corresponding inputs. In limit $w_i = 1$ eliminates the relevance of x_i. With all w_i set to 0, the output of the AND neuron is just an *and* aggregation of the inputs

$$y = x_1 \text{ and } x_2 \text{ and} \ldots \text{and } x_n \tag{3.23}$$

Let us conclude that the neurons are highly nonlinear processing units whose nonlinear mapping depends upon the specific realizations of the logic connectives. They also come with potential plasticity whose usage becomes critical when learning the networks including such neurons.

3.11.2 Architectures of Logic Networks

The logic neurons (aggregative and referential) can serve as building blocks of more comprehensive and functionally appealing architectures. The diversity of the topologies one can construct with the aid of the proposed neurons is surprisingly high. This architectural multiplicity is important from the application point of view as we can fully reflect the nature of the problem in a flexible manner. It is essential to capture the problem in a logic format and then set up the logic skeleton – conceptual blueprint (by forming the structure and finally refine it parametrically through a thorough optimization of the connections. Throughout the entire development process we are positioned quite comfortably by monitoring the optimization of the network as well as interpreting its semantics.

3.11.2.1 Logic Processor in the Processing of Fuzzy Logic Functions: A Canonical Realization

The typical logic network that is at the center of logic processing originates from the two-valued logic and comes in the form of the famous Shannon theorem of decomposition of Boolean functions. Let us recall that any Boolean function $\{0,1\}^{\mathrm{n}} \rightarrow \{0,1\}$ can be represented as a logic sum of its corresponding miniterms or a logic product of maxterms. By a minterm of "*n*" logic variables $x_1, x_2, \ldots, x_{\mathrm{n}}$ we mean a logic product involving all these variables either in direct or complemented form. Having "*n*" variables we end up with 2^{n} minterms starting from the one involving all complemented variables and ending up at the logic product with all direct variables. Likewise by a maxterm we mean a logic sum of all variables or their complements. Now in virtue of the decomposition theorem, we note that the first representation scheme involves a two-layer network where the first layer consists of AND gates whose outputs are combined in a single OR gate. The converse topology occurs for the second decomposition mode: there is a single layer of OR gates followed by a single AND gate aggregating *or*-wise all partial results.

The proposed network (referred here as a logic processor) generalizes this concept as shown in Fig. 3.11. The OR–AND mode of the logic processor comes with the two types of aggregative neurons being swapped between the layers. Here the first (hidden) layer is composed of the OR neuron and is followed by the output realized by means of the AND neuron.

The logic neurons generalize digital gates. The design of the network (viz. any fuzzy function) is realized through learning. If we confine ourselves to Boolean

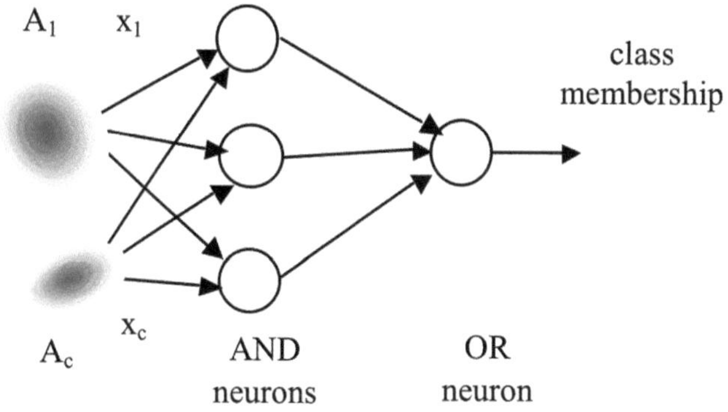

Fig. 3.11 A topology of the logic processor in its AND-OR realization mode

{0,1} values, the network's learning becomes an alternative to a standard digital design, especially a minimization of logic functions. The logic processor translates into a compound logic statement (we skip the connections of the neurons to underline the underlying logic content of the statement)

- if (input_1 *and*... *and* input_j) *or* (input_d *and*... *and* input_f) then class membership

The logic processor's topology (and underlying interpretation) is standard. Two LPs can vary in terms of the number of AND neurons, their connections but the format of the resulting logic expression stays quite uniform (as a sum of generalized minterms) and this introduces a significant level of interpretability.

3.12 Computational Intelligence Methods in ECG Signal Analysis and Interpretation

Computational Intelligence has assumed a visible position in studies on processing, interpretation and classification of ECG signals. A representative set of examples is collected in Table 3.4. Here it is worth stressing the synergistic nature of algorithms involved. This synergy becomes particularly visible when dealing with a variety of ways neurocomputing and fuzzy sets become involved in the design of classification and interpretation schemes.

3.13 Conclusions

A wealth of problems of signal processing (filtering, discrimination, interpretation) can be effectively formulated and solved in the setting of Computational Intelligence. CI provided new, attractive opportunities by bringing a facet of nonlinear

Table 3.4 The technology of computational intelligence in ECG signal classification and interpretation: a collection of selected examples

Study	Technologies of CI	Category of problem
Mitra et al. (2006)	Rough sets	Classification
Ozbay et al. (2011)	Type-2 fuzzy sets	Clustering of signals and classification
Yeh et al. (2010)	Fuzzy clustering	Classification
Chua et al. (2011)	Genetic algorithms, fuzzy sets	Arrhythmia classification
Yeh et al. (2010)	Fuzzy sets	Feature selection (signal description)
Lee et al. (2008)	Fuzzy sets (ontology)	Signal description
Meau et al. (2006)	Neural networks and fuzzy sets (neurofuzzy system)	Signal classification
Engin (2004)	Neural networks and fuzzy sets	Signal classification
Acharya et al. (2003)	Fuzzy sets and neural networks	Classification of heart rate
Kundu et al. (2000)	Fuzzy sets, neural networks, knowledge-based systems	Signal interpretation
Presedo et al. (1996)	Fuzzy sets	Ischemia detection
Gacek and Pedrycz (2003)	Genetic segmentation of signals	Preprocessing of ECG signals
Gacek and Pedrycz (2006)	Granulation of signals	Representation (compactification) of ECG signals
Pedrycz and Gacek (2001, 2002)	Fuzzy automata	Classification of ECG signals
Barro et al. (1991)	Fuzzy sets (fuzzy grammars)	Arrhythmia classification
Barro et al. (1981, 1990)	Fuzzy sets (rule-based systems)	Classification (beat labeling)
Korurek and Dogan (2010)	Particle swarm optimization and neural networks	Beat classification
Fei (2010)	Particle swarm optimization and neural networks (support vector machines)	Arrhytmia detection
Moavenian and Khorrami (2010)	Neural networks	Arrhytmia classification
Osowski et al. (2008)	Neural networks	Arrhytmia classification

processing (supported by neural networks) and deliver a realization of a variable perspective at the problem description through information granularity. Furthermore evolutionary computing helps approach the system design from the perspective of structural optimization – a unique opportunity not commonly available when dealing with the "standard" methods of signal processing or classification.

We outlined the fundamentals of Computational Intelligence showing that the synergy of the technologies of fuzzy sets becomes a vital component of the design of intelligent systems.

With this regard, fuzzy sets or, being more general, information granules form an important front- and back-end of constructs of CI. By forming the front end, they help develop a suitable view at ECG data, incorporate available domain knowledge, and come up with a feature space that supports the effectiveness of ensuing processing, quite commonly engaging various schemes of neurocomputing or evolutionary neurocomputing. Equally important role is played by fuzzy sets in the realization of the back end of the overall processing scheme: they strengthen the interpretability of classification results as well as provide useful interpretation faculties to neural networks or help develop logic mappings in the form fuzzy logic neural networks.

Our intention was to highlight the main ideas and the principles of research agenda of Computational Intelligence as well as show that they are well aligned with the challenges we witness in ECG signal processing and interpretation. There have been a number of promising studies at the junction of CI and ECG classifier; they form a solid starting point for further progression.

References

Acharya, U.R., Bhat, P.S., Iyengar, S.S., Rao, A., Dua, S.: Classification of heart rate data using artificial neural network and fuzzy equivalence relation. Pattern Recognit. **36**, 61–68 (2003)

Bargiela, A., Pedrycz, W.: Granular Computing: An Introduction. Kluwer Academic, Dordrecht (2002)

Bargiela, A., Pedrycz, W.: Recursive information granulation: aggregation and interpretation issues. IEEE Trans. Syst. Man Cybern. B **33**(1), 96–112 (2003)

Barro, S., Ruiz, R., Mirai, J.: Fuzzy beat labeling for intelligent arrhythmia monitoring. Comput. Biomed. Res. **2**, 240–258 (1981)

Barro, S., Ruiz, R., Presedo, J., Mirai, J.: Grammatic representation of beat sequences for fuzzy arrhytmia diagnosis. Int. J. Biomed. Comput. **21**, 245–259 (1991)

Bezdek, J.C.: Pattern Recognition with Fuzzy Objective Function Algorithms. Plenum Press, New York (1981)

Bezdek, J.C.: On the relationship between neural networks, pattern recognition and intelligence. Int. J. Approx. Reason. **6**(2), 85–107 (1992)

Bezdek, J.C.: What is computational intelligence, In: Zurada, J.M., Marks II, R.J., Robinson, C.J. (eds.) Computational Intelligence Imitating Life, pp. 1–12. IEEE Press, Piscataway (1994)

Chua, T.W., Tan, W.: Non-singleton genetic fuzzy logic system for arrhythmias classification. Eng. Appl. Artif. Intell. **24**(2), 251–259 (2011)

Duda, R.O., Hart, P.E., Stork, D.G.: Pattern Classification, 2nd edn. Wiley, New York (2001)

Engelbrecht, A.P.: Fundamentals of Computational Swarm Intelligence. Wiley, London (2005)

Engin, M.: ECG beat classification using neuro-fuzzy network. Pattern Recognit. Lett. **25**, 1715–1722 (2004)

Fei, S.W.: Diagnostic study on arrhythmia cordis based on particle swarm optimization-based support vector machine. Exp. Syst. Appl. **37**, 6748–6752 (2010)

Fukunaga, K.: Introduction to Statistical Pattern Recognition, 2nd edn. Academic, New York (1990)

Fulcher, J., Jain, L.C. (eds.): Computational Intelligence: A Compendium. Springer, Berlin (2008)

Gacek, A., Pedrycz, W.: A genetic segmentation of ECG signals. IEEE Trans. Biomed. Eng. **50**(10), 1203–1208 (2003)

Gacek, A., Pedrycz, W.: A granular description of ECG signals. IEEE Trans. Biomed. Eng. **53**(10), 1972–1982 (2006)

Goldberg, D.E.: Genetic Algorithms in Search, Optimization, and Machine Learning. Addison Wesley, Reading (1989)

Haykin, S.: Neural Networks: A Comprehensive Foundation, 2nd edn. Prentice Hall Upper Saddle River (1999)
Hirota, K.: Concepts of probabilistic sets. Fuzzy Sets Syst. **5**(1), 31–46 (1981)
Hirota, K., Pedrycz, W.: Logic based neural networks. Inform. Sci. **71**, 99 130 (1993)
Hoppner, F., et al.: Fuzzy Cluster Analysis. Wiley, Chichester (1999)
Klement, E., Mesiar, R., Pap, E.: Triangular Norms. Kluwer Academic, Dordrecht (2000)
Korurek, M., Dogan, B.: ECG beat classification using particle swarm optimization and radial basis function neural network. Exp. Syst. Appl. **37**, 7563–7569 (2010)
Kundu, M., Nasipuri, M., Basu, D.K.: Knowledge-based ECG interpretation: a critical review. Pattern Recognit. **33**, 351–373 (2000)
Lee, C.S., Wang, M.H.: Ontological fuzzy agent for electrocardiogram application. Exp. Syst. Appl. **35**, 1223–1236 (2008)
Loia, V., Pedrycz, W., Senatore, S.: P-FCM: a proximity-based fuzzy clustering for user-centered web applications. Int. J. Approx. Reason. **34**, 121–144 (2003)
Meau, Y.P., et al.: Intelligent classification of electrocardiogram (ECG) signal using extended Kalman Filter (EKF) based neuro fuzzy system. Comput. Methods Prog. Biomed. **8**(2), 157–168 (2006)
Mitra, S., Mitra, M., Chaudhuri, B.B.: A rough-set-based inference engine for ECG classification. IEEE Trans. Instrum. Meas. **55**(6), 2198–2206 (2006)
Moavenian, M., Khorrami, H.: A qualitative comparison of artificial neural networks and support vector machines in ECG arrhythmias classification. Exp. Syst. Appl. **37**, 3088–3093 (2010)
Moore, R.: Interval analysis. Prentice-Hall, Englewood Cliffs (1966)
Mumford, C.L., Jain, L.C. (eds.): Computational Intelligence. Springer, Berlin (2009)
Osowski, S., Markiewicz, T., Tran Hoai, L.: Recognition and classification system of arrhythmia using ensemble of neural networks. Measurement **41**, 610–617 (2008)
Özbay, Y., Ceylan, R., Karlik, B.: Integration of type-2 fuzzy clustering and wavelet transform in a neural network based ECG classifier. Exp. Syst. Appl. **38**, 1004–1010 (2011)
Pawlak, Z.: Rough sets. Int. J. Comput. Inform. Sci. **11**, 341–356 (1982)
Pawlak, Z.: Rough Sets. Theoretical Aspects of Reasoning About Data. Kluwer Academic, Dordercht (1991)
Pawlak, Z., A. Skowron, rough sets and boolean reasoning. Inform. Sci. **177**(1), 41–73 (2007)
Pedrycz, W.: Fuzzy sets in pattern recognition: methodology and methods. Pattern Recognit. **23**(1–2), 121–146 (1990)
Pedrycz, W.: Computational Intelligence: An Introduction. CRC Press, Boca Raton (1997)
Pedrycz, W.: Shadowed sets: representing and processing fuzzy sets. IEEE Trans. Syst. Man Cybern. Part B **28**, 103–109 (1998)
Pedrycz, W.: Knowledge-Based Clustering: From Data to Information Granules. Wiley, Hoboken (2005)
Pedrycz, W., Bargiela, A.: Granular clustering: a granular signature of data. IEEE Trans. Syst. Man Cybern. **32**(2), 212–224 (2002)
Pedrycz, W., Gacek, A.: Learning of fuzzy automata. Int. J. Comput. Intell. Appl. **1**, 19–33 (2001)
Pedrycz, W., Gacek, A.: Temporal granulation and its application to signal analysis. Inform. Sci. **143**(1–4), 47–71 (2002)
Pedrycz, W., Gomide, F.: Fuzzy Systems Engineering. Wiley, Hoboken (2007)
Pedrycz, W., Rocha, A.: Knowledge-based neural networks. IEEE Trans. Fuzzy Syst. **1**, 254–266 (1993)
Pedrycz, W., Waletzky, J.: Neural network front-ends in unsupervised learning. IEEE Trans. Neural Netw. **8**, 390–401 (1997a)
Pedrycz, W., Waletzky, J.: Fuzzy clustering with partial supervision. IEEE Trans. Syst. Man Cybern. **5**, 787–795 (1997b)
Presedo, J., et al.: Fuzzy modelling of the expert's knowledge in ECG-based ischaemia detection. Fuzzy Sets Syst. **77**, 63–75 (1996)
Yeh, Y.C., Wang, W.J., Chiou, C.W.: A novel fuzzy c-means method for classifying heartbeat cases from ECG signals. Measurement **43**, 1542–1555 (2010)

Yeh, Y.C., Wang, W.J., Chiou, C.W.: Feature selection algorithm for ECG signals using range-overlaps method. Exp. Syst. Appl. **37**, 3499–3512 (2010)

Wassermann, P.D.: Neural Computing: Theory and Practice. Van Nostrand, Reinhold, New York (1989)

Zadeh, L.A.: Fuzzy sets. Inf. Control, **8**, 338–353 (1965)

Zadeh, L.A.: Towards a theory of fuzzy information granulation and its centrality in human reasoning and fuzzy logic. Fuzzy Sets Syst. **90**, 111–117 (1997)

Zadeh, L.A.: Toward a generalized theory of uncertainty (GTU) – –an outline. Inf. Sci. **172**, 1–40 (2005)

Chapter 4
A Generic and Patient-Specific Electrocardiogram Signal Classification System

Turker Ince, Serkan Kiranyaz, and Moncef Gabbouj

4.1 Introduction

Each individual heartbeat in the cardiac cycle of the recorded electrocardiogram (ECG) waveform shows the time evolution of the heart's electrical activity, which is made of distinct electrical depolarization–repolarization patterns of the heart. Any disorder of heart rate or rhythm, or change in the morphological pattern is an indication of an arrhythmia, which could be detected by analysis of the recorded ECG waveform. Real-time automated ECG analysis in clinical settings is of great assistance to clinicians in detecting cardiac arrhythmias, which often arise as a consequence of a cardiac disease and may be life-threatening and require immediate therapy. However, automated classification of ECG beats is a challenging problem as the morphological and temporal characteristics of ECG signals show significant variations for different patients and under different temporal and physical conditions (Hoekema et al. 2001). Many algorithms for automatic detection and classification of ECG heartbeat patterns have been presented in the literature including signal processing techniques such as frequency analysis (Minami et al. 1999), wavelet transform (Shyu et al. 2004; Inan et al. 2006), and filter banks (Alfonso and Nguyen 1999), statistical (Willems and Lesaffre 1987) and heuristic approaches (Talmon 1983), hidden Markov models (Coast et al. 1990), support vector machines (Osowski et al. 2004), artificial neural networks (ANNs) (Hu et al. 1994), and mixture-of-experts method (Hu et al. 1997). In general, ECG classifier systems based on past approaches have not performed well in

T. Ince (✉)
Faculty of Engineering and Computer Sciences, Izmir University of Economics, Balcova-Izmir, Turkey
e-mail: turker.ince@ieu.edu.tr

S. Kiranyaz · M. Gabbouj
Department of Signal Processing, Tampere University of Technology, Tampere, Finland
e-mail: serkan.kiranyaz@tut.fi; moncef.gabbouj@tut.fi

A. Gacek and W. Pedrycz (eds.), *ECG Signal Processing, Classification and Interpretation: A Comprehensive Framework of Computational Intelligence*,
DOI 10.1007/978-0-85729-868-3_4, © Springer-Verlag London Limited 2012

practice because of their important common drawback of having an inconsistent performance when classifying a new patient's ECG waveform. This makes them unreliable to be widely used clinically, and causes severe degradation in their accuracy and efficiency for larger databases, (Lee 1989; de Chazal and Reilly 2006). Moreover, the *Association for the Advancement of Medical Instrumentation* (AAMI) provides standards and recommended practices for reporting performance results of automated arrhythmia detection algorithms (AAMI 1987). However, despite quite many ECG classification methods proposed in the literature, only few (Hu et al. 1997; de Chazal et al. 2004; Jiang and Kong 2007) have in fact used the AAMI standards as well as the complete data from the benchmark MIT-BIH arrhythmia database.

The performance of ECG pattern classification strongly depends on the characterization power of the features extracted from the ECG data and on the design of the classifier (classification model or network structure and parameters). Due to its time–frequency localization properties, the wavelet transform is an efficient tool for analyzing non-stationary ECG signals (Li et al. 1995). The wavelet transform can be used to decompose an ECG signal according to scale, allowing separation of the relevant ECG waveform morphology descriptors from the noise, interference, baseline drift, and amplitude variation of the original signal. Several researchers have previously used the wavelet transform coefficients at the appropriate scales as morphological feature vectors rather than the original signal time series and achieved good classification performance (Shyu et al. 2004; Inan et al. 2006). Accordingly in the current work the proposed feature extraction technique employs the translation-invariant dyadic wavelet transform (TI-DWT) in order to extract effectively the morphological information from ECG data. Furthermore, the dimension of the input morphological feature vector is reduced by projecting it onto a lower-dimensional feature space using principal component analysis (PCA) in order to significantly reduce redundancies in such a high dimensional data space. The lower-dimensional morphological feature vector is then combined with two critical temporal features related to inter-beat time interval (the R-R time interval and R-R time interval ratio) to improve accuracy and robustness of classification as suggested by the results of previous studies (de Chazal et al. 2004).

Artificial neural networks (ANNs) are powerful tools for pattern recognition as they have the capability to learn complex, nonlinear surfaces among different classes, and such ability can therefore be the key for ECG beat recognition and classification (Silipo and Marchesi 1998). Although many promising ANN-based techniques have been applied to ECG signal classification, (Silipo and Marchesi 1998; Osowski and Linh 2001; Lagerholm et al. 2000; Silipo et al. 1995) the global classifiers based on a static (fixed) ANN have not performed well in practice. On the other hand, algorithms based on patient-adaptive architecture have demonstrated significant performance improvement over conventional global classifiers (Hu et al. 1997; de Chazal and Reilly 2006; Jiang and Kong 2007). Among all, one particular approach, a personalized ECG heartbeat pattern classifier based on evolvable block-based neural networks (BbNN) using *Hermite* transform coefficients (Jiang and Kong 2007), achieved such a performance that is significantly higher than the others. Although this recent work clearly demonstrates the advantage of using evolutionary ANNs, which can be automatically designed according to the problem (patient's ECG data), serious drawbacks and limitations can also be observed. For instance, there are around 10–15 parameters/thresholds that needed to be set empirically with respect to the dataset used and this obviously brings about the issue of robustness when it is used for a different database. Another drawback can occur due to the specific ANN structure proposed, i.e., the BbNN, which requires equal sizes for input and output layers. Even more critical is the Back Propagation (BP) method, used for training, and Genetic Algorithm (GA), for evolving the network structure, both have certain deficiencies (Yao and Liu 1997). In particular, the BP most likely gets trapped into a local minimum, making it entirely dependent on the initial (weight) settings.

In order to address such deficiencies and drawbacks, in this chapter we propose a multi-dimensional particle swarm optimization (MD PSO) technique, which automatically designs the optimal ANNs (both network structure and connection weights with respect to the training mean square error) specifically for each patient and according to the patient's ECG data. On the contrary to the specific BbNN structure used in (Jiang and Kong 2007) with the aforementioned problems, MD PSO is used to evolve traditional ANNs and so the focus is particularly drawn on automatic design of the multilayer perceptrons (MLPs). This evolutionary operator makes the proposed system *generic*, that is no assumption is made about the number of (hidden) layers and in fact none of the network properties (e.g., feed-forward or not, differentiable activation function or not, etc.) is an inherent constraint. As long as the potential network configurations are transformed into a hash (dimension) table with a proper hash function where indices represent the solution space dimensions of the particles, MD PSO can then seek both positional and dimensional optima in an interleaved PSO process. The optimum dimension found corresponds to a distinct ANN architecture where the network parameters (connections, weights and biases) can be resolved from the positional optimum reached on that dimension. Earlier work on detection of premature ventricular contractions (PVCs) demonstrated performance improvement of the proposed approach over conventional techniques (Ince et al. 2008). Moreover, we aim to achieve a high level of *robustness* with respect to the variations of the dataset, since the proposed system is designed with a minimum set of parameters, and in such a way that their significant variations should not show a major impact on the overall performance. Above all, using standard ANNs such as traditional MLPs, instead of specific architectures [e.g., BbNN in (Jiang and Kong 2007)] further contributes to the generic nature of the proposed system and in short, all these objectives are meant to make it applicable to any ECG dataset without any modifications (such as tuning the parameters or changing the feature vectors, ANN types, etc.). The overview of the proposed system is shown in Fig. 4.1.

The rest of this chapter is organized as follows. Section 4.2 outlines the ECG dataset used in this study and provides a detailed description of the feature extraction methodology for the proposed patient-specific heartbeat classification system. MD PSO and its application over the automatic ANN design are presented in Sect. 4.3. In Sect. 4.4, the optimality, performance and robustness of the proposed classifier

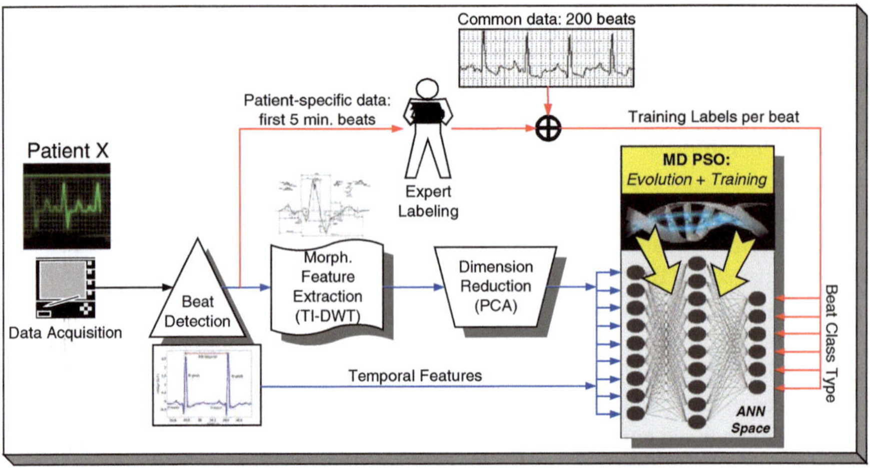

Fig. 4.1 Patient-specific training process of the proposed ECG classification system

are evaluated over the MIT/BIH arrhythmia database using standard performance metrics and the results are compared with previously published work. Finally, Sect. 4.5 concludes the chapter.

4.2 ECG Data Processing

4.2.1 ECG Data

In this study, the MIT/BIH arrhythmia database (Mark and Moody 1980) is used for training and performance evaluation of the proposed patient-specific ECG classifier. The database contains 48 records, each containing two-channel ECG signals for 30-min duration selected from 24-h recordings of 47 individuals. Continuous ECG signals are band-pass filtered at 0.1–100 Hz and then digitized at 360 Hz. The database contains annotation for both timing information and beat class information verified by independent experts. In the current work, so as to comply with the AAMI ECAR-1987 recommended practice (AAMI 1987), we used 44 records from the MIT/BIH arrhythmia database, excluding 4 records which contain paced heartbeats. The first 20 records (numbered in the range of 100–124), which include representative samples of routine clinical recordings, are used to select representative beats to be included in the common training data. The remaining 24 records (numbered in the range of 200–234) contain ventricular, junctional, and supraventricular arrhythmias. A total of 83,648 beats from all 44 records are used as test patterns for performance evaluation. AAMI recommends that each ECG beat be classified into the following five heartbeat types: N (beats originating in the sinus mode), S (supraventricular ectopic beats), V (ventricular ectopic beats), F (fusion beats), and Q (unclassifiable beats). For all records, we used the modified-lead II signals and utilized the labels to locate beats in ECG data. The beat detection process is beyond the scope of this work, as many highly accurate (>99%) beat detection algorithms have been reported in literature (Pan and Tompkins 1985; Li et al. 1995).

4.2.2 Feature Extraction Methodology

As suggested by the results from previous works (Hu et al. 1994, 1997; de Chazal et al. 2004), both morphological and temporal features are extracted and combined into a single feature vector for each heartbeat to improve accuracy and robustness of the proposed classifier. The wavelet transform is used to extract morphological information from the ECG data. The time-domain ECG signatures were first normalized by subtracting the mean voltage before transforming into time-scale domain using the dyadic wavelet transform (DWT). According to wavelet transform theory, the multiresolution representation of the ECG signal is achieved by convolving the signal with scaled and translated versions of a mother wavelet. For practical applications, such as processing of sampled and quantized raw ECG signals, the discrete wavelet transform can be computed by scaling the wavelet at the dyadic sequence $(2^j)_{j \in Z}$ and translating it on a dyadic grid whose interval is proportional to 2^{-j}. The discrete WT is not only complete but also non-redundant unlike the continuous WT. Moreover, the wavelet transform of a discrete signal can be efficiently calculated using the decomposition by a two-channel multirate filter bank (the pyramid decomposition). However, due to the rate-change operators in the filter bank, the discrete WT is not time-invariant but actually very sensitive to the alignment of the signal in time (Mallat 1999).

To address the time-varying problem of wavelet transforms, Mallat proposed a new algorithm for wavelet representation of a signal, which is invariant to time shifts (Mallat and Zhong 1992). According to this algorithm, which is called a translation-invariant dyadic wavelet transform (TI-DWT), only the scale parameter is sampled along the dyadic sequence $(2^j)_{j \in Z}$ and the wavelet transform is calculated for each point in time. TI-DWTs pioneered by Mallat have been successfully applied to pattern recognition (Mallat and Zhong 1992). The fast TI-DWT algorithm, whose computational complexity is $O(N \log N)$, can be implemented using a recursive filter tree architecture (Mallat and Zhong 1992). In this study, we selected a quadratic spline wavelet with compact support and one vanishing moment, as defined in (Mallat and Zhong 1992). The same wavelet function has already been successfully applied to QRS detection in (Li et al. 1995), achieving a 99.8% QRS detection rate for the MIT/BIH arrhythmia database. In the proposed ECG classification system, using a wavelet-based beat detector such as in (Li et al. 1995) allows the same wavelet transform block to operate directly on the raw input ECG signal for beat detection and then morphological feature extraction, thus making the system more efficient and robust.

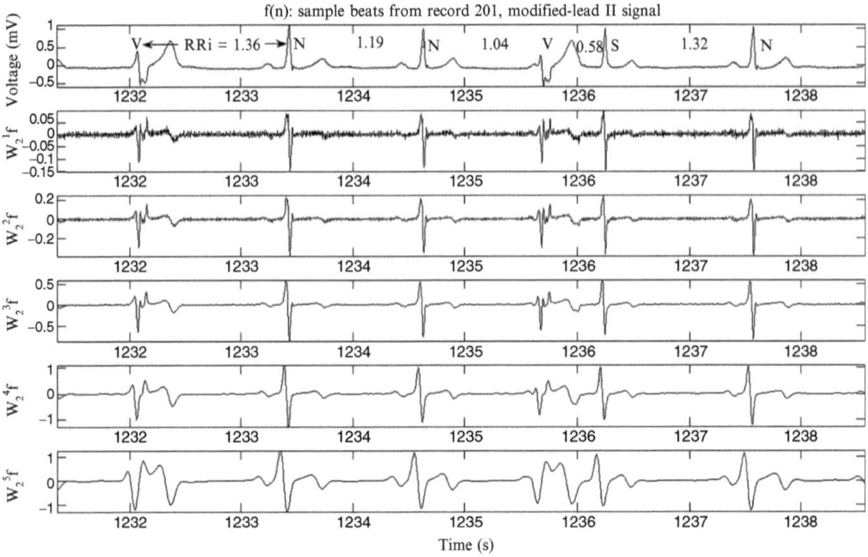

Fig. 4.2 Sample beat waveforms, including Normal (*N*), PVC (*V*), and APC (*S*) AAMI heartbeat classes, selected from record 201 modified-lead II from the MIT/BIH arrhythmia database and corresponding TI DWT decompositions for the first five scales

Figure 4.2 shows sample beat waveforms, including Normal (N), PVC (V), and APC (S) AAMI heartbeat classes, selected from record 201, modified-lead II from the MIT/BIH arrhythmia database and their corresponding translation-invariant DWT decompositions computed for the first five scales. While wavelet-based morphological features provide effective discrimination capability between normal and some abnormal heartbeats (i.e., PVC beats), two temporal features (i.e., the R-R time interval and R-R time interval ratio) contribute to the discriminating power of wavelet-based features, especially in discriminating morphologically similar heartbeat patterns (i.e., Normal and APC beats).

In Fig. 4.3 (top), the estimated power spectrum of windowed ECG signal (a 500-ms long *Hanning* window is applied before FFT to suppress high-frequency components due to discontinuities in the end-points) from record 201 for N, V, and S beats is plotted, while equivalent frequency responses of FIR filters, $Q_j(w)$, for the first five scales at the native 360-Hz sampling frequency of the MIT/BIH data are illustrated at the bottom part of the figure. After analyzing the DWT decompositions of different ECG waveforms in the database, and according to the power spectra of ECG signal (the QRS complex, the P- and T-waves), noise, and artifact in Thakor et al. (1984), we selected $W_{2^4}f$ (at scale 2^4) signal as morphological features of each heartbeat waveform. Based on the -3-dB bandwidth of the equivalent $Q_4(w)$ filter (3.9–22.5 Hz) in Fig. 4.3 (bottom), $W_{2^4}f$ signal is expected to contain most of QRS complex energy and the least amount of high-frequency noise and low-frequency baseline wander. The fourth scale decomposition together with RR-interval timing

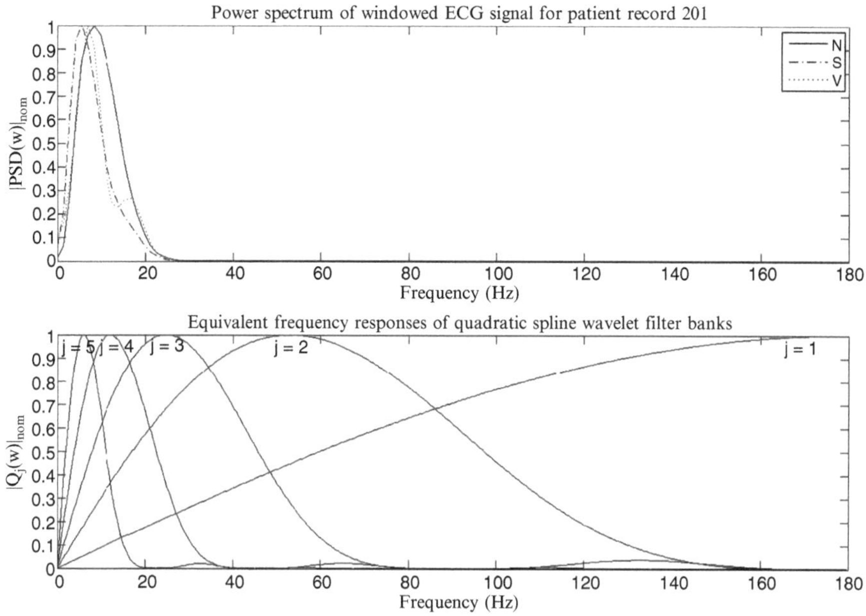

Fig. 4.3 Power spectrum of windowed ECG signal from record 201 for Normal (*N*), PVC (*V*), and APC (*S*) AAMI heartbeat classes, and equivalent frequency responses of FIR digital filters for a quadratic spline wavelet at 360-Hz sampling rate

information was previously shown to be the best performing feature set for DWT-based PVC beat classification in (Inan et al. 2006). Therefore, a 180-sample morphological feature vector is extracted per heartbeat from DWT of ECG signal at scale 2^4 by selecting a 500-ms window centered at the R-peak (found by using the beat annotation file). Each feature vector is then normalized to have a zero-mean and a unit variance to eliminate the effect of dc offset and amplitude biases.

4.2.3 Preprocessing by Principal Component Analysis

The wavelet-based morphological features in the training set are post-processed using principal component analysis (PCA) to reduce dimensionality (and redundancy) of input feature vectors. PCA, also known as the Karhunen-Loéve transform (KLT), is a well-known statistical method that has been used for data analysis, data compression, redundancy and dimensionality reduction, and feature extraction. PCA is the optimal linear transformation, which finds a projection of the input pattern vectors onto a lower-dimensional feature space that retains the maximum amount of energy among all possible linear transformations of the pattern space. To describe the basic procedure of PCA, let F be a feature matrix of size $K \times N$, whose

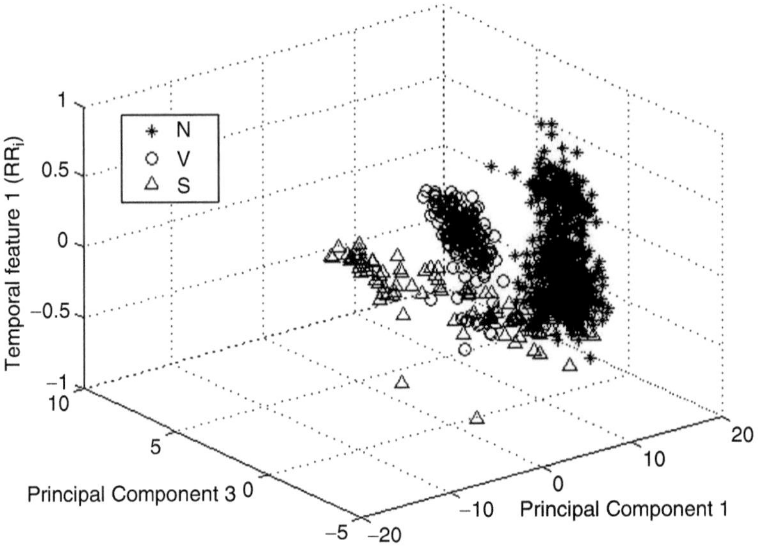

Fig. 4.4 Scatter plot of Normal (*N*), PVC (*V*), and APC (*S*) beats from record 201 in terms of the first and third principal components and RR_i time interval

rows are wavelet features of size $1 \times N$ each belonging to one of K heartbeats in the training data. First, the covariance matrix C_{F} of this feature matrix is computed as,

$$C_{\mathrm{F}} = E\left\{(F-m)(F-m)^t\right\}, \tag{4.1}$$

where m is the mean pattern vector. From the eigen-decomposition of C_F, which is a $K \times K$ symmetric and positive-definite matrix, the principal components taken as the eigenvectors corresponding to the largest eigenvalues are selected, and the morphological feature vectors are then projected onto these principal components (KL basis functions). In this work, nine principal components which contain about 95% of overall energy in the original feature matrix are selected to form a resultant compact morphological feature vector for each heartbeat signal. In this case, the PCA reduced the dimensionality of morphological features by a factor of 20. Figure 4.4 shows a scatter plot of Normal, PVC, and APC beats from record 201 in terms of the first and third principal components and inter-beat time interval. It is worth noting that dimensionality reduction of the input information improves efficiency of the learning for a NN classifier due to a smaller number of input nodes (Pittner and Kamarthi 1999).

The data used for training the individual patient classifier consists of two parts: global (common to each patient) and local (patient-specific) training patterns. While patient-specific data contains the first 5-min segment of each patient's ECG record and is used as part of the training data to perform patient adaptation, the global data set contains a relatively small number of representative beats from each class in the training files and helps the classifier learn other arrhythmia patterns that are not included in the patient-specific data. This practice conforms to the AAMI-recommended procedure allowing the usage of at most 5-min section from the beginning of each patient's recording for training (AAMI 1987).

4.3 MD PSO Technique for Automatic ANN Design

As mentioned earlier, evolutionary ANNs are used for the classification of ECG data from each individual patient in the database. In this section, the MD PSO technique, which is developed for evolving ANNs, will be introduced first and we shall present its application for evolving the feed-forward ANNs next.

4.3.1 MD PSO Algorithm

The behavior of a single organism in a swarm is often insignificant but their collective and social behavior is of paramount importance. The particle swarm optimization (PSO) was introduced by Kennedy and Eberhart in 1995 as a population-based stochastic search and optimization process (Kennedy and Eberhart 1995). It is originated from the computer simulation of the individuals (particles or living organisms) in a bird flock or fish school, which basically shows a natural behavior when they search for some target (e.g., food). In the basic PSO algorithm, the particles are initially distributed randomly over the search space with a random velocity and the goal is to converge to the global optimum (according to a given fitness score) of a function or a system. Each particle keeps track of its position in the search space and its best solution (i.e., lowest fitness score) so far achieved. This is the personal best value (the so-called *pbest*) and the PSO process also keeps track of the global best solution so far achieved by the swarm with its particle index (the so called *gbest*). So during their journey with discrete time iterations, the velocity of each particle in the next iteration is computed by the best position of the swarm (position of the particle *gbest* as the *social* component), the best personal position of the particle (*pbest* as the *cognitive* component), and its current velocity (the *memory* term). Both *social* and *cognitive* components contribute randomly to the position of the particle in the next iteration. In principle, PSO follows the same path of the other evolutionary algorithms (EAs) such as Genetic Algorithm (GA), Genetic Programming (GP), Evolutionary Strategies (ES), and Evolutionary Programming (EP). The common point of all is that EAs are in population-based nature and thus they can avoid being trapped in a local optimum. Thus, they can find the optimum solutions; however, this is never guaranteed.

Instead of operating at a fixed dimension N, the MD PSO algorithm is designed to seek both positional and dimensional optima within a dimension range, ($D_{\min} \leq N \leq D_{\max}$). In order to accomplish this, each particle has two sets of components, each of which has been subjected to two independent and consecutive processes. The first one is a regular positional PSO, i.e., the traditional velocity updates and due positional shifts in N dimensional search (solution) space. The second one is a dimensional PSO, which allows the particle to navigate through a range of dimensions. Accordingly, each particle keeps track of its last position, velocity, and personal best position (*pbest*) in a particular dimension so that when it revisits that same dimension at a later time, it can perform its regular "positional" fly using this information. The dimensional PSO process of each particle may then move the particle to another dimension where it will remember its positional status and keep "flying" within the positional PSO process in this dimension, and so on. The swarm, on the other hand, keeps track of the *gbest* particles in all dimensions, each of which respectively indicates the best (global) position so far achieved and can thus be used in the regular velocity update equation for that dimension. Similarly, the dimensional PSO process of each particle uses its personal best dimension in which the personal best fitness score has so far been achieved. Finally, the swarm keeps track of the global best dimension, *dbest*, among all the personal best dimensions. The *gbest* particle in *dbest* dimension represents the optimum solution and dimension, respectively. The details and the pseudo-code of the MD PSO algorithm can be found in (Kiranyaz et al. 2010).

4.3.2 MD PSO for Evolving ANNs

As a stochastic search process in a multi-dimensional search space, MD PSO seeks for (near-)optimal (with respect to the training error) networks in an architecture space, which can be defined by any type of ANNs with any properties. All network configurations in the architecture space are enumerated into a (dimensional) hash table with a proper hash function, which basically ranks the networks with respect to their complexity, i.e., associates higher hash indices to networks with higher complexity. MD PSO can then use each index as a unique dimension of the search space where particles can make inter-dimensional navigations to seek an optimum dimension (*dbest*) and the optimum solution on that dimension, $x\hat{y}^{dbest}$. As mentioned earlier, the former corresponds to the optimal architecture and the latter encapsulates the (optimum) network parameters (connections, weights, and biases).

In this section, we apply MD PSO technique for evolving fully-connected, feed-forward ANNs, or the so-called MLPs. As mentioned earlier, the reasoning behind this choice is that MLP is the most widely used in this field and so our aim is to show that a superior performance as in (Jiang and Kong 2007) can also be achieved without using such specific ANN structures. MD PSO can evolve any MLP type and thus the architecture space can be defined over a wide range of configurations, i.e., say from a single-layer perceptron (SLP) to complex MLPs with many hidden layers. Suppose for the sake of simplicity, a range is defined for the minimum and maximum number of layers, $\{L_{\min}, L_{\max}\}$ and number of neurons for hidden layer l, $\{N^l_{\min}, N^l_{\max}\}$.Without loss of generality, assume that the size of both input and output layers is determined by the problem, and hence, fixed. As a result, the architecture space can now be defined only by two range arrays, $R_{\min} = \{N_{\rm I}, N^1_{\min}, \ldots, N^{L_{\max}-1}_{\min}, N_{\rm O}\}$ and $R_{\max} = \{N_{\rm I}, N^1_{\max}, \ldots, N^{L_{\max}-1}_{\max}, N_{\rm O}\}$, one for the minimum and the other for the maximum number of neurons allowed for each layer of a MLP. The size of both arrays is naturally $L_{\max} + 1$ where corresponding entries define the range of the lth hidden layer for all those MLPs, which can have an lth hidden layer. The size of input and output layers, $\{N_{\rm I}, N_{\rm O}\}$, is fixed and remains the same for all configurations in the architecture space within which any l-layer MLP can be defined provided that $L_{\min} \le l \le L_{\max}$. $L_{\min} \ge 1$ and $L_{\max}$ can be set to any meaningful value for the problem at hand. The hash function then enumerates all potential MLP configurations into hash indices, starting from the simplest MLP with $L_{\min} - 1$ hidden layers, each of which has a minimum number of neurons given by $R_{\min}$, to the most complex network with $L_{\max} - 1$ hidden layers, each of which has a maximum number of neurons given by $R_{\max}$.

Let $N^l_{\rm h}$ be the number of hidden neurons in layer l of a MLP with input and output layer sizes $N_{\rm I}$ and $N_{\rm O}$, respectively. The input neurons are merely fan-out units since no processing takes place. Let F be the activation function applied over the weighted inputs plus a bias, as follows:

$$y^{p,l}_k = F\left(s^{p,l}_k\right) \quad \text{where} \quad s^{p,l}_k = \sum_j w^{l-1}_{jk} y^{p,l-1}_j + \theta^l_k \tag{4.2}$$

where $y^{p,l}_k$ is the output of the kth neuron of the lth hidden/output layer when the pattern p is fed, w^{l-1}_{jk} is the weight from the jth neuron in layer $(l-1)$ to the kth neuron in layer l, and θ^l_k is the bias value of the kth neuron of the lth hidden/output layer, respectively. The cost function under which optimality is sought is the training mean square error, *MSE*, formulated as,

$$\text{MSE} = \frac{1}{2PN_{\rm O}} \sum_{p \in T} \sum_{k=1}^{N_{\rm O}} \left(t^p_k - y^{p,O}_k\right)^2 \tag{4.3}$$

where t^p_k is the target (desired) output and $y^{p,O}_k$ is the actual output from the kth neuron in the output layer, $l = O$, for pattern p in the training set T with size P, respectively. At time t, suppose that the particle a in the swarm, $\xi = \{x_1, \ldots, x_a, \ldots, x_S\}$, has the positional component formed as, $xx^{xd_a(t)}_a(t) = \{\{w^0_{jk}\}, \{w^1_{jk}\}, \{\theta^1_k\}, \{w^2_{jk}\}, \{\theta^2_k\}, \ldots, \{w^{O-1}_{jk}\}, \{\theta^{O-1}_k\}, \{\theta^O_k\}\}$ where $\{w^l_{jk}\}$ and $\{\theta^l_k\}$ represent the sets of weights and biases of the layer l. Note that the input layer $(l = 0)$ contains only weights whereas the output layer $(l = O)$ has only biases. By means of such a direct encoding scheme, a particle a in the swarm represents all potential network parameters of the MLP architecture at the dimension (hash index) $xd_a(t)$. As mentioned earlier, the dimension range, $D_{\min} \le xd_a(t) \le D_{\max}$, where MD PSO particles can make inter-dimensional jumps, is determined by the architecture space defined. Apart from the regular limits such as (positional) velocity range, $\{V_{\min}, V_{\max}\}$, dimensional velocity range, $\{VD_{\min}, VD_{\max}\}$, the data space can also be limited with some practical range, i.e., $X_{\min} < xx_a^{xd_a(t)}(t) < X_{\max}$. In short, only some meaningful boundaries should be defined in advance for a MD PSO process, as opposed to other GA-based methods, which use several parameters, thresholds and some other (alien) techniques (e.g., simulated annealing (SA), back-propagation (BP), etc.) in a complex process. Setting *MSE* in Eq. 4.3 as the fitness function enables MD PSO to perform *evolutions* of both network parameters and architectures within its native process.

4.4 Experimental Results

In this section, we shall first demonstrate the *optimality* of the networks [with respect to the training mean square error as in Eq. 4.3], which are automatically evolved by the MD PSO method according to the training set of an individual patient record in the benchmark database. We shall then present the overall results obtained from the ECG classification experiments and perform comparative evaluations against several state-of-the-art techniques in this field. Finally the robustness of the proposed system against variations of major parameters will be evaluated.

4.4.1 MD PSO Optimality Evaluation

In order to determine which network architectures are optimal (whether it is global or local) for a particular problem, we apply exhaustive BP training over every network configuration in the architecture space defined. As mentioned earlier, BP is a gradient descent algorithm, and thus, for a single run, it is susceptible to get trapped to the nearest local minimum. However, performing it a large number of times (e.g., $K = 500$) with randomized initial parameters eventually increases the chance of converging to (a close vicinity of) the global minimum of the fitness function. Note that even though K is kept quite high, there is still no guarantee of converging to the global optimum with BP; however, the idea is to obtain the "trend" of best performances achievable with every configuration under equal training conditions. In this way, the optimality of the networks evolved by MD PSO can be justified under the assumed criterion.

Due to the reasoning given earlier, the architecture space is defined over MLPs (possibly including one SLP) with the following activation function: *hyperbolic tangent* ($\tanh(x) = \frac{e^x - e^{-x}}{e^x + e^{-x}}$). The input and output layer sizes are determined by the problem. We use a learning parameter for BP as $\lambda = 0.001$ and iteration number is 10,000. We kept the default PSO parameters for MD PSO with a swarm size, $S = 100$, and velocity ranges are empirically set as $V_{\max} = -V_{\min} = X_{\max}/2$, and

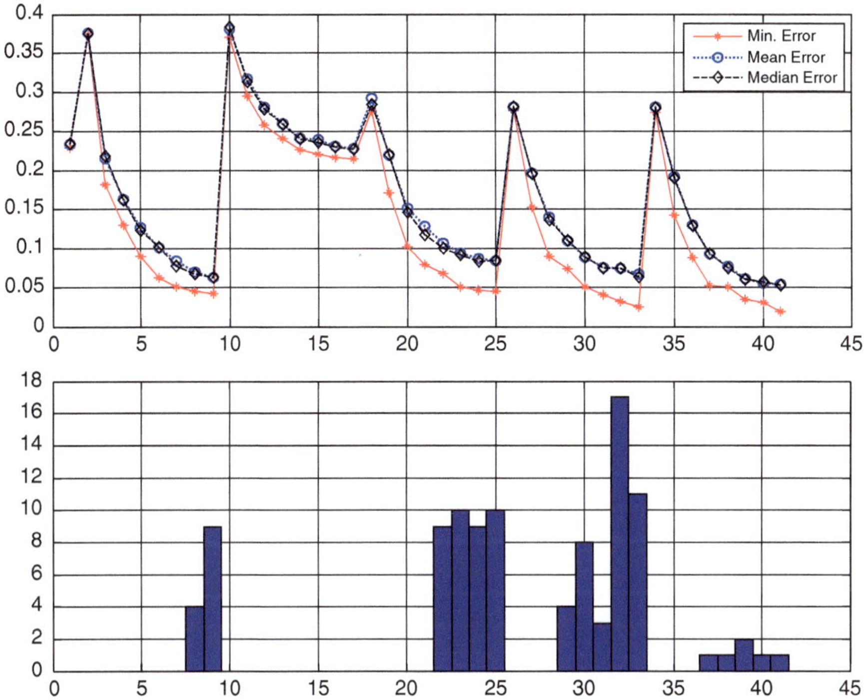

Fig. 4.5 Error statistics (MSE vs. hash index) from exhaustive BP training (*top*) and *dbest* histogram from 100 MD PSO evolutions (*bottom*) for patient record 222

$VD_{\max} = -VD_{\min} = D_{\max}/2$. The dimension range is determined by the architecture space defined and the position range is set as $X_{\max} = -X_{\min} = 2$. Unless stated otherwise, these parameters are used in all experiments presented in this section.

In order to show the optimality of the network configurations evolved by MD PSO with respect to the MSE criterion, we first use the "limited" architecture space with 41 ANNs ($R^1 : R^1_{\min} = \{N_I, 1, 1, N_O\}$ and $R^1_{\max} = \{N_I, 8, 4, N_O\}$) containing the simplest 1, 2, or 3 layers MLPs with $L^1_{\min} = 1$, $L^1_{\max} = 3$, and $N_I = 11$, $N_O = 5$. We then select one of the most challenging records among MIT/BIH arrhythmia database, belonging to the patient record 222. For this record, we perform 100 MD PSO runs with 100 particles, each of which terminates at the end of 1,000 epochs (iterations). At the end of each run, the best fitness score (minimum MSE) achieved, $f(x\hat{y}^{dbest})$, by the particle with the index *gbest(dbest)* at the optimum dimension *dbest* is stored. The histogram of *dbest*, which is a hash index indicating a particular network configuration in R^1, eventually provides the crucial information about the (near-) optimal configuration(s).

Figure 4.5 shows *dbest* histogram and the error statistics plot from the exhaustive BP training the data of patient record 222. From the minimum (mean-square) error (*mMSE*) plot of the exhaustive BP training on top, it is clear that only four distinct sets of network configurations can achieve training *mMSEs* below 0.1. The corresponding indices (dimensions) to these four optimal networks are $dbest = 9, 25, 33$, and 41, where MD PSO managed to evolve either to them or to a neighbor (near-optimal) configuration. MD PSO can in fact achieve the best (lowest) training *MSEs* for two sets of configurations: $dbest = 33$ and 41 (including their 3 close neighbors). These are three-layer MLPs; $dbest = 33$ is for $11 \times 8 \times 3 \times 5$ and $dbest = 41$ is for $11 \times 8 \times 4 \times 5$. All MD PSO runs evolved either to $dbest = 25$ (corresponding to configuration $11 \times 8 \times 2 \times 5$) or to its neighbors, performed slightly worse than the best configurations. MD PSO runs, which evolved to the simplest MLPs with single hidden layer (i.e., $dbest = 8$ and 9 are for the MLPs $11 \times 7 \times 5$ and $11 \times 8 \times 5$) achieved the worst *mMSE, about 15% higher than for* $dbest = 33$ and 41. The reason of MD PSO evolutions to those slightly worse configurations (for $dbest = 25$ and particularly for $dbest = 9$) is that MD PSO or PSO in general performs better in low dimensions. Furthermore, premature convergence is still a problem in PSO when the search space is in high dimensions (Van den Bergh 2002). Therefore, MD PSO naturally favors a low-dimension solution when it exhibits a competitive performance compared to a higher dimension counterpart. Such a natural tendency eventually yields the evolution process to compact network configurations in the architecture space rather than the complex ones, as long as optimality prevails.

4.4.2 Classification Performance

We performed classification experiments on all 44 records of the MIT/BIH arrhythmia database, which includes a total of 100,389 beats to be classified into five heartbeat types following the AAMI convention. For the classification experiments in this work, the common part of the training data set contains a total of 245 representative beats, including 75 from each type N, -S, and -V beats, and all (13) type-F and (7) type-Q beats, *randomly* sampled from each class from the first 20 records (picked from the range 100–124) of the MIT/BIH database. The patient-specific training data includes the beats from the first 5 min of the corresponding patient's ECG record. Patient-specific feed-forward MLP networks are trained with a total of 245 common training beats and a variable number of patient-specific beats depending on the patient's heart rate, so only less than 1% of the total beats are used for training each neural network. The remaining beats (25 min) of each record, in which 24 out of 44 records are completely new to the classifier, are used as test patterns for performance evaluation.

Table 4.1 summarizes beat-by-beat classification results of ECG heartbeat patterns for all test records. Classification performance is measured using the four standard metrics found in the literature (Hu et al. 1997): classification accuracy (*Acc*), sensitivity (*Sen*), specificity (*Spe*), and positive predictivity (*Ppr*). While accuracy measures the overall system performance over all classes of beats, the other metrics are specific to each class and they measure the ability of the classification

Table 4.1 Summary table of beat-by-beat classification results for all 44 records in the MIT/BIH arrhythmia database

		Classification result				
		N	S	V	F	Q
Ground Truth	N	73019 (40532)	991 (776)	513 (382)	98 (56)	29 (20)
	S	686 (672)	1568 (1441)	205 (197)	5 (5)	6 (5)
	V	462 (392)	333 (299)	4993 (4022)	79 (75)	32 (32)
	F	168 (164)	28 (26)	48 (46)	379 (378)	2 (2)
	Q	8 (6)	1 (0)	3 (1)	1 (1)	1 (0)

Classification results for the testing dataset only (24 records from the range 200–234) are shown in parenthesis.

algorithm to distinguish certain events (i.e., VEBs or SVEBs) from nonevents (i.e., non-VEBs or non-SVEBs). The respective definitions of these four common metrics using true positive (*TP*), true negative (*TN*), false positive (*FP*), and false negative (*FN*) are as follows: *Accuracy* is the ratio of the number of correctly classified patterns to the total number of patterns classified, $\text{Acc} = (\text{TP}+\text{TN})/(\text{TP}+\text{TN}+\text{FP}+\text{FN})$; *Sensitivity* is the rate of correctly classified events among all events, $\text{Sen} = \text{TP}/(\text{TP}+\text{FN})$; *Specificity* is the rate of correctly classified nonevents among all nonevents, $\text{Spe} = \text{TN}/(\text{TN}+\text{FP})$; and *Positive Predictivity* is the rate of correctly classified events in all detected events, $\text{Ppr} = \text{TP}/(\text{TP}+\text{FP})$. Since there is a large variation in the number of beats from different classes in the training/testing data (i.e., 39,465/50,354 type-N, 1,277/5,716 type-V, and 190/2,571 type-S beats), sensitivity, specificity, and positive predictivity are more relevant performance criteria for medical diagnosis applications.

The proposed system is compared with three existing algorithms, (Hu et al. 1997; de Chazal and Reilly 2006; Jiang and Kong 2007), which comply with the AAMI standards and use *all* records from the MIT/BIH arrhythmia database. For comparing the performance results, the problem of VEB and SVEB detection is considered individually. The VEB and SVEB classification results of the proposed technique over all 44 records are summarized in Table 4.2. The performance results for VEB detection in the first four rows of Table 4.2 are based on 11 test recordings (200, 202, 210, 213, 214, 219, 221, 228, 231, 233, and 234) that are common to all four methods. For SVEB detection, comparison results are based on 14 common recordings (with the addition of records 212, 222, and 232) between the proposed technique and the methods in (de Chazal and Reilly 2006; Jiang and Kong 2007). Several interesting observations can be made from these results. First, for SVEB detection, sensitivity and positive predictivity rates are comparably lower than VEB detection, while a high specificity performance is achieved. The reason for the worse classifier performance in detecting SVEBs is that SVEB class is under-represented in the training data and hence more SVEB beats are misclassified as normal beats. Overall, the performance of the proposed technique in VEB and SVEB detection is significantly better than (Hu et al. 1997; de Chazal and Reilly 2006) for all measures and is comparable to the results obtained with evolvable BbNNs in (Jiang

Table 4.2 VEB and SVEB classification performance of the proposed method and comparison with the three major algorithms from the literature

	VEB				SVEB			
Methods	Acc	Sen	Spe	Ppr	Acc	Sen	Spe	Ppr
Hu et al. (1997)[a]	94.8	78.9	96.8	75.8	N/A	N/A	N/A	N/A
de Chazal and Reilly (2006)[a]	96.4	77.5	98.9	90.6	92.4	76.4	93.2	38.7
Jiang and Kong (2007)[a]	98.8	94.3	99.4	95.8	97.5	74.9	98.8	78.8
Proposed[a]	97.9	90.3	98.8	92.2	96.1	81.8	98.5	63.4
Jiang and Kong (2007)[b]	98.1	86.6	99.3	93.3	96.6	50.6	98.8	67.9
Proposed[b]	97.6	83.4	98.1	87.4	96.1	62.1	98.5	56.7
Proposed[c]	98.3	84.6	98.7	87.4	97.4	63.5	99.0	53.7

[a]The comparison results are based on 11 common recordings for VEB detection and 14 common recordings for SVEB detection
[b]The VEB and SVEB detection results are compared for 24 common testing records only
[c]The VEB and SVEB detection results of the proposed system for all training and testing records

Table 4.3 Performance comparison of PVC detection (in percent)

		Normal		PVC		Other	
Method	A	Se	Pp	Se	Pp	Se	Pp
Proposed	97.0	99.4	98.9	93.4	93.3	87.5	97.8
Inan et al. (2006)	95.2	98.1	97.0	85.2	92.4	87.4	94.5

and Kong 2007). Moreover, it is observed that the proposed classifier achieves comparable performance over the training and testing set of patient records. It is worth noting that the number of training beats used for each patient's classifier was less than 2% of all beats in the training data set and the resulting classifiers designed by the MD PSO process have improved generalization ability, i.e., the same low number of design parameters are used for all networks.

4.4.3 Detection of Premature Ventricular Contractions

The proposed technique is also tested on a separate problem of distinguishing premature ventricular contraction beats from the others. Accurate detection of PVCs from the ventricular group (V) in a long-term ECG data is essential for patients with heart disease since it may lead to possible life-threatening cardiac conditions (Iwasa et al. 2005). From the summarized results in Table 4.3, the proposed systematic approach performed with very high accuracy for detection of PVC, Normal and other groups of beats. The results are compared with the other recent major technique by Inan et al. (2006) using the same standard metrics: accuracy (A), sensitivity (Se), and positive predictivity (Pp). Overall, the proposed classifier achieved high average detection accuracy of 97.0% with average standard deviation of 0.5% during the tests, and average accuracy of 98.6% with average standard deviation of 0.3% during the training phase.

Table 4.4 VEB and SVEB classification accuracy of the proposed method for different PSO parameters and architecture spaces

(%)	I	II	III	IV
VEB	98.3	98.2	98.3	98.0
SVEB	97.4	97.3	97.1	97.4

$\mathrm{I}: R^1_{\min} = \{11,8,4,5\}, R^1_{\max} = \{11,16,8,5\}, S = 100, I = 500$
$\mathrm{II}: R^1_{\min} = \{11,8,4,5\}, R^1_{\max} = \{11,16,8,5\}, S = 250, I = 200$
$\mathrm{III}: R^1_{\min} = \{11,8,4,5\}, R^1_{\max} = \{11,16,8,5\}, S = 80, I = 200$
$\mathrm{IV}: R^1_{\min} = \{11,6,6,3,5\}, R^1_{\max} = \{11,12,10,5,5\}, S = 400, I = 500$

4.4.4 Robustness

In order to investigate the robustness of the proposed technique against the variations of the few PSO parameters used, such as the swarm size S, the iteration number I, and to evaluate the effect of the architecture space (and hence the characteristics of the ANNs used), we performed four classification experiments over the MIT/BIH arrhythmia database (I–IV) and their classification accuracy results per VEB and SVEB, are presented in Table 4.4. Experiments I–III are performed over the same architecture space, with 1-, 2-, and 3-layer MLP architectures defined by $R^1_{\min} = \{11, 8, 4, 5\}$, $R^1_{\max} = \{11, 16, 8, 5\}$. Between I and II, the swarm size, and between II and III, the iteration number are changed significantly, whereas in IV an entirely different architecture space containing four-layer MLPs is used. From the table, it is quite evident that the effects of such major variations over the classification accuracy are insignificant. Therefore, any set of common PSO parameters within a reasonable range can be conveniently used within the proposed technique. Furthermore, for this ECG database, the choice of the architecture space does not affect the overall performance, yet any other ECG dataset containing more challenging ECG data might require the architecture spaces such as in IV in order to obtain a better generalization capability.

4.4.5 Computational Complexity

The computational complexity of the proposed method depends on three distinct processes: the DWT-based feature extraction stage, the PCA-based pre-processing, and the MD PSO evolutionary process. In the first stage, as explained in Sect. 4.2.2, the fast TI-DWT algorithm has a computational complexity of $O(N \log N)$ for an N-sample (i.e., 180 samples of) ECG beat waveform. The complexity of the pre-processing stage based on PCA approximately follows $O(N^2)$. It is not feasible to accomplish a precise computational complexity analysis of the MD PSO evolutionary process since this mainly depends on the networks that the particles converge and in a stochastic process such as PSO this cannot be determined. However, there are certain attributes which directly affect the complexity such as swarm size (S), the number of iteration (*IterNo*) to terminate the MD PSO process, and the dimensions of data space (D). While the problem determines D, the computational complexity can still be controlled by S and *IterNo* settings. The further details of computational complexity analysis for the MD PSO process can be found in (Kiranyaz et al. 2009).

4.5 Conclusions

In this work, we proposed an automated patient-specific ECG heartbeat classifier, which is based on an efficient formation of morphological and temporal features from the ECG data and evolutionary neural network processing of the input patterns individually for each patient. The translation-invariant DWT and the PCA are the principal signal processing tools employed in the proposed feature extraction scheme. The wavelet-based morphology features are extracted from the ECG data and are further reduced to a lower-dimensional feature vector using PCA technique. Then, by combining compact morphological features with the two critical temporal features, the resultant feature vector to represent each ECG heartbeat is used as the input to MLP classifiers, which are automatically designed (both network structure and connection weights are optimized) using the proposed MD-PSO technique.

With the proper adaptation of the native MD PSO process, the proposed method can thus evolve to the optimum network within an architecture space, and for a particular problem, according to a given error function. It is furthermore generic as it is applicable to any type of ANNs in an architecture space with varying size and properties, as long as a proper hash function enumerates all possible configurations in the architecture space with respect to their complexity into proper hash indices representing the dimensions of the solution space over which a MD PSO process seeks for the optimal solution. MD PSO evolutionary process has a simple and unique structure for evolving ANNs without any significant parameter dependency or interference of any other method. It also has a native characteristic of having better and faster convergence to optimum solution in low dimensions, and consequently leads to *compact* networks.

The results of the classification experiments, which are performed over the benchmark MIT/BIH arrhythmia database, show that the proposed classifier technique can achieve average accuracies and sensitivities better than most of the existing algorithms for classification of ECG heartbeat patterns according to the AAMI standards. An overall average accuracy of 98.3% and an average sensitivity of 84.6% for VEB detection, and an average accuracy of 97.4% and an average sensitivity of 63.5% for SVEB detection were achieved over all 44 patient records from the MIT/BIH database. The overall results promise a significant improvement over other major techniques in the literature with the exception of the BbNN-based personalized ECG classifier in (Jiang and Kong 2007), which gave comparable results over the test set of 24 records. However, it used many critical parameters,

BP and a specific ANN architecture, which may not suit feature vectors in higher dimensions. The proposed method is based only on well-known, standard techniques such as DWT and PCA, whilst using the most typical ANN structure, the MLPs. Experimental results approve that its performance is not affected significantly by variations of the few parameters used. Therefore, the resulting classifier successfully achieves the main design objectives, i.e., maintaining a robust and generic architecture with superior classification performance. As a result, it can be conveniently applied to any ECG database "as is," alleviating the need of human "expertise" and "knowledge" for designing a particular ANN.

References

Alfonso, X., Nguyen, T.Q.: ECG beat detection using filter banks. IEEE Trans. Biomed. Eng. **46**(2), 192–202 (1999)

Coast, D.A., Stern, R.M., Cano, G.G., Briller, S.A.: An approach to cardiac arrhythmia analysis using hidden Markov models. IEEE Trans. Biomed. Eng. **37**(9), 826–836 (1990)

de Chazal, P., Reilly, R.B.: A patient-adapting heartbeat classifier using ECG morphology and heartbeat interval features. IEEE Trans. Biomed. Eng. **53**(12), 2535–2543 (2006)

de Chazal, P., O'Dwyer, M., Reilly, R.B.: Automatic classification of heartbeats using ECG morphology and heartbeat interval features. IEEE Trans. Biomed. Eng. **51**(7), 1196–1206, (2004)

Hoekema, R., Uijen, G.J.H., Oosterom, A.V.: Geometrical aspects of the interindividual variability of multilead ECG recordings. IEEE Trans. Biomed. Eng. **48**(5), 551–559 (2001)

Hu, Y.H., Tompkins, W.J., Urrusti, J.L., Afonso, V.X.: Applications of artificial neural networks for ECG signal detection and classification. J. Electrocardiol. **26**, 66–73 (1994)

Hu, Y., Palreddy, S., Tompkins, W.J.: A patient-adaptable ECG beat classifier using a mixture of experts approach. IEEE Trans. Biomed. Eng. **44**(9), 891–900 (1997)

Inan, O.T., Giovangrandi, L., Kovacs, G.T.A.: Robust neural-networkbased classification of premature ventricular contractions using wavelet transform and timing interval features. IEEE Trans. Biomed. Eng. **53**(12), 2507–2515 (2006)

Ince, T., Kiranyaz, S., Gabbouj, M.: Automated patient-specific classification of premature ventricular contractions. In: IEEE Proceedings on International Conference on EMBS, Vancouver, pp. 5474–5477 (2008)

Iwasa, A., Hwa, M., Hassankhani, A., Liu, T., Narayan, S.M.: Abnormal heart rate turbulence predicts the initiation of ventricular arrhythmias. Pacing Clin. Electrophysiol. **28**(11), 1189–1197 (2005)

Jiang, W., Kong, S.G.: Block-based neural networks for personalized ECG signal classification. IEEE Trans. Neural Netw. **18**(6), 1750–1761 (2007)

Kennedy, J., Eberhart, R.: Particle swarm optimization. Proceedings of IEEE International Conference on Neural Networks, vol. **4**, pp. 1942–1948, Perth (1995)

Kiranyaz, S., Ince, T., Yildirim A., Gabbouj, M.: Evolutionary artificial neural networks by multi-dimensional particle swarm optimization. Neural Netw. **22**, 1448–1462 (2009)

Kiranyaz, S., Ince, T., Yildirim, A., Gabbouj, M.: Fractional particle swarm optimization in multi-dimensional search space. IEEE Trans. Syst. Man Cybern. – Part B, **40**, 298–319 (2010)

Lagerholm, M., Peterson, C., Braccini, G., Edenbrandt, L., Sörnmo, L.: Clustering ECG complexes using Hermite functions and self-organizing maps. IEEE Trans. Biomed. Eng. **47**(7), 838–848 (2000)

Lee, S.C.: Using a translation-invariant neural network to diagnose heart arrhythmia. In: IEEE Proceedings Conference on Neural Information Processing Systems, Seattle (1989)

Li, C., Zheng, C.X., Tai, C.F.: Detection of ECG characteristic points using wavelet transforms. IEEE Trans. Biomed. Eng. **42**(1), 21–28 (1995)

Mallat, S.: A Wavelet Tour of Signal Processing, 2nd edn. Academic Press, San Diego (1999)

Mallat, S.G., Zhong, S.: Characterization of signals from multiscale edges. IEEE Trans. Pattern Anal. Mach. Intell. **14**, 710–732 (1992)

Mark, R., Moody, G.: MIT-BIH Arrhythmia Database Directory. Available: http://ecg.mit.edu/dbinfo.html

Minami, K., Nakajima, H., Toyoshima, T.: Real-Time discrimination of ventricular tachyarrhythmia with Fourier-transform neural network. IEEE Trans. Biomed. Eng. **46**(2), 179–185 (1999)

Osowski, S., Linh, T.L.: ECG beat recognition using fuzzy hybrid neural network. IEEE Trans. Biomed. Eng. **48**, 1265–1271 (2001)

Osowski, S., Hoai, L.T., Markiewicz, T.: Support vector machine based expert system for reliable heartbeat recognition. IEEE Trans. Biomed. Eng. **51**(4), 582–589 (2004)

Pan, J., Tompkins, W.J.: A real-time QRS detection algorithm. IEEE Trans. Biomed. Eng. **32**(3), 230–236 (1985)

Pittner, S., Kamarthi, S.V.: Feature extraction from wavelet coefficients for pattern recognition tasks. IEEE Trans. Pattern Anal. Mach. Intell. **21**, 83–88 (1999)

Recommended practice for testing and reporting performance results of ventricular arrhythmia detection algorithms. Association for the Advancement of Medical Instrumentation, Arlington (1987)

Shyu, L.Y., Wu, Y.H., Hu, W.C.: Using wavelet transform and fuzzy neural network for VPC detection from the holter ECG. IEEE Trans. Biomed. Eng. **51**(7), 1269–1273 (2004)

Silipo, R., Marchesi, C.: Artificial neural networks for automatic ECG analysis. IEEE Trans. Signal Process. **46**(5), 1417–1425 (1998)

Silipo, R., Laguna, P., Marchesi, C., Mark, R.G.: ST-T segment change recognition using artificial neural networks and principal component analysis. Computers in Cardiology, 213–216 (1995)

Talmon, J.L.: Pattern Recognition of the ECG. Akademisch Proefscrift, Berlin (1983)

Thakor, N.V., Webster, J.G., Tompkins, W.J.: Estimation of QRS complex power spectra for design of a QRS filter. IEEE Trans. Biomed. Eng. **31**, 702–705 (1984)

Van den Bergh, F.: An analysis of particle swarm optimizers. Ph.D. thesis, Department of Computer Science, University of Pretoria, Pretoria (2002)

Willems, J.L., Lesaffre, E.: Comparison of multigroup logisitic and linear discriminant ECG and VCG classification. J. Electrocardiol. **20**, 83–92 (1987)

Yao, X., Liu, Y.: A new evolutionary system for evolving artificial neural networks. IEEE Trans. Neural Netw. **8**(3), 694–713 (1997)

Chapter 5
Model-Based Atrial Fibrillation Detection

Paulo de Carvalho, Jorge Henriques, Ricardo Couceiro, Matthew Harris, Manuel Antunes, and Joerg Habetha

5.1 Introduction

The World Health Organization estimates that 17.5 million people died of cardiovascular diseases in 2005, representing 30% of all global deaths. Among cardiovascular disorders, Atrial Fibrillation (AF) is the most common clinically significant cardiac arrhythmia (Alan et al. 2001). AF leads to several patient risks and is a major risk factor for ischemic stroke. It has significant implications on the patient's quality of life, since it typically is associated to the reduction of the functional and cardiac performance, as well as increased medical costs and increased risk of death. According to Alan et al. (2001), it is projected that the disease will increase two-and-a-half-fold until 2050.

The use of new continuous tele-monitoring solutions and specialized processing methodologies based on wearable and information technologies provide professionals with adequate information that allows the evaluation of cardiovascular conditions and symptoms progression, enabling the prompt detection of forthcoming clinical severe conditions. In this context, personal Health systems (*pHealth*) are a new and fast growing concept. The patient is at the center of the health delivery process and, through remote monitoring and management applications, pHealth systems aim the

P. de Carvalho (✉) · J. Henriques · R. Couceiro
Center for Informatics and Systems, University of Coimbra, 3030-290 Coimbra, Portugal
e-mail: carvalho@dei.uc.pt; jh@dei.uc.pt; rcouceir@dei.uc.pt

M. Antunes
Cardio-thoracic Surgery Center, University Hospital of Coimbra, Coimbra, Portugal

Faculty of Medicine, University of Coimbra, Portugal
e-mail: antunes.cct.huc@sapo.pt

M. Harris · J. Habetha
Philips Research Laboratories, Aachen, Germany
e-mail: matthew.harris@philips.com; joerg.habetha@philips.com

A. Gacek and W. Pedrycz (eds.), *ECG Signal Processing, Classification and Interpretation: A Comprehensive Framework of Computational Intelligence*,
DOI 10.1007/978-0-85729-868-3_5, © Springer-Verlag London Limited 2012

continuity of care at all levels of health care delivery. Several potential benefits might be achieved using this new health delivery paradigm, ranging from better adjustment of pharmacological treatments to higher patient survival rates (Cleland et al. 2005). In particular, when considering AF, tele-monitoring applications might lead to a better up-titration and dynamic titration of potentially harmful medications, such as arrhythmic drugs and blood thinners. This perspective is being explored by several research projects over the past few years, e.g., the MyHeart (Habetha 2006) and the HeartCycle (Reiter and Maglaveras 2009) research projects. In this type of application scenarios, it is decisive to grant high levels of sensitivity and specificity of diagnosis algorithms, since high rates of false positives have a significant impact on user acceptance, motivation, and long-term adherence to the system, whereas a high rate of false negatives has an impact on user safety. Another important requirement for these types of applications is low computational complexity, since most of the systems perform processing on the patient side where low-power/performance systems are deployed.

From the clinical point of view, AF is a result of multiple re-entrant excitations of the atria, which conducts to its partial disorganization. One of the characteristics of AF episodes is the absence of defined P waves before the QRS-T complex of the electrocardiogram (ECG), which presents a *sawtooth*-like pattern waves along the cardiac cycle. Additionally, AF is usually associated with irregular cardiac frequency. During the last years, these two features (P wave presence/absence and heart rate irregularities), together with the atrial activity, have been object of intense research for the detection and prediction of AF. Moody and Mark (1983) constructed a Hidden Markov model of heart cycle duration states (RR duration) and used the related transition probabilities to detect AF episodes. Cerutti et al. (1997) proposes the use of linear and non-linear indexes for characterization of RR series and consequent AF detection. Tateno and Glass (2000) estimate the similarity between standard and test RR interval histograms to reveal the presence or absence of AF episodes. Extraction of atrial activity is of crucial importance in the detection of AF. Techniques like Blind Source Separation, Spatio-Temporal Cancellation, and Artificial Neural Networks (ANNs) are the most promising in this field of research. Despite the satisfactory results achieved by those approaches, most of them need several ECG leads to be implemented – a serious drawback for pHealth applications, where usually only one ECG lead is available. Senhadji et al. (2002) presents an algorithm for QRS-T interval cancellation based on dyadic wavelet transform, enabling the analysis of the atrial activity. Similarly, Sanchez et al. (2002), proposes an algorithm where Discrete Packet Wavelet Transform is used for the extraction of atrial activity. Shkurovich et al. (1998) uses a median template-based approach to cancel ventricular activity.

Patients with AF usually exhibit Premature Ventricular Contractions (PVCs), which by itself are a relevant cardiac arrhythmia occurrence. These PVCs episode cycles have to be removed from the ECG prior to AF analysis, since they typically exhibit highly disturbing morphologies and highly interfere with RR regularity. Most of the algorithms reported in literature for PVC detection share the same characteristic: they are based on features derived from the QRS complex, independently from the surrounding ECG morphological characteristics. However, patients can exhibit several physical, clinical, and cardiac conditions, which can affect the ECG morphology in numerous ways. For example, a wide QRS complex may be considered a non-PVC (normal beat) in one patient, while it may suggest the presence of a PVC in another patient (Couceiro et al. 2008). Since most of the algorithms proposed in literature are based on unrelated features and classifiers are trained with limited datasets, correct identification of PVC events in patients with unexpected conditions can become a difficult task.

Although the algorithms reported in the literature cover the most important characteristics of AF, a robust algorithm for AF detection has not yet been presented. Furthermore, the most significant existing methods usually concentrate on only one of the physiological characteristics of AF. In this chapter we introduce the AF detection algorithm that has been developed in the context of the MyHeart project (Habetha 2006). In this project the algorithm developed for real-time AF detection is based on a novel architecture that combines the three principal characteristics of AF that are applied by cardiologists in their daily reasoning (P wave presence/absence, heart rate irregularity, and atrial activity analysis). Moreover, it takes into account the presence of PVC events. This has the advantage of increasing interpretability of the results to the medical community, while improving detection robustness. The method profits from the complementary information provided by the features, which allow increased resilience toward distinct interferences that disturb the ECG's morphology. This is particularly important in non-controlled settings such as those found in long-term ambulatory patients follow-up.

This chapter is organized as follows: in the next section relevant AF characteristics, including epidemiology- and ECG-based diagnosis, are presented. In Sect. 5.3 the proposed methodology is described and, in Sect. 5.4, validation results, using public databases (MIT-BIH Arrhythmia and QT databases from Physionet) and European MyHeart project database are carried out. Finally, in Sect. 5.5 some conclusions are drawn.

5.2 Atrial Fibrillation Background Information

5.2.1 Atrial Fibrillation Epidemiology and Therapies

Atrial fibrillation (AF) is the single most common dysrhythmia in the general population. Hemodynamic impairment and thromboembolic events related to AF result in significant morbidity, mortality, and costs.

AF prevalence increases with age. Currently, the median age of the AF population is 75 years. Being a disease related to aging, it is observed that it does not have a homogeneous distribution in the population. In adults younger than 55 years AF exhibits a prevalence of 0.1% (Alan et al. 2001). As the population ages, AF becomes an increasingly prevalent disorder. It is estimated to be present in 5% of the population older than age 65 and to increase to 13.7% in persons aged 80 years or older (Wolf et al. 1991). The number of patients with AF is projected to increase 2.5-fold in the next 50 years, reflecting the growing proportion of elderly individuals, with more than 50% of affected individuals aged 80 years or older (Cleland et al. 2005).

Atrial fibrillation is most commonly (approximately 70% of all AF situations) triggered as a result of some cardiac condition. This is usually called secondary atrial fibrillation. The remaining cases, the so-called lone atrial fibrillation, which occurs in about 30% of the AF patients, refers to AF that occurs without evidence of any underlying heart problems (Lévy et al. 1998). The latter is more commonly observed in younger populations (Fuster et al. 2001) (50% of AF situation in younger populations are lone AF). Some of the most significant non-heart related AF triggering sources are related to hyperthyroidism, pulmonary embolism, pneumonia, acute pericarditis, acute myocarditis, and alcohol intake (Lévy et al. 1998). Lone AF is less likely to recur, once the precipitating condition has been resolved. AF is a common complication of cardiac surgery (e.g., coronary bypass surgery, mitral valvulotomy, and valve replacement) or thoracic surgery, but typically reverts after some days.Regarding cardiac triggers of AF, the most prevalent sources are hypertension and left ventricle hypertrophy, which is most often related to untreated hypertension. Heart valve diseases usually related to degenerations and calcifications of valve cusps with age, deterioration of the heart muscle (hypertrophic or dilated cardiomyopathy), coronary artery disease related to atherosclerosis, constrictive pericarditis, as well as sick sinus syndrome are other relevant sources of AF. It should be mentioned that heart diseases are highly interrelated, i.e., sometimes they are triggering sources and sometimes they might be triggered by some of the aforementioned sources. As was mentioned by Lévy et al. (1998), AF may be associated with a variety of arrhythmias including atrioventricular reentrant tachycardias, atrioventricular nodal reentrant tachycardias, or atrial tachycardia.

AF is normally associated to highly perceivable and disturbing symptoms that have a negative impact on quality of life and increased patient anxiety. Symptomatic manifestations of paroxysmal AF are palpitations (a sensation of rapid and irregular heart beat). When AF is persistent or permanent, patient suffer more often non-specific symptoms like dizziness and fainting, chest pain, poor effort tolerance, lack of energy, and shortness of breath. AF is by itself a major risk factor of several severe cardiac conditions. The loss of atrial contraction leads to the enlargement of the atria, thus increasing the stasis of blood in the atria, which promotes clot formation and embolic stroke. AF is the single most important cause of ischaemic stroke in population over 75 years old. As was mentioned in (Sherman 2007), 2.9–7.9% of AF patients under treatment suffer an embolic stroke episode and about 15% of all ischemic strokes are attributed to an embolus generated from a left atria thrombus (Sherman 2007). This is two to seven times higher than that of people without AF (Fuster et al. 2001). AF is also a high risk for mortality. The mortality rate of patients with AF is about double that of patients in normal sinus rhythm and is linked with the severity of underlying heart disease. Several AF studies, e.g. (Sherman 2007), report mortality rates ranging from 1% to 23.8%, attributable to AF. It is also observed that AF can by itself cause congestive heart failure after

Table 5.1 AF classification (Levy et al. 2003; Fuster et al. 2001)

Terminology	Clinical feature	Arrhythmia pattern
Initial event	Symptomatic	May not recur
	Asymptomatic (first detected)	
	Onset unknown (first detected)	
Paroxysmal	Spontaneous termination <7 days and most often <48 h	Recurrent
Persistent	Not self-terminating	Recurrent
Permanent	Not terminated or terminated but relapsed	Established
	Cardioversion failed or not attempted	

several weeks to months. In fact, as was observed by Fuster et al. (2001), there are studies that clearly show that the increased mortality risk in AF patients is due to increased number of deaths due to heart failure rather than to thromboembolism.

Episodes of AF dysrhythmia may be self-terminating or non-self-terminating. The terms chronic and paroxysmal have been utilized in the biomedical literature to characterize states of AF. However, clinicians utilize a more detailed classification scheme to delineate effective treatment and therapeutic strategies. It is important for clinicians to ascertain whether an incident of AF is the very first episode, the so-called initial event, whether it is symptomatic or not and whether it is self-terminating or not. If the patient has experienced more than one episode, AF is said recurrent. The usual clinical classification of AF is described in Table 5.1.

There are several treatment options for AF, depending on age, type of AF, and co-mobidity (Fuster et al. 2001). The main treatment strategies are rate control, rhythm control, and anti-coagulation. In rate control, the heart rate is brought down to normal so that the heart regains efficiency. In rate control, irregularity of the rhythm might persist. Rhythm control, also known as cardioversion, may be applied using an electric shock or through medication. In this treatment strategy, the goal is to regain normal regular rhythm. This treatment option is more likely to be considered when AF has developed recently, for lone AF, for patients under 65 years when the patient has acute heart failure or unstable angina which is being made worse by the irregular heart beat of AF. Finally, as already mentioned, ischemic stroke is the main risk associated to AF. In order to reduce the risk of clot formation, usually an anticoagulation therapy is followed in AF patients.

5.2.2 *Mechanisms of ECG and Atrial Fibrillation*

A precise understanding of the mechanism(s) of AF in patients is not yet available (Waldo 2003). There are two main concurrent theories: the multiple reentrant wavelet hypotheses and a more recent theory that regards the AF mechanism to be related to stable or unstable reentrant circuits of short cycle length.

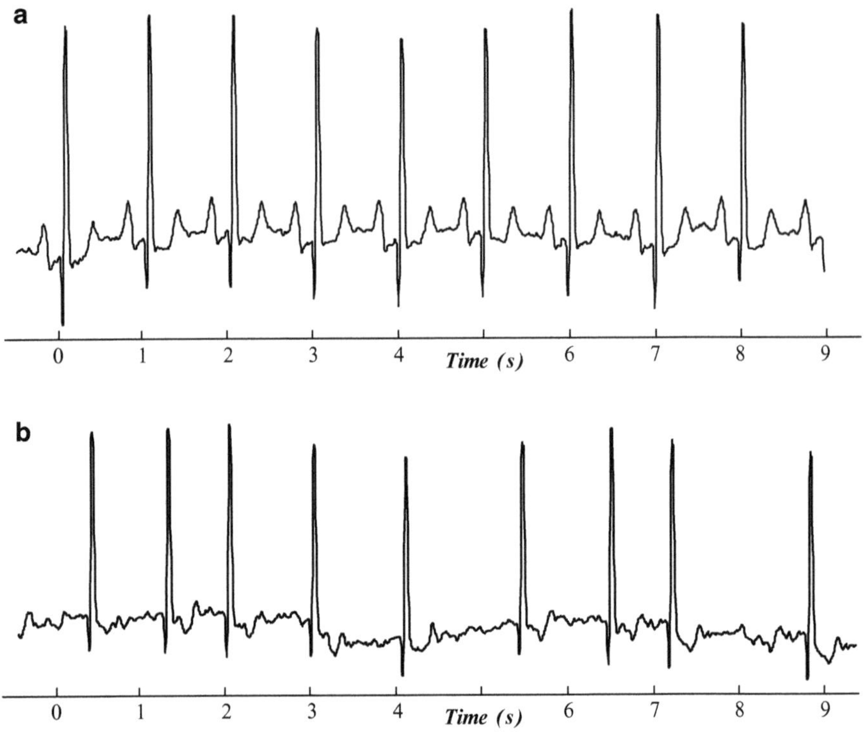

Fig. 5.1 Typical ECG signals. **(a)** Regular rate ECG signal; **(b)** AF signal

Moe and Abildskov (1964) first proposed the classical multiple-wavelet theory in the 1950s. Moe hypothesized that AF was sustained by multiple randomly wandering wavelets that either collided with each other and were extinguished or divided into daughter wavelets that continually re-excited the atria. More recently, Jalife (2003) observed that AF is not random. It exhibits a high degree of spatiotemporal periodicity. This has led to the hypothesis that maintenance of AF may depend on the uninterrupted periodic activity of a small number of discrete reentrant sites, established by the interaction of propagating waves with anatomical heterogeneities in the atria.

Whatever the actual triggering mechanism(s) of AF, this supraventricular tachyarrhythmia is characterized by uncoordinated excitation of the atria which results in highly characteristic morphology and timing signatures in the electrocardiogram (ECG). In regular hearts, the P wave reflects the depolarization of the atria (Fig. 5.1a). As can be observed in Fig. 5.1b, in AF due to the chaotic depolarization of the atria the ECG is described by the replacement of consistent P waves by rapid oscillations or fibrillatory waves that vary in size, shape, and timing, associated with irregular, frequently rapid ventricular response when atrioventricular conduction is intact (Fuster et al. 2001). The irregular and frequently rapid ventricular response manifests itself on the short duration and irregular nature of the RR intervals. In the presence of atrioventricular block or interference induced by ventricular tachycardia, the irregular RR characteristic might disappear.

5.3 Methods

Figure 5.2 depicts the schematic diagram of the methodology followed in this work. As already mentioned, the proposed algorithm assumes that based on the three main ECG morphological characteristics (P wave presence/absence, heart rate irregularity, and atrial activity analysis), it is possible to detect an AF episode. The input consists of a discrete one-lead ECG signal, which is passed through a set of pre-processing stages for noise reduction, baseline removal, and segmentation (identification of the main ECG waves). Then, premature ventricular contractions (PVCs) are identified. Following this, the algorithm involves two processing steps: first, feature extraction methods are applied to derive specific parameters related to the three main ECG morphological characteristics. The second step consists of a classifier where features determined in the previous step are fed into a classifier in order to categorize ECG data into two classes, i.e., with/without AF.

Real-time AF detection is one of the main priority aspects of the proposed algorithm. Since the information contained in single beat is not sufficient to discriminate AF episodes, a sliding window analysis is used. Thus, a minimum of 12 beats per analysis window is established. For real time applications, the length of the present analysis window is estimated based on the heart rate frequency observed in the previous window. For offline operation, each window length is set according to the established number of beats. As referred, in each analysis window a set of features is extracted, to evaluate one of the three AF characteristics. Basically, P wave absence is quantified by measuring the correlation of the detected

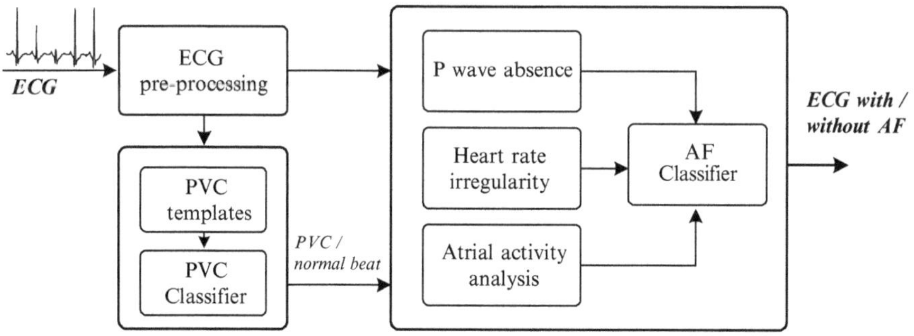

Fig. 5.2 Scheme of the proposed AF detection algorithm

P waves to a P wave model; heart rate variability is accessed by assuming that the observed ECG is a nonlinear transformed version of a model and the statistical similarity determined using the Kullback-Leibler divergence measure; atrial activity is processed through frequency analysis, using a wavelet approach.

The proposed classifiers consist of feedforward ANNs (both for PVC and AF classification), trained with the Levenberg-Marquardt algorithm. In both cases, normalization of the input feature vector has been performed in order to fit into the dynamic range of the used log-sigmoid transfer function.

5.3.1 *ECG Pre-processing*

One of the essential tasks in arrhythmia detection is the detection of major characteristic waves, namely the QRS complexes, P and T waves. Difficulties in this task are mainly due to oscillation in the baseline, presence of noise, artifacts, and frequency overlapping. To avoid these situations noise filtering and baseline removal are essential. For ECG segmentation, the algorithm proposed by Sun et al. (2005) has been adopted. These steps are performed using morphologic transform concepts, such as multiscale morphological transform, opening and closing operators.

5.3.1.1 Morphological Operators

Mathematical morphology, which is based on operation sets, provides an approach to the development of non-linear signal processing methods. Fundamentally, in mathematical morphology operations, a set is transformed by another set, where the result depends on the shapes of the two sets involved. There are mainly two basic morphological operators: erosion (Θ) and dilation ($\oplus$). Denoting a discrete signal, consisting of N points, by $f(n)$, $\{n = 0, 1, \ldots, N-1\}$, and a symmetric structuring element of M points by $B(m)$, $\{m = 0, 1, \ldots, M-1\}$, the erosion and dilation operators are defined, respectively, by (5.1) and (5.2).

$$(f\Theta B)(n) = \min_{m=0,\ldots,M-1}\left\{f\left(n - \frac{M-1}{2} + m\right) - B(m)\right\} \quad \text{for } n = \left\{\frac{M-1}{2}, \ldots, N - \frac{M+1}{2}\right\} \tag{5.1}$$

$$(f \oplus B)(n) = \max_{m=0,\ldots,M-1}\left\{f\left(n - \frac{M-1}{2} + m\right) + B(m)\right\} \quad \text{for } n = \left\{\frac{M-1}{2}, \ldots, N - \frac{M+1}{2}\right\} \tag{5.2}$$

Based on these morphological operators, it is possible to define the concept of morphology derivative. Considering a one-dimensional signal, $f(x)$, it is possible to define left, $D_f^-(x)$, and right, $D_f^+(x)$, derivatives according to (5.3) and (5.4).

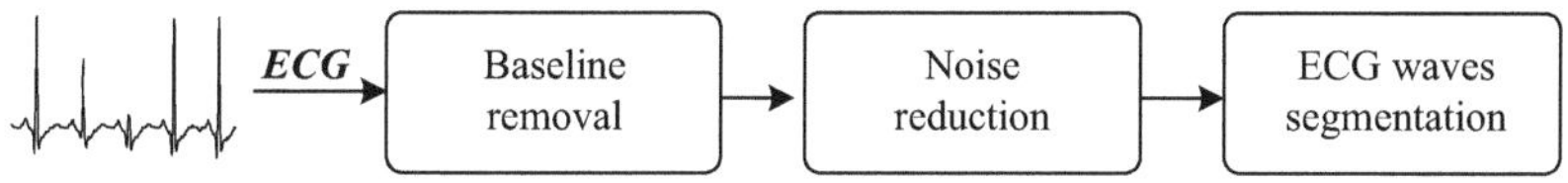

Fig. 5.3 ECG pre-processing phases

$$D_f^-(x) = \lim_{h\to 0} \frac{f(x)-f(x-h)}{h} \tag{5.3}$$

$$D_f^+(x) = \lim_{h\to 0} \frac{f(x+h)-f(x)}{h} \tag{5.4}$$

Similarly, the derivative on the left (right) can be represented by morphological inf-derivative (sup-derivative), as described by (5.5) and (5.6).

$$M_f^-(x) = \lim_{s\to 0} \frac{f(x)-(f\Theta g_s)(x)}{s} \tag{5.5}$$

$$M_f^+(x) = \lim_{s\to 0} \frac{(f\oplus g_s)(x)-f(x)}{s} \tag{5.6}$$

A multiscale morphological derivative difference, $M_f^d(x)$, used to characterize the difference between the left and right derivatives, is then obtained by (5.7):

$$\begin{aligned} M_f^d(x) &= M_f^+(x) - M_f^-(x) \\ &= \lim_{s\to 0} \frac{(f\oplus g_s)(x)-f(x)}{s} - \lim_{s\to 0} \frac{f(x)-(f\Theta g_s)(x)}{s} \\ &= \lim_{s\to 0} \frac{(f\oplus g_s)(x)+(f\Theta g_s)(x)-2f(x)}{s} \end{aligned} \tag{5.7}$$

The scaled version of $M_f^d(x)$ at scale s, M_f^{ds} is defined according to (5.8).

$$M_f^{ds}(x) = \lim_{s\to 0} \frac{(f\oplus g_s)(x)+(f\Theta g_s)(x)-2f(x)}{s} \tag{5.8}$$

5.3.1.2 Processing Steps

The algorithm proposed here follows the approach introduced by Sun et al. (2005). It consists of two preliminary stages of signal pre-processing (baseline removal and noise reduction) and a last phase, ECG segmentation, as depicted in Fig. 5.3.

Basically, the characteristic points of ECG, such as QRS complex, the P wave, and the T wave are detected using the morphological derivative transform concept, Eq. 5.8. For ECG signals, the Q, R, and S peaks correspond to the local minima of the M_f^{ds}. In effect, at a peak its left derivative is positive and its right derivative

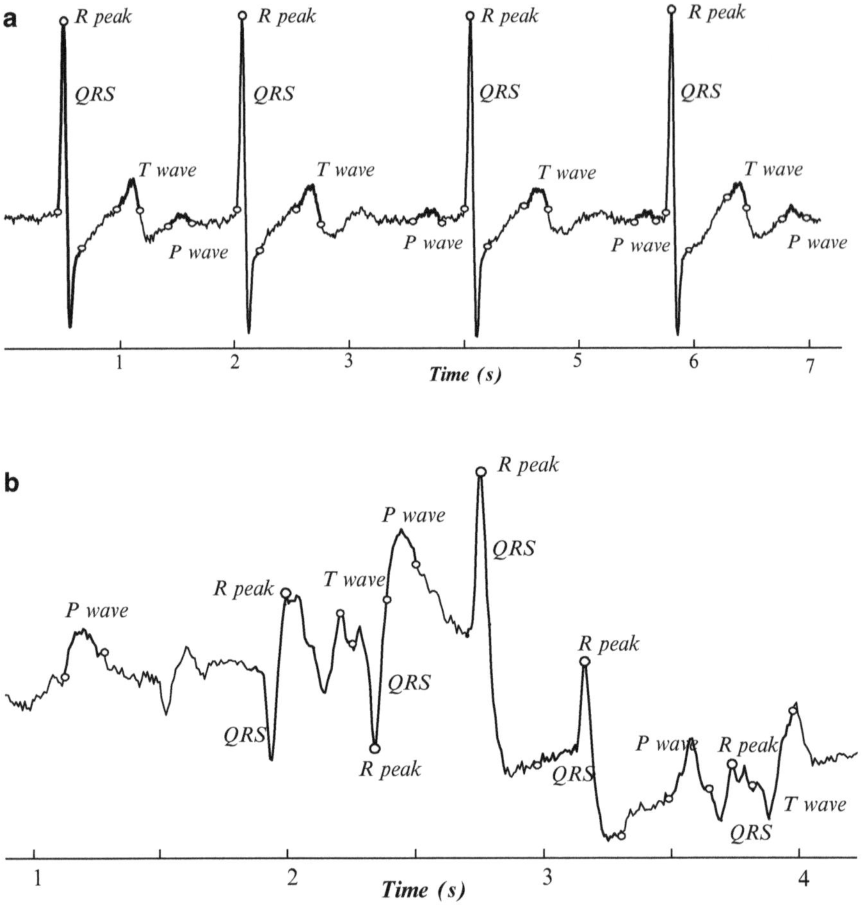

Fig. 5.4 ECG segmentation. **(a)** ECG typical segmentation; **(b)** ECG uncharacteristic segmentation

is negative. Therefore, peaks in the ECG signal correspond to the local minima in M_f^{ds}, while the onsets and offsets of the P wave and T wave correspond to the local maxima of the M_f^{ds}.

The baseline removal, as well as noise reduction, is accomplished by means of opening and closing operations, using appropriate structuring elements B (Sun et al. 2005). Opening and closing operations are described using erosion and dilation operators, respectively, Eqs. 5.9 and 5.10.

$$f \circ B = f \Theta B \oplus B \tag{5.9}$$

$$f \bullet B = f \oplus B \Theta B \tag{5.10}$$

The next two figures depict two typical situations related to the ECG segmentation process. The first (Fig. 5.4a) presents a situation where the relevant parameters

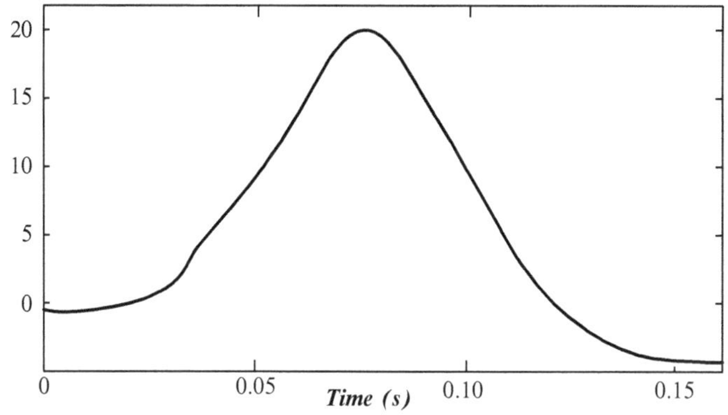

Fig. 5.5 P wave template

were effectively computed; the second (Fig. 5.4b) illustrates a situation where the algorithms reveal some difficulties to obtain these parameters. This is mainly due to the uncharacteristic morphology of the signal.

5.3.2 P Wave Detection

The detection of P wave's absence during the fibrillation process before the QRS complexes is an important characteristic of AF episodes. Although ECG segmentation methods can be very accurate in the detection of ECG fiducial points for regular patterns, it is observed that these algorithms present some difficulties when dealing with the detection of P waves during AF episodes. To reduce these misclassification errors, a template-based approach is proposed here. The proposed approach exhibits a reduced computational complexity and significant sensitivity and specificity, compared to current state-of-the-art methods. First, a P wave template is extracted by averaging all annotated *P* waves found in the*Physionet QT* Database. The resulting template is shown in Fig. 5.5. Note that, since the extraction of the P waves is performed after a pre-processing step, where the ECG signal is normalized, no units were attributed to the y-axis of the P-wave model.

The likelihood of the existence of a P wave in an ECG signal is then assessed by computing the correlation coefficient between the current P wave candidate and the P wave template. Defining $\overline{P_{\text{wave}}}$ as the aforementioned template (Fig. 5.5) and $P_{\text{wave}}(i)$ as the *P* wave under analysis, where $i = 1, \ldots, n\text{beats}$. The likelihood of the existence of a *P* wave is assessed by (5.11).

$$P_w(i) = \max(\text{cc}) - \text{cc}(i), \quad i = 1, \ldots, n\text{beats} \tag{5.11}$$

The variable $\text{cc}(i)$, $i = 1, \ldots, n\text{beats}$, defined by Eq. 5.12, denotes the absolute value of correlation coefficient between $P_{\text{wave}}(i)$ and $\overline{P_{\text{wave}}}$, which is computed by (5.13).

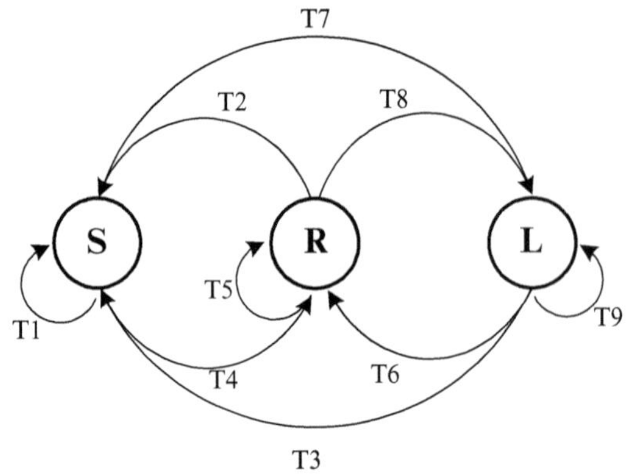

Fig. 5.6 States and transitions in the considered Markov model

$$\mathrm{cc}(i) = \left|\mathrm{corr\ coef}\left(P_{\mathrm{wave}}(i), \overline{P_{\mathrm{wave}}}\right)\right|, \quad i = 1, \ldots, n\mathrm{beats} \tag{5.12}$$

$$\mathrm{corr\ coef}(x,y) = \frac{\sum_{i=1}^{n}(x(i)-\bar{x})(y(i)-\bar{y})}{\cdot\sqrt{\sum_{i=1}^{n}(x(i)-\bar{x})^2}\sqrt{\sum_{i=1}^{n}(y(i)-\bar{y})^2}} \tag{5.13}$$

Finally, the absence or presence of P waves is estimated by the rate of P waves in each window, defined by Eq. 5.14. This rate is assessed by relating the number of selected P waves, N_{pw}, whose index $P_{\mathrm{w}}(i)$ is greater than a predefined threshold, with the number of cardiac beats, N_{CB}. In the present work the value of 0.2 was used for the threshold.

$$R = \frac{N_{\mathrm{pw}}}{N_{\mathrm{CB}}} \tag{5.14}$$

5.3.3 *Heart Rate Analysis*

The second characteristic used for AF detection relates to the variability of the RR interval. Basically, the RR interval sequence is modeled as a three-state Markov process being each interval classified as one of the three states S, R, L (short, regular, or long) (Moody and Mark 1983). Intervals are called short if they do not exceed 85% of the mean interval duration, long if they exceed 115% of the mean interval duration, and regular otherwise. Thus, the RR interval sequence can be assumed as a stationary first-order Markov process, as illustrated in Fig. 5.6, characterized by its state transition probability matrix.

In the current approach, the regularity of the heart rate is characterized by the probability of transition from state R to itself, since this transition is more likely to

Table 5.2 Probabilistic distributions

(a) Normal sinus rhythm				(b) AF episode			
	S	R	L		S	R	L
S	0.005	0.023	0.006	S	0.056	0.114	0.062
R	0.007	0.914	0.013	R	0.101	0.350	0.096
L	0.019	0.006	0.003	L	0.060	0.114	0.035

occur when the RR intervals present approximately the same length. Note that since PVCs induce large variability in heart rate, they are excluded from the computation of the transition matrix in the Markov model. Based on the transitions between states $T_i, i = 1,\ldots,9$, a transition probability matrix is derived, describing the probability of cardiac rhythm. In particular, the probability of transition from state R to itself is computed by (5.15).

$$P(R|R) = \frac{P(R,R)}{P(R)} \tag{5.15}$$

The complete matrix of transition probabilities is built by using all probabilistic distribution $P(E_i,E_j) = P(E_i|E_j) \times P(E_i)$ where $\{E_1,E_2,E_3\} = \{S,R,L\}$. In Table 5.2 the probabilistic distributions of a normal rhythm (left) and an AF episode rhythm (right) are presented. The high regularity of normal rhythms is represented by a Dirac-impulse-like distribution centered in the transition between two regular states (R). In this kind of rhythms almost no transition between other states can be observed. On the other hand, when studying AF episodes (right), the presence of various RR interval lengths result in a flatter probabilistic distribution.

Based on this observation the concentration/dispersion of the RR interval variability is estimated using the entropy of the distribution, as described by (5.16) and (5.17).

$$H = \sum_{i=1}^{3} P(E_i)H(E_i) \tag{5.16}$$

$$H(E_i) = -\sum_{j=1}^{3} P(E_j|E_i)\log_2 P(E_j|E_i) \tag{5.17}$$

The specificity of probabilistic distributions for both normal rhythms and AF episodes is also object of study. The objective is to determine the similarity between a probabilistic distribution under analysis and a model that represents AF episodes. Based on MIT-BIH Atrial Fibrillation database, a model for the AF episode probability distribution (defined by $\overline{P_{\mathrm{AF}}(E_i,E_j)}$) was extracted (see Table 5.2b). Using Kullback–Leibler divergence, D_{KL}, the similarity between the distribution

$\overline{P_{\mathrm{AF}}(E_i,E_j)}$ and the distribution under analysis $(P(E_i,E_j))$ is evaluated. This feature is described by (5.18).

$$D_{\mathrm{KL}}\left(P(E_i,E_j),\overline{P_{\mathrm{AF}}(E_i,E_j)}\right)=\sum_{i=1}^{3}\sum_{j=1}^{3}P(E_i,E_j)\log\left(\frac{P(E_i,E_j)}{\overline{P_{\mathrm{AF}}(E_i,E_j)}}\right) \tag{5.18}$$

5.3.4 Atrial Activity Analysis

Extraction of atrial activity is of crucial importance in the detection of AF. AF episodes are characterized by a fibrillatory wave with specific frequency between 4 and 10 Hz. To obtain a valid frequency domain characterization of AF episodes the extraction or cancellation of the signal components associated to ventricular activity is needed, that is, the QRS complex and the T wave (QRS-T). For this propose, the methods reported by Senhadji et al. (2002) and Sanchez et al. (2002), have been followed. The QRS-T cancellation is conducted in the frequency domain by excluding the values corresponding to the QRS-T segments and the values above a predefined threshold. This approach guaranties the minimization of the influence of miss-segmented QRS-T complexes in the cancelled signal. Spectral analysis is performed on the residual ECG signal using a Fast Fourier Transform. Once the frequency spectrum has been calculated, it should be parameterized in order to find specific characteristics for AF episodes. The main characteristic of AF episodes, observed in the frequency spectrums, is the concentration around the main peak, which is positioned in the interval [4, 10] Hz. The concentration of each spectrum is assessed by calculating the entropy of each normalized cancelled ECG window spectrum.

Following a similar approach, a scheme based on a spectrum model extracted from the MIT-BIH Atrial Fibrillation database was used. The resulting template is shown in Fig. 5.7.

Using a similar approach as in the heart rate analysis, the first feature extracted from atrial activity consists of entropy of the analyzed spectrum distribution $AA(x)$, Eq. 5.19.

$$H(x)=\sum_{x\in X}AA(x)\log\left(AA(x)\right) \tag{5.19}$$

The second feature addresses the similarity between the probabilistic distribution under analysis and the frequency spectrum model that represents AF episodes. Let $AA(i)$ be the spectrum under analysis and $\overline{AA}$ be the aforementioned model. The similarity between $AA(i)$ and $\overline{AA}$ is related to the likelihood of the time window under analysis to be an AF episode. This similarity is evaluated by the Kullback–Leibler divergence between the two distributions, obtained using Eq. 5.20.

$$D_{KL}\left(AA(i),\,\overline{AA}\right)=\sum_{i}AA(i)\log\left(\frac{AA(i)}{\overline{AA}}\right) \tag{5.20}$$

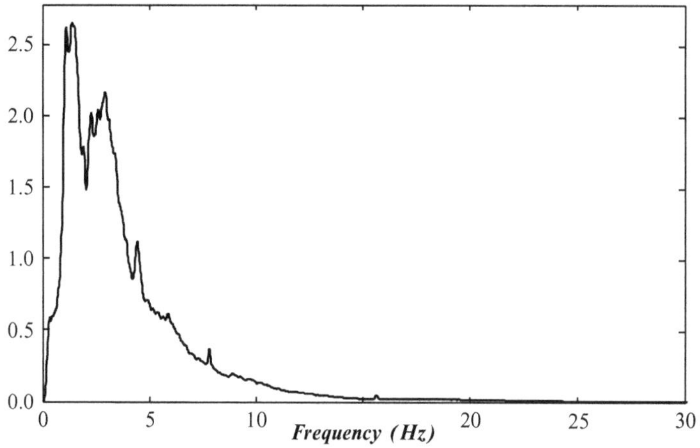

Fig. 5.7 Normalized frequency spectrum model of an AF episode

5.3.5 PVC Detection

Most of the algorithms reported in literature share the same characteristic: they are based on features derived from the QRS complex, independently from the surrounding ECG morphological characteristics. However, patients can exhibit several physical, clinical, and cardiac conditions, which can affect the ECG morphology in numerous ways. For example, a wide QRS complex may be considered normal in one patient, while it may suggest the presence of a PVC in another patient. Since most of the algorithms proposed in literature are based on unrelated features and classifiers are trained with limited datasets, correct identification of PVC events in patients with unexpected conditions can become a difficult task. The proposed algorithm approaches this problem by assuming that measurements extracted from PVC characteristics can be compared to normal, patient-specific ECG beat characteristics and that these exhibit inter-individual resilience, i.e., in order to capture patient-specific ECG characteristics, for each beat the measurements are compared with those extracted from the neighboring beats.

Figure 5.8 illustrates the potential of the proposed methodology for a particular QRS complex morphology feature, the QRS center of mass. Figure 5.8a and b present, respectively, the achieved results by means of an absolute procedure (feature computed independently from the adjacent ECG beats) and by using the proposed technique (feature computed taking into account the neighboring beats). As can be observed, the proposed technique improves feature's discrimination properties.

It has been established that every analysis window must contain at least 10 beats. In order to meet this constraint for real time applications the length of the present analysis window is estimated based on the heart rate frequency observed

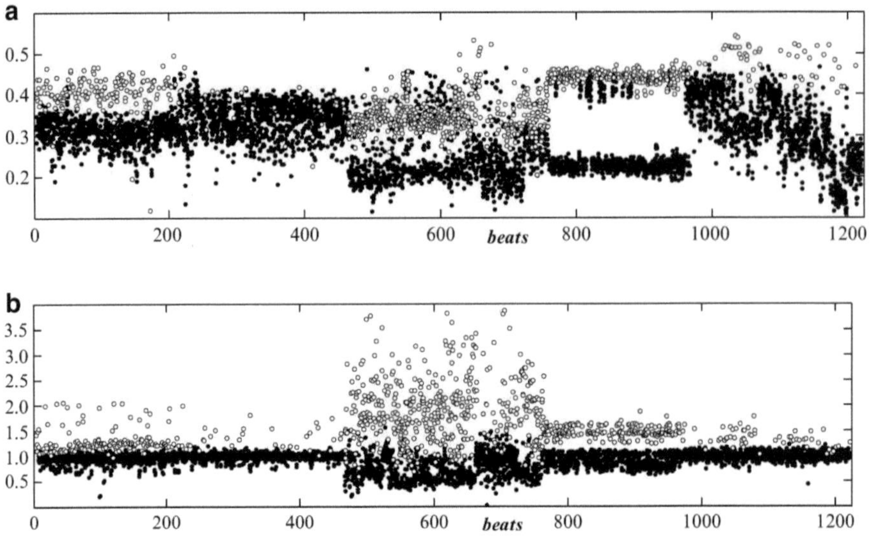

Fig. 5.8 QRS center of mass amplitudes. Symbol (•) denotes a normal beat, while symbol (o) denotes an abnormal (PVC) beat. **(a)** Absolute amplitude; **(b)** relative amplitude, with respect to neighboring beats

in the previous window. For each beat in a given time window a set of 13 features $(f_i, i = 1 \ldots 13)$ is extracted. Some of the features are directly related to well-defined characteristics of PVCs: *R* wave length, area and centre of mass of QRS complex, *T* wave deflection and amplitude, *P* wave absence and *RR* interval variability. The remaining features have been defined using feature extraction methods such as morphological derivative, Fourier transform, and information theory concepts.

5.3.5.1 ECG Morphology

Figure 5.9 depicts the beats corresponding to normal beats and to abnormal beats (PVC). These two types of beats can be distinguished by using a set of characteristics.

QRS Complex Length and Area

PVCs have a wider QRS complex and therefore greater area than normal beats. Two features are based on the PVC characteristics. In each beat, QRS complex length, QRS_{length}, the time interval from Q peak to S peak (Fig. 5.9), is compared to the average length of the two adjacent QRS complexes, $\overline{QRS_{length}}$, according to

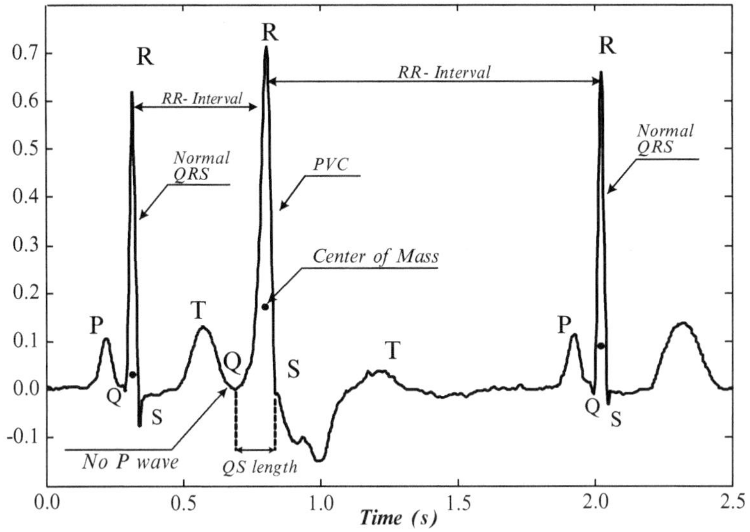

Fig. 5.9 Features extracted directly connected to ECG characteristics

(5.21). Analogously, using (5.22), the area of each QRS complex (QRS_{area}), defined from Q peak to S peak, is compared to the adjacent QRS complexes' areas average ($\overline{QRS_{area}}$).

$$f_1(i) = QRS_{length}(i) \log \frac{QRS_{length}(i)}{\overline{QRS_{length}}}, \quad i = 1, \ldots, n\text{beats} \tag{5.21}$$

$$f_2(i) = QRS_{area}(i) \log \frac{QRS_{area}(i)}{\overline{QRS_{area}}}, \quad i = 1, \ldots, n\text{beats} \tag{5.22}$$

R Peak Amplitude

PVCs do not always present the same R peak amplitude. This characteristic is combined with the previous ones and is used to derive two other features based on the centre of mass of QRS complexes. The first one is the centre of mass ordinate's absolute value (CoM_y) of each QRS complex, as in Eq. 5.23, while the other one is the logarithmic comparison with the average value of the QRS complex centre of mass ordinates ($\overline{CoM_y}$), according to (5.24).

$$f_3(i) = CoM_y(i), \quad i = 1, \ldots, n\text{beats} \tag{5.23}$$

$$f_4(i) = CoM_y(i) \log \frac{CoM_y(i)}{\overline{CoM_y}}, \quad i = 1, \ldots, n\text{beats} \tag{5.24}$$

T Waves

The next two features are related to the characteristics of the waves that precede/succeed the QRS complex under analysis. When a PVC occurs, the T wave after the respective QRS exhibits a more elevated peak (T_{peak}) with opposite curvature to the main deflection of QRS complex (see Fig. 5.9). On the other hand, no P wave precedes the PVCs' QRS complex. The amplitude of each T wave, Eq. 5.24, is compared with the average amplitude, $|\overline{T_{\text{peak}}}|$, of all T waves inside the analysis window, resulting in the feature described in (5.25). The main deflection of T wave is identified by the signal of the second derivative of the ECG at the peak.

$$f_5(i) = T_{\text{peak}}(i), \quad i = 1, \ldots, n\text{beats} \tag{5.25}$$

$$f_6(i) = T_{\text{peak}}(i) \log \frac{|T_{\text{peak}}(i)|}{|\overline{T_{\text{peak}}}|}, \quad i = 1, \ldots, n\text{beats} \tag{5.26}$$

P Waves

Typically, a PVC does not exhibit a preceding P wave. Therefore the methodology proposed for P wave absence detection (Sect. 5.3.2) was used here. As a result the existence of a P wave is assessed by (5.11).

RR Regularity

As already mentioned, the main characteristic of PVCs is its premature occurrence. This characteristic is measured by relating the RR interval lengths of heart cycles adjacent to the PVC. In case of a PVC, these lengths should be notoriously different (see Fig. 5.9).

$$f_8(i) = \frac{RR(i)}{RR(i+1)}, \quad i = 1, \ldots, n\text{beats} \tag{5.27}$$

5.3.5.2 Morphological Derivative

The remaining features have been defined using feature extraction methods based on the morphological derivative, spectral and information content. Figure 5.10 depicts the morphological derivatives (top) (Eq. 5.8) corresponding to a normal and a abnormal (PVC) beat (bottom).

The next two features are based on the ECG signal's morphological derivative. It is observed that PVC complexes present lower slop before or/and after an R peak. The slop from the Q peak to the R peak can be measured by calculating the morphological derivative's peak amplitudes in this segment (QR_{amp}, see Fig. 5.10 bottom). Analogously, the slop after the R peak can be represented by the amplitude of the

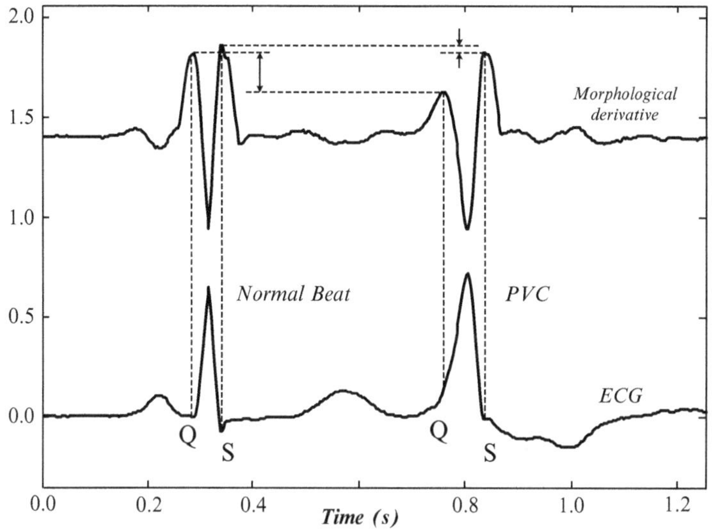

Fig. 5.10 Comparison of amplitude differences between normal beats and PVCs morphologic

RS peak segment (RS_{amp}). An approximation to the normal beat R wave left and right slopes can be estimated by calculating the averages of QR and RS amplitudes. Denote these by $\overline{\mathrm{QR}_{\mathrm{amp}}}$ and $\overline{\mathrm{RS}_{\mathrm{amp}}}$, respectively. The relations between $\mathrm{QR}_{\mathrm{amp}}$ and $\overline{\mathrm{QR}_{\mathrm{amp}}}$, and the relation between RS_{amp} and $\overline{\mathrm{RS}_{\mathrm{amp}}}$, provide two original features:

$$f_9(i) = \mathrm{QR}_{\mathrm{amp}}(i) \times \log \frac{\mathrm{QR}_{\mathrm{amp}}(i)}{\overline{\mathrm{QR}_{\mathrm{amp}}}}, \quad i = 1, \ldots, n\text{beats} \tag{5.28}$$

$$f_{10}(i) = \mathrm{RS}_{\mathrm{amp}}(i) \times \log \frac{\mathrm{RS}_{\mathrm{amp}}(i)}{\overline{\mathrm{RS}_{\mathrm{amp}}}}, \quad i = 1, \ldots, n\text{beats} \tag{5.29}$$

5.3.5.3 Spectral Analysis

Chikh et al. (2003) proposed that the QRS complexes' morphology differences between PVCs and normal beats may be evaluated using frequency spectrum signatures. Namely, PVC spectrums tend to be more concentrated in lower frequencies, while spectrums from normal beats tend to be more dispersed. The following features are based on this observation. The concentration of each spectrum is assessed by calculating the entropy of each normalized QRS spectrum. The logarithmic comparison between the entropy (H) and the average of all entropies ($\overline{H}$) leads to the feature presented in (5.30).

$$f_{11}(i) = H(i) \log \frac{H(i)}{\overline{H}}, \quad i = 1, \ldots, n\text{beats} \tag{5.30}$$

One other feature is calculated using the Kullback–Leibler divergence (D_{KL}). This measure is computed between every normalized spectrum (S_{p}) and the average of all spectrums ($\overline{S_{\mathrm{p}}}$), according to Eq. 5.31.

$$f_{12}(i) = D_{\mathrm{KL}}\left(S_{\mathrm{p}}(i), \overline{S_{\mathrm{p}}}\right), \quad i = 1, \ldots, n\mathrm{beats} \tag{5.31}$$

The last feature is assessed by calculating the quotient between the sum of first and second half of the QRS complex spectrum.

$$f_{13}(i) = \frac{\sum_{k=k_1+1}^{ns_{\mathrm{p}}} S_{\mathrm{p}}(i,k)}{\sum_{k=1}^{ns_{\mathrm{p}}} S_{\mathrm{p}}(i,k)}, \quad i = 1, \ldots, n\mathrm{beats}, \quad k1 = \frac{ns_{\mathrm{p}}}{2} \tag{5.32}$$

where ns_{p} is the length of the QRS complex spectrum.

5.3.5.4 PVC Classifier

The proposed PVC classifier consists of a three layer $13 \times 6 \times 1$, (input layer, hidden layer, output layer) sigmoidal feedforward neural network, trained with the Levenberg-Marquardt algorithm.

5.3.6 Atrial Fibrillation Classifier

The AF detection algorithm is based on a sliding window approach, where a minimum of 12 beats is imposed for each window. For real time applications, the length of the present analysis window is estimated based on the heart rate frequency observed in the previous window. The overlap between two consecutive windows was set to be one beat, as depicted in Fig. 5.11.

For each window six features are computed:

Type	Feature
P wave absence	Ratio of P waves in each window, Eq. 5.14
One feature	
Heart rate regularity	Transition probability from R to R state, Eq. 5.15
	Entropy of the distribution $P(E_i, E_j)$, Eq. 5.16
Three features	KL divergence between current and RR model distribution, (5.18).
Atrial activity analysis	Entropy of the spectrum distribution $AA(i)$, Eq. 5.19
Two features	KL divergence between current and AF model spectrum distribution, (5.20)

These features are used as inputs to the classifier, a feedforward Neural Network (NN) structure, which provides the global result of the AF algorithm (ECG window with/without AF). The NN structure consists of three layer architecture, where the

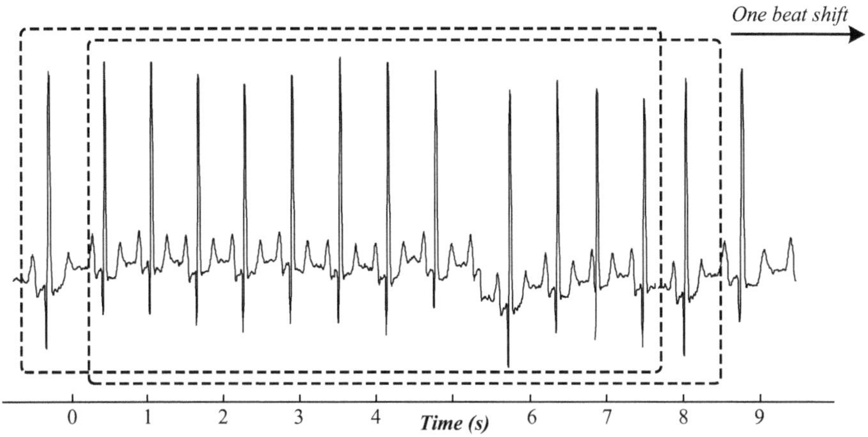

Fig. 5.11 Features are calculated in the sliding windows contain 12 heart beats

number of hidden neurons has been determined experimentally. In particular a $6 \times 6 \times 1$ (input layer, hidden layer, output layer) architecture was used. The activation function consists of a sigmoidal type and the parameters (weights and bias), that characterize the NN trained using the Levenberg Marquardt algorithm.

5.4 Results and Discussion

5.4.1 Applied Databases

Performance evaluation of the algorithms was conducted using the available database from Physionet and ECG signals collected in the MyHeart observational study. Currently it is observed that the databases from Physionet are the standard information source for algorithm performance comparability in the research area. The Physionet databases have been collected using wet electrode ECG technology. The MyHeart database was collected using dry textile electrode technology. Hence, it enables to test the performance of the algorithms with a technology that opens new application scenarios in personal health systems – continuous disease management.

5.4.1.1 MIT-BIH Public Databases

To assess the performance of the PVC detection method the MIT-BIH Arrhythmia database from Physionet was utilized. This database consists of 48 annotated records collected from 47 subjects studied by the Boston's Beth Israel Hospital (BIH)

Arrhythmia Laboratory. The database contains a mixture of 23 recordings chosen at random from a set of 4,000 24-h ambulatory ECG recordings collected from a mixed population of about 60% of inpatients and about 40% of outpatients at BIH, and the remaining recordings selected from the same set to include less common but clinically significant arrhythmias. Each record is 30-min long and was recorded at 360 Hz. To preserve coherence in the morphological characteristics of the ECG applied for training and validation, two records that do not include the MLII lead ECG configuration have been excluded. Hence, validation and testing was performed on 46 complete records. The training set was composed of 1,965 PVCs and 11,250 non-PVC QRS complexes, whereas the validation set was formed by 6,595 PVCs and 95,893 non-PVC beats.

Regarding the assessment of the AF detection algorithm the MIT-BIH Atrial Fibrillation database long-term records were applied. This database is composed of 25 long-term ECG recordings of human subjects with AF (mostly paroxysmal). From these 25 records, only 23 records have the raw ECG signal (original sampled ECGs). The two records where this signal is not available have been excluded. Each recording is 10 h in duration and is composed of two leads ECG sampled at 250 Hz. These 23 records have been utilized for the training and validation phases of the algorithm. More specifically, 19,161 and 29,893 randomly selected windows of 12 s of ECG signal, corresponding to AF and non AF episodes, composed the training dataset. Validation has been performed using 238,321 and 59,785 AF and non-AF episodes of the aforementioned 23 records of the database.

5.4.1.2 MyHeart Database

The MyHeart project (Habetha 2006) is a European funded research project where the main goal was to research wearable solutions for continuous patient home telemonitoring for cardiac disease prevention and early diagnosis, enabling intervention when appropriate. The approach of the MyHeart project is to monitor Vital Body Signs with wearable technology, particularly textile sensors embedded into garments, to process the measured data, and to give (therapy) recommendations to the user of the system. Many new sensors and much algorithmic work has been researched and developed in the MyHeart project and assembled into four distinct concepts which target different groups of medical needs, from primary prevention to therapy support.

One of the developed concepts inside MyHeart is aimed at secondary prevention in the heart failure management context. The goal of this concept is to detect heart failure decompensation symptoms at incipient states, through regular vital body signs measurement (bio-impedance, heart rate, heart rate profile during exercise, arrhythmia, respiratory rate, blood pressure, and weight) and diagnosis algorithms. As can be observed in Fig. 5.12, in this concept, each heart failure patient is equipped with a system composed of two off-the-shelf sensors (weight scale and blood pressure cuff) and two sensors developed inside the project – the

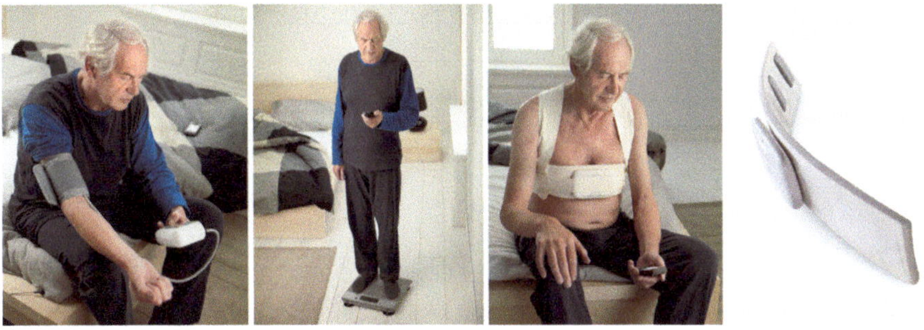

Fig. 5.12 The MyHeart Heart Failure Management system. From left to right: daily blood pressure; daily weight measurement; daily measurements of ECG, and bio-impedance with the MyHeart Bio-Impedance Monitor and vest; MyHeart Bio-Impedance Monitor sensor and electronics

bio-impedance monitor and bed-side ECG-respiration monitor, and a PDA (Personal Digital Assistant) that implements the user interface, runs diagnosis algorithm, and communicates with the medical server.

In order to assess the effectiveness of the developed sensors and algorithms, measurement data was required from heart failure patients using the developed sensors and algorithms. The MyHeart project ended with a clinical observational study where such data was collected. In this trial, a total of 148 chronic heart failure patients, enrolled in 6 different cities in Germany and Spain, were followed during 1 year in their homes. These patients performed a daily measurement protocol composed of measurements of vital signs at rest. Vital signs measurement always included the measurement of a one-lead ECG signal using the textile electrodes depicted in Fig. 5.11. It should be mentioned that at the time of writing the observational study has not been finalized and that only some snapshots of the data are available for analysis.

5.4.2 PVC Detection Results Using Public Databases

Table 5.3 presents a comparative analysis of the achieved results using the described PVC method (Sect. 5.3.5) and the reference state of the art algorithms described in the literature, based on the available MIT-BIH Arrhythmia databases. The reference state-of-the-art algorithms for PVC have not been implemented by the team for comparison. The results presented are those reported by authors. Furthermore, it should be stressed that the results in Table 5.3 have not been achieved under similar conditions. Some of the PVC detection algorithms have been tested using a subset

Table 5.3 PVC detection, sensitivity (SE) and specificity (SP)

			Num records	
	SE (%)	SP (%)	T. set	V. set
Proposed algorithm	96.35	99.15	46	46
Jekova et al. (2004)	93.30	97.30	48	48
Christov et al. (2005)	96.90	96.70	48	48
Christov and Bortolan (2004)	98.50	99.70	48	48
Ham and Han (1996)[b]	99.88	97.43	4	2
Chikh et al. (2004)	99.93	98.30	4	5
Millet et al. (1997)[b]	94.60	97.30	7	7
Ribeiro et al. (2007)	94.13	99.76	24	24
Moraes et al. (2002)[a]	90.34	96.55	44	44
Wang et al. (1999)[a]	94.39	97.09	44	44
Wieben et al. (1999)[a]	85.29	85.23	43	43
Al-Nashash (2000)[a]	98.10	94.30	14	14
Omer et al. (2006)[a]	82.57	93.42	18	40

Right column presents the reported number of records used by the authors: Training set (T. set) and validation set (V. set)
[a]These values refer to positive predictiveness (+P)
[b]Values of SE and SP are not obtained with the standard metrics: SE = TP/(TP + FN) and SP = TN/(TN + FP)

of the available data in the MIT-BIH Arrhythmia database. To clarify the conditions applied in each test, the two last columns have been added. These present the number of records used for training and validation in each method.

As can be observed in Table 5.3, sensitivity (SE) and specificity (SP) achieved using the proposed strategy for PVC detection are 96.35% and 99.15%, respectively. The comparison of these performance indexes with those achieved by the competing reference methods suggests that the proposed method reveals very accurate and robust detection behavior. Namely, comparing with the methods evaluated under similar test conditions, i.e., the methods introduced by Christov et al. (2005), Jekova et al. (2004), Christov and Bortolan (2004), Moraes et al. (2002), Wang et al. (1999), Wieben et al. (1999) and Omer et al. (2006), it is observed that the proposed algorithm reveals the highest sensitivity and specificity of all, with exception to Christov et al. (2005) and Christov and Bortolan (2004). Christov et al. (2005) report slightly higher sensitivity (+0.55%), however lower specificity (−2.45%) than the proposed algorithm. Christov and Bortolan (2004) present higher sensitivity (+2.15%) and slightly higher specificity (+0.55%) than the proposed algorithm. It should be noted that the algorithm proposed by these authors is based on two ECG leads and 26 features, while the proposed algorithm is based in only one ECG lead and 13 features. The use of a smaller number of features and only one lead, increases the applicability of the proposed algorithm in general environments, such as for personnel health (pHealth) systems, where usually only a one lead ECG and lower processing capabilities are available. The remaining results were reported by Ham and Han (1996), Chikh et al. (2004), and Millet et al. (1997). Really optimistic

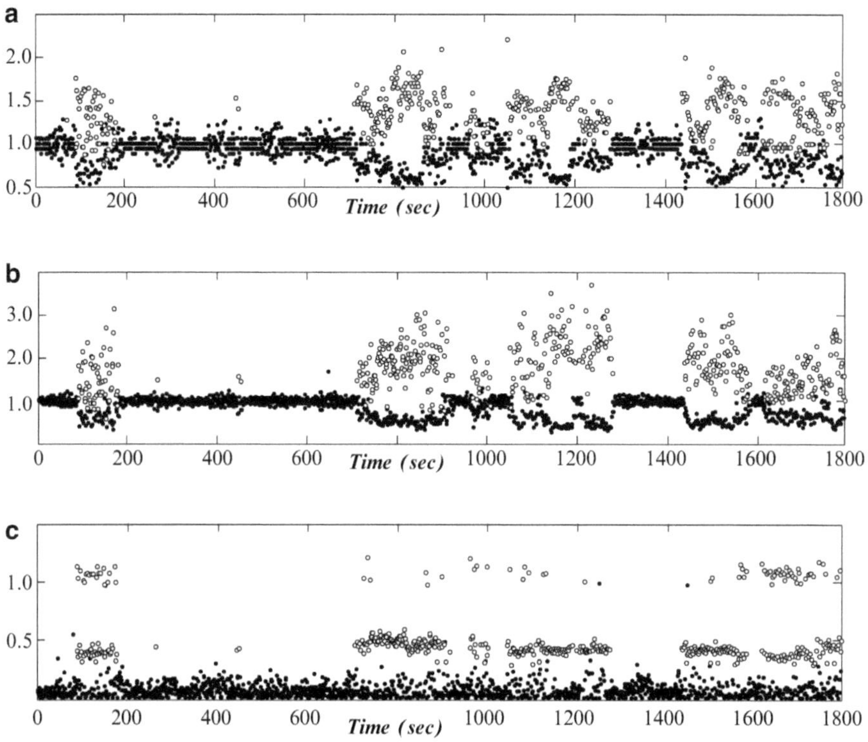

Fig. 5.13 Typical PVC features. Symbol (•) denotes a normal beat, while symbol (o) denotes an abnormal (PVC) beat. **(a)** QRS length ratio; **(b)** QRS area ratio; **(c)** P wave correlation

results were presented by some of these authors; however, a small dataset has been used for training and validation purposes. This scenario prevents a realistic comparison with the proposed method.

One of the main innovative aspects of the proposed algorithms is that it considers, additionally to the features derived from the current QRS complex, ECG morphological characteristics from the neighbor beats. Figure 5.13 presents three of these features that are employed by the PVC classifier. The first two, associated with the QRS complex morphology, QRS length ratio (feature f_1 - Eq. 5.21) and QRS area ratio (feature f_2 - Eq. 5.22) are shown, respectively, in Fig. 5.13a and b. The absence of P waves, corresponding to the feature f_7, is presented in Fig. 5.13c. As can be observed, the features derived using this approach achieve notable discrimination properties.

Based on those features, an illustrative ECG signal and the correspondent beat classification (normal/PVC) are depicted in Fig. 5.14. It reveals the algorithm's capacity to differentiate normal from abnormal beats.

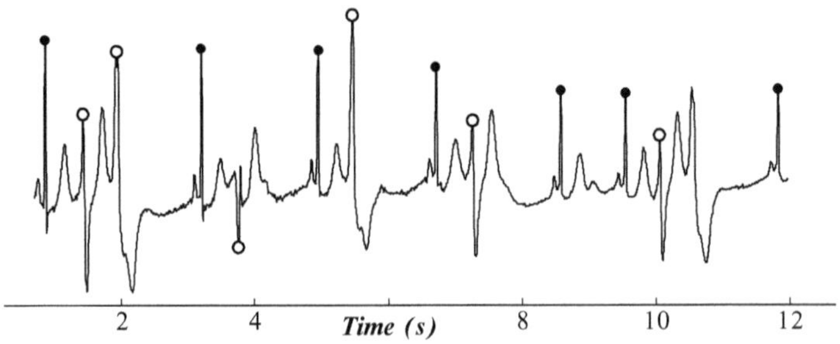

Fig. 5.14 PVC classification results. Symbol (•) denotes a normal beat, while symbol (o) denotes an abnormal (PVC) beat

Table 5.4 AF detection, sensitivity (SE), and specificity (SP)

	SE (%)	SP (%)
Proposed algorithm	93.80	96.09
Moody and Mark (1983)	93.58	85.92[a]
Cerutti et al. (1997)	93.3	94[a]
Tateno and Glass (2000)	93.2	96.7
Shkurovich et al. (1998)	78	92.65

[a] Values corresponding to positive predictiveness (+P)

5.4.3 AF Classification Results Using Public Databases

Table 5.4 present a comparative analysis of the achieved results using the described AF detection methodology, as well as results for reference state of the art algorithms described in literature using the Atrial Fibrillation database. As in the case of PVC, the state of the art algorithms for AF detection have not been implemented by the team. The results presented are those reported in their respective published papers.

From the comparative detection performance analysis reported in Table 5.4, it is observed that the proposed method presents 93.80% and 96.09% of sensitivity and specificity, respectively. Moody and Mark (1983) introduced an algorithm whose sensitivity is similar to the proposed method. Tateno and Glass (2000) algorithm achieved slightly higher specificity (+0.61%), however a slightly lower sensitivity (−0.6%) than the proposed algorithm. Although this method presents similar results, it is observed that it requires ECG segments composed of at least 100 heart beats to perform the classification. This significantly limits the method for real time applications. When comparing with the remaining algorithms, it is seen that the proposed AF method achieves higher sensitivity and specificity values. These results outline the accuracy of the proposed method, suggesting its reliability for the detection of AF.

In order to characterize the feasibility of the individual features, as well as to analyze their specific clinical relevance, a set of experiments was carried out

Table 5.5 Performance using specific groups of features – complete ECG signal

Performance (Se/Sp)	P wave analysis	Heart rate analysis	Atrial activity analysis
Train 1	0.8316/0.8624	0.8521/ 0.9262	0.7938/ 0.9107
Train 2	0.8241/0.8716	0.8584/ 0.9220	0.7972/ 0.9101
Train 3	0.8296/0.8624	0.8499/ 0.9326	0.7905/ 0.9139
Average	0.8284/0.8655	0.8535/0.9269	0.7938/0.9116
Std	0.0039/0.0053	0.0044/0.0053	0.0034/0.0020

Table 5.6 Performance using specific groups of features – window ECG analysis

Performance (Se/Sp)	P wave analysis	Heart rate analysis	Atrial activity analysis
Train 1	0.7761/0.8307	0.8349/0.9176	0.8309/0.9011
Train 2	0.7629/0.8431	0.8226/0.9131	0.8373/0.9002
Train 3	0.7754/0.8307	0.8320/0.9250	0.8237/0.9037
Average	0.7715/0.8348	0.8298/0.9186	0.8306/0.9017
Std	0.0074/0.0072	0.0064/0.0060	0.0068/0.0018

assessing sensitivity and specificity values considering several independent groups of features. Table 5.5 presents the AF classification results based on the individual analysis of three particular feature groups, associated to: (1) P wave absence, (2) heart rate regularity, and (3) atrial activity analysis. These results correspond to the sensitivity and specificity average of all MIT-BIH Atrial Fibrillation Database records. Moreover, three appropriate NN classifiers were derived for each group of features, reported as train1 through to train3.

As can be observed, when comparing with the simultaneously use of all features, the employment of each group of features independently (P wave, heart rate analysis, and atrial activity analysis) presents a lower capacity to differentiate AF episodes. In particular, features related to heart rate analysis provide the highest sensitivity and specificity results, respectively 85.35% and 92.69%. From the clinical perspective these results are consistent. In effect, heart rate regularity is considered the most important clinical signal employed by clinicians when detecting AF episodes. It should be mentioned that these results tend to drop when a window analysis, required for real-time processing, on the ECG is performed (see Table 5.6).

In a second set of experiments the combination of the aforementioned group of features was performed. Table 5.7 presents the classification results based on three pairs of feature group combinations: (1) P wave analysis + heart rate analysis; (2) P wave analysis + atrial activity analysis; (3) Heart rate analysis + atrial activity analysis. As in the previous experiment, the presented performance results correspond to the average of sensitivity and specificity of all MIT-BIH Atrial Fibrillation Database records, considering adequate classifiers (feedforward neural networks) for the complete ECG signals (Table 5.7) and using an ECG-based window analysis (Table 5.8).

Table 5.7 Combination of group of features – complete ECG signal

Performance (Se/Sp)	P-wave analysis + heart rate analysis	P-wave analysis + atrial activity analysis	Heart rate analysis + atrial activity analysis
Train 1	0.9064/0.9558	0.9114/0.9440	0.8726/0.9278
Train 2	0.8887/0.9520	0.8638/0.9378	0.8929/0.9306
Train 3	0.9168 /0.9508	0.7698/0.9603	0.8612/0.9350
Average	0.9039/0.9528	0.8483/0.9473	0.8755/0.9311
Std	0.0142/0.0026	0.0720/0.0116	0.0160/0.0036

Table 5.8 Combination of group of features – window ECG analysis

Performance (Se/Sp)	P-wave analysis + heart rate analysis	P-wave analysis + atrial activity analysis	Heart rate analysis + atrial activity analysis
Train 1	0.8912/0.9508	0.9103/0.9320	0.8966/0.9227
Train 2	0.8787/0.9514	0.8860/0.9312	0.8934/0.9240
Train 3	0.9003/0.9459	0.7916/0.9590	0.8713/0.9313
Average	0.8900/0.9493	0.8626/0.9407	0.8871/0.9260
Std	0.0108/0.0030	0.0627/0.0158	0.0137/0.0046

From Tables 5.7 and 5.8 it is possible to conclude that this combination enables to improve the performance of the classification results, when considering each individual group of features. It can also be concluded that the higher results are achieved when the features correspondent to P wave analysis are combined with those relative to heart rate analysis, respectively 90.39% and 95.28% of sensitivity and specificity. Again, these results are consistent with the clinical practice. Actually, AF is typically assessed by a clinician based on these two aspects: heart rate regularity/irregularity and absence of P waves. It should be noted that these results drop when a window ECG analysis is performed.

Finally, in a third set of experiments, the discrimination properties of individual features representative of each group (P wave, heart rate, and atrial activity analysis) were assessed, respectively as the (1) P wave ratio, (2) the regularity of the RR interval (entropy), and (3) the spectrum of the atrial activity analysis (entropy). Figure 5.15 illustrates the discrimination significance of those features, during an AF episode (approximately from window 1,000 to window 2,750).

5.4.4 AF Classification Using MyHeart Database

This section reports part of the results achieved by running the developed algorithms on the ECG data gathered with the MyHeart vest during the MyHeart trial. It is important to note that there was no extra ECG measurement taken in parallel during the MyHeart study, and, due to ethical reasons, the ECG measurements carried out with the Bio-Impedance Monitor will be evaluated by clinical experts when the trial is completed. As a result, it is not possible to currently adequately assess the performance of the algorithms (sensitivity and specificity values).

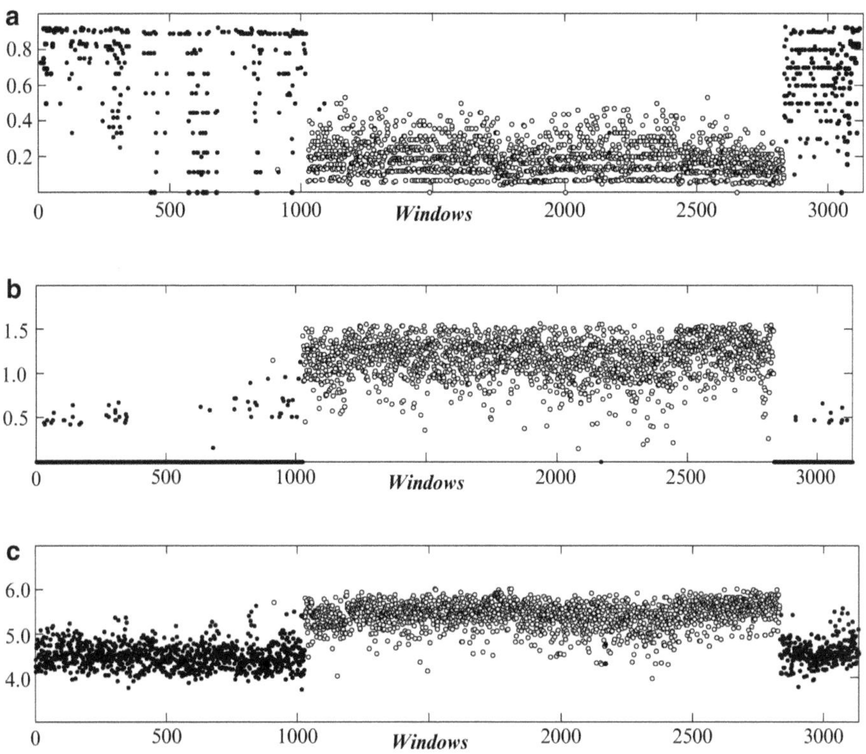

Fig. 5.15 Individual AF features. Symbol (•) denotes a normal ECG, while symbol (o) denotes an AF episode. **(a)** P waves ratio; **(b)** Hidden Markov entropy; **(c)** Spectrum entropy

The present methodology was employed to segment the ECG and to determine the RR interval, the QRS width, the PR interval, the PQ interval, and the QT interval. The following figure, Fig. 5.16, depicts one example of the segmentation parameters obtained from a typical patient along 192 sessions using the Bio-Impedance Monitor and textile vest. The parameters presented for each session results from the average of all values acquired during the session (a session is performed during 5 min).

As mentioned, although it is not possible to compare/validate the obtained results, the computed values are consistent with expected clinical parameters (QRS complex width and RR, QT, PQ, and PR intervals). Additionally, for each patient the number of PVCs and AF episodes was computed using the proposed algorithms. Figure 5.17a and b presents, respectively, the PVC and AF episodes detected in each session.

As can be observed, the algorithms have identified a relatively large number of PVCs (in session 174 a maximum number of 39 PVCs was achieved), as well as some AF episodes (the maximum number was 3 episodes in a session). Two main aspects may justify these figures. First, the morphology of the ECG signal, which

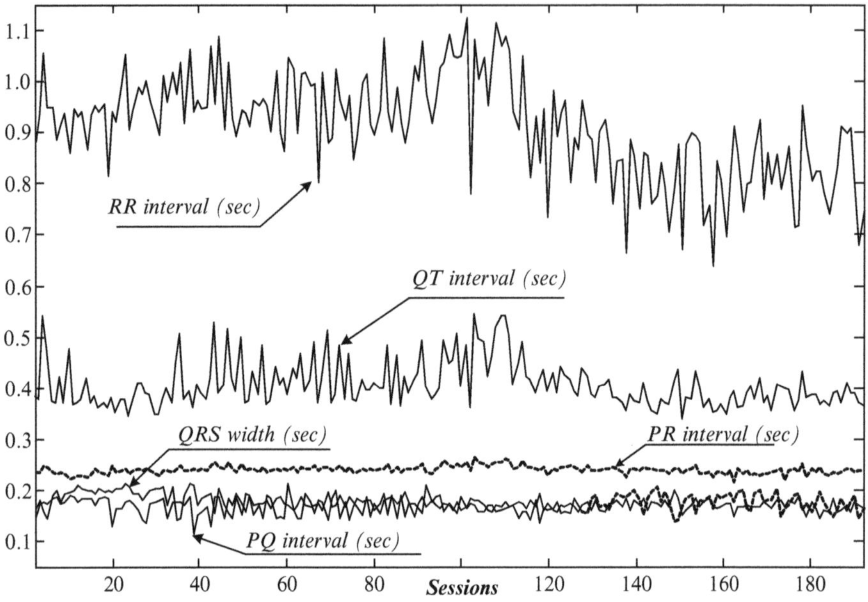

Fig. 5.16 Typical ECG segmentation results (MyHeart trial). The parameters presented for each session results from the average of all values acquired during the session (5 min)

presents some differences from the ones used in the training phase (MIT-BIH public databases), may be the origin of such results. On the other hand, patients involved in MyHeart study are heart failure patients. Therefore, when considering this clinical condition, the occurrence of PVC and AF episodes can be considered common. When the MyHeart trial is completed, the possible adjustment of the algorithms for the specific signals collected should be considered.

Two illustrative examples relative to ECG segmentation, PVC detection, and AF classification are presented in Fig. 5.18. Figure 5.18a shows part of the ECG collected during the session number 13 (where 22 PVC beats and 3 AF episodes were detected). Figure 5.18b shows part of the ECG signal corresponding to session 33, where no PVC or AF episodes were identified. Although it is not possible to validate the presented results, the figures suggest the correctness of the developed algorithms.

5.4.5 Processing Time

Table 5.9 presents the average processing time of the ECG segmentation, PVC detection algorithm, and AF classification for each window of 10 s of ECG signal. These average processing times have been obtained using a C-language

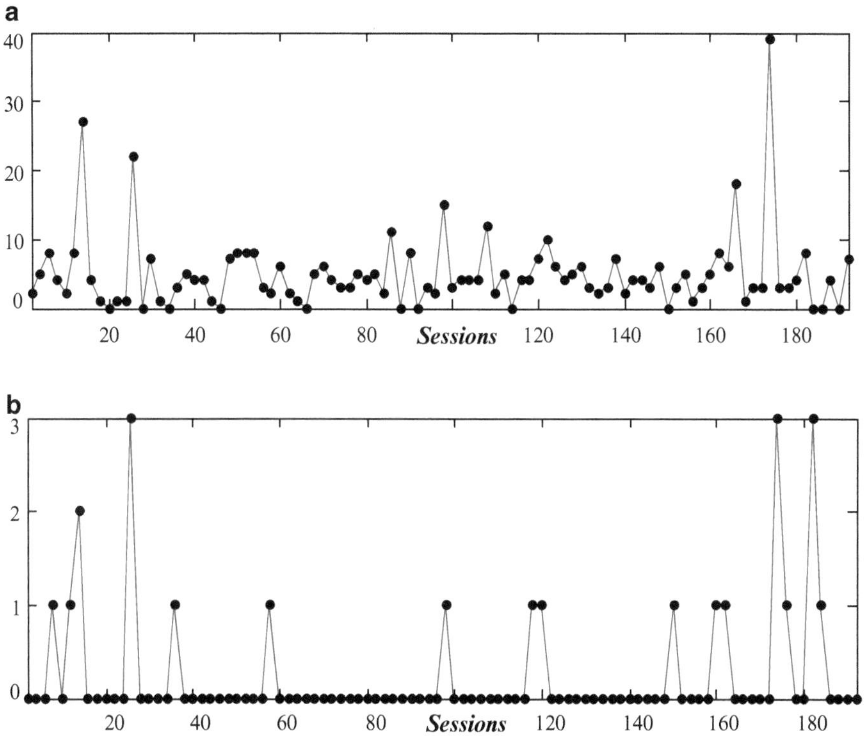

Fig. 5.17 PVC and AF detection results. The parameters presented for each session results from the average of all values acquired during the session (5 min). **(a)** PVC episodes; **(b)** AF episodes

implementation of the algorithm running on a QTek S200 PDA with Windows Mobile 5 and 195 MHz OMAP850 processor. This device was the equipment used by patients in the MyHeart clinical trial.

Furthermore, the indicated times have been achieved on the MIT-BIH Arrhythmia database. As can be observed, the proposed PVC method takes on average 0.4 s to process each window of 10 s of ECG. This is significantly shorter compared to the processing time required to fully segment the ECG, i.e., to identify all fiducial points (Q, R, and S) and characteristic waves (T and P-waves), with the implemented ECG segmentation method on the same platform with the same implementation language.

The results obtained, by implementing the algorithm in a PDA with a standard CPU, demonstrate that it is possible to run the algorithms in real-time, if required. In our current implementation this is clearly not possible (nor was it the goal of the application), since processing time is larger than the analysis window duration. However, it should be stressed that there is a considerable margin for code optimization (e.g., in our implementation floating point arithmetic was used instead of fixed point or integer arithmetic), which could enable real-time execution if required.

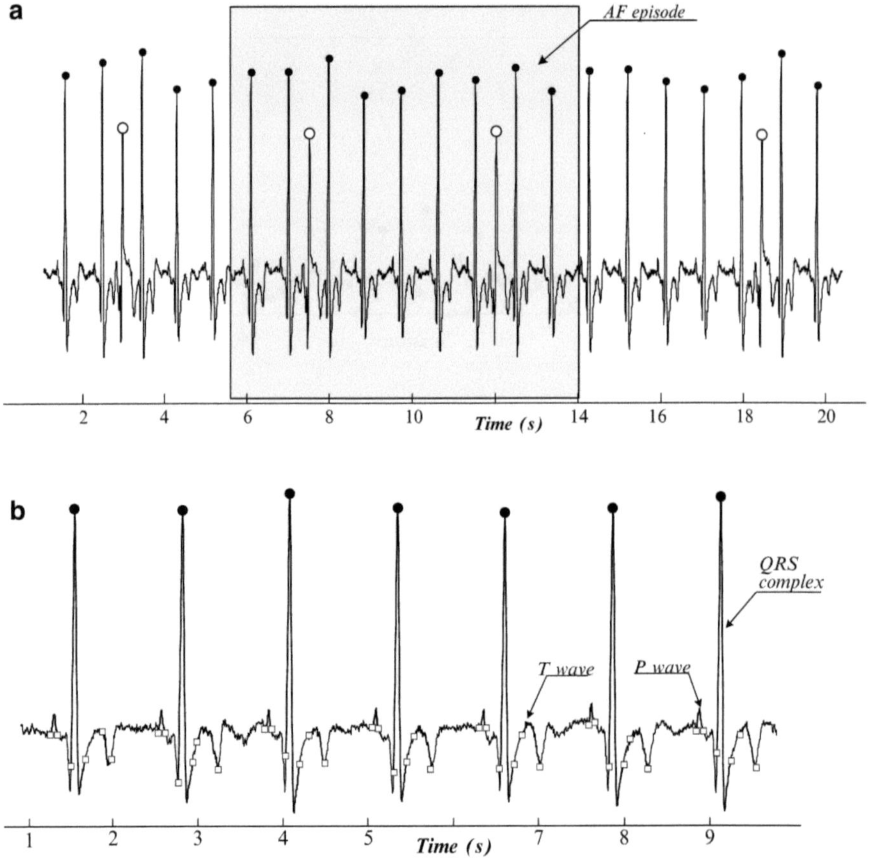

Fig. 5.18 Illustrative examples of PVC and AF detection results from Myheart database. Symbol (•) denotes a normal ECG, while symbol (o) denotes an AF episode. Symbol (□) denotes the delimitation of a QRS, P, and T waves. (**a**) Session 13– irregular ECG (22 PVC beats and 3 AF episodes); (**b**) Session 33– regular ECG

Table 5.9 Processing times

Algorithm	Time (s)
ECG segmentation	4.8
PVC detection	0.4
AF detection	7.9

5.5 Conclusions

In this chapter the integrated ECG analysis algorithm for atrial fibrillation detection, developed in the context of European research project MyHeart, was presented. This algorithm is based on a novel architecture that combines the three main physiological characteristics of AF that support cardiologist's diagnosis in their daily reasoning: P wave absence, heart rate irregularity, and atrial activity analysis. Moreover, it takes into account the occurrence of PVC events to be removed from the ECG prior to AF analysis. New features, based on estimated models using data-driven approaches and a new approach to achieve patient invariance constitute the main innovative aspects of the proposed algorithms. The proposed architecture is modular and the modules of the algorithm have been designed to operate on short signal windows (typically in the order of 10 s). This has the potential to enable real-time operation, which is a significant aspect for home monitoring pHealth applications.

Experimental results using public databases (Physionet MIT-BIH Arrhythmia and QT databases) revealed that the proposed algorithm presents overall better discrimination performance, when compared to the state-of-the-art methods reported in literature. Although currently a true validation cannot be performed using MyHeart project database (based on data collected using wearable ECG sensors), the results achieved so far by the algorithms suggest their correctness. Nevertheless, some modules probably have to be improved, to maintain/increase the obtained sensitivity and specificity and to assure robustness to changes in real measurement conditions (inc. noise). This will be performed in the very near future, after the observational study of MyHeart.

Acknowledgments This project was partially financed by the IST FP6 MyHeart project, IST-2002-507816 supported by the European Union.

References

Alan, G., Hylek, E., Phillips, K., Chang, Y., Henault, L., Selby, J., Singer, D.: Prevalence of diagnosed atrial fibrillation in adults: national implications for rhythm management and stroke prevention: the nticoagulation and risk factors in atrial fibrillation (ATRIA) study. JAMA. **285**, 2370–2375 (2001)

Al-Nashash, H.: Cardiac arrhythmia classification using neural networks. Technol. Health Care. **8**(6), 363–372 (2000)

Cerutti, S., Mainardi, L.T., Porta, A., Bianchi, A.: Analysis of the dynamics of RR interval series for the detection of atrial fibrillation episodes. IEEE Comput. Cardiol. **24**, 77–80 (1997)

Chikh, M., Gbelgacem, N., Reguig, F.: The use of artificial neural networks to detect PVC beats. Lab. de Génie Biomédical. Dép. d'électronique, Univ. Abou Bekr Belkaïd (2003)

Chikh, M., Belgacem, N., Chikh, A., Reguig, F.: The use of artificial neural network to detect the premature ventricular contraction (PVC) beats. Electron. J. Tech. Acoust. **2**, 1–14 (2004)

Christov, I., Bortolan, G.: Ranking of pattern recognition parameters for premature ventricular contractions classification by neural networks. Physiol. Meas. **25**, 1281–1290 (2004)

Christov, I., Jekova, I., Bortolan, G.: Premature ventricular contraction classification by the Kth nearest-neighbours rule. Physiol. Meas. **26**, 123–130 (2005)

Cleland, J., Louis, A., Rigby, A., Janssens, U., Balk, A.: Noninvasive home telemonitoring for patients with heart failure at high risk of recurrent admission and death. J. Am. Coll. Cardiol. **45**, 1654–1664 (2005)

Couceiro, R., Carvalho, P., Henriques, J., Antunes, M.: On the detection of premature ventricular contractions. Conf. Proc. IEEE Eng. Med. Biol. Soc. **2008**:1087–1091 (2008)

Fuster, V., Rydén, L., Asinger, R., Cannom, D., Crijns, H., Frye, R., Halperin, J., Kay, G., Klein, E., Lévy, S., MCNamara, R., Prysowsky, E., Wann, L., Wyse, D.: ACC/AHA/ESC guidelines for the management of patients with atrial fibrillation. J. Am. Coll. Cardiol. **38**(4), 1231–1265, 765 (2001)

Habetha, J.: The myheart project – fighting cardiovascular diseases by prevention and early diagnosis. Conf. Proc. IEEE Eng. Med. Biol. Soc. 6746–6749 (2006)

Ham, F., Han, S.: Classification of cardiac arrhythmias using Fuzzy ARTMAP. IEEE Trans. Biomed. Eng. **43**(4), 425–430 (1996)

Jalife, J.: Experimental and clinical AF mechanisms: bridging the divide. J. Intervent. Card. Electrophysiol. **9**, 85–92 (2003)

Jekova, I., Bortolan, G., Christov, I.: Pattern recognition and optimal parameter selection in premature ventricular contraction classification. IEEE Comput. Cardiol. **31**, 357–360 (2004)

Levy, A., Camm, J., Saksena, S.: International consensus on nomenclature and classification of atrial fibrillation: a collaborative of the working group an arrhythmias and the work group of cardiac pacing of the European society of cardiology and the north American society of pain and electrophysiology. Cardiovasc. Electrophysiol. **14**, 443–445 (2003)

Lévy, S., Breithardt, G., Campbell, R., Camm, A., Daubert, J., Allessie, M., Aliot, E., Capucci, A., Cosio, F., Crijns, H., Jordaens, L., Hauer, R., Lombardi, F., Lüderitz, B.: Atrial fibrillation: current knowledge and recommendations for management. Eur. Heart J. **19**(9), 1294–1320 (1998)

Millet, J., Perez, M., Joseph, G., Mocholi, A., Chorro, J.: Previous identification of QRS onset and offset is not essential for classifying QRS complexes in a single lead. IEEE Comput. Cardiol. **24**, 299–302 (1997)

Moe, G., Abildskov, J.: Observations on the ventricular dysrhythmia associated with atrial fibrillation in the dog heart. Circ. Res. **4**, 447–460 (1964)

Moody, B., Mark, R.: A new method for detecting atrial fibrillation using RR intervals. IEEE Comput. Cardiol. **10**, 227–230 (1983)

Moraes, J., Seixas, M., Vilani, F., Costa, E.: A real time QRS complex classification method using Mahalanobis distance. IEEE Comput. Cardiol. **29**, 201–204 (2002)

Omer, T., Giovangrandi, L., Kovacs, G.: Robust neural-network-based classification of premature ventricular contraction using wavelet transform and timing interval features. IEEE Trans. Biomed. Eng. **53**(12), 2507–2515 (2006)

Reiter, H., Maglaveras, N.: HeartCycle: compliance and effectiveness in HF and CAD closed-loop management. Conf. Proc. IEEE Eng. Med. Biol. Soc. 299–302 (2009)

Ribeiro, B., Marques, A., Henriques, J.: Choosing real-time predictors for ventricular arrhythmia detection. Int. J. Pattern Recog. Artifi. Intell. **21**(8), 1–15 (2007)

Sanchez, C., Millet, J., Rieta, J., Castells, F., Ródenas, J., Ruiz-Granell, R., Ruiz, V.: Packet wavelet decomposition: an approach for atrial activity extraction. IEEE Comput. Cardiol. **29**, 33–36 (2002)

Senhadji, L., Wang, F., Hernandez, A., Carrault, G.: Wavelets extrema representation for QRS-T cancellation and P wave detection. IEEE Comput. Cardiol. **29**, 37–40 (2002)

Sherman, D.: Pharmacological rate versus rhythm control. Stroek. **38**, 615 (2007)

Shkurovich, S., Sahakian, A., Swiryn, S.: Detection of atrial activity from high-voltage leads of implantable ventricular fibrillators, using a cancellation technique. IEEE Trans. Biomed. Eng. **45**(2), 229–234 (1998)

Sun, Y., Chan, K., Krishnan, S.: Characteristic wave detection in ECG signal using morphological transform. BMC Cardiovasc. Disord. **5**, 28 (2005)

Tateno, K., Glass, L.: A method for detection of atrial fibrillation using RR intervals. IEEE Comput. Cardiol. **27**, 391–394 (2000)

Waldo, A.: Mechanisms of atrial fibrillation. J. Cardiovasc. Electrophysiol. **14**(12), 267–274 (2003)

Wang, J., Yeo, C., Aguire, A.: The design and evaluation of a new multi-lead arrhythmia monitoring algorithm. IEEE Comput. Cardiol. **26**, 675–678 (1999)

Wieben, O., Afonso, V., Tompkinks, W.: Classification of premature ventricular complexes using filter bank features, induction of decision trees and a fuzzy rule-based system. Med. Biol. Eng. Comput. **37**(1), 560–565 (1999)

Wolf, P., Abbott, R., Kannel, W.: Atrial fibrillation as an independent risk factor for stroke: the Framingham Study. Stroke. **22**, 983–988 (1991)

Chapter 6
An Introduction to the Use of Evolutionary Computation Techniques for Dealing with ECG Signals

Guillermo Leguizamón and Carlos A. Coello

6.1 Introduction

Evolutionary Computation (EC) techniques have reached an impressive level of development, both from the point of view of basic research as well as from the perspective of practical applications. This has also triggered an important amount of research on other bio-inspired metaheuristics such as Particle Swarm Optimization (PSO), Ant Colony Optimization (ACO), Differential Evolution (DE), and Artificial Immune Systems (AIS), which have also been extensively applied in many real-world problems.

Biomedical signals (biosignals) processing has become a very appealing area for developing and applying Computational Intelligence (CI) techniques. CI can be defined as a broad class of bio-inspired approaches normally used for classification and optimization, which includes EC techniques, artificial neural networks, and fuzzy logic. Among the most relevant biosignals are those represented by raw data collected by different medical instruments such as Electrocardiograms (ECG), Electroencephalograms (EEG), and Electromyogram (EMG); however, in this chapter we will focus specifically on ECG signals.

It is worth emphasizing that the use of CI-based techniques for medical applications is a vast and promising research area that has been kept under continuous development in the last few years. Although (Begg et al. 2008) have observed that neural networks and fuzzy logic are the most developed CI techniques used for

G. Leguizamón (✉)
UMI LAFMIA 3175 CNRS at CINVESTAV-IPN, Departmento de Computación, México D.F., MÉXICO and LIDIC - Universidad Nacional de San Luis, San Luis, Argentina
e-mail: legui@unsl.edu.ar

C.A. Coello
CINVESTAV-IPN (Evolutionary Computation Group), Departamento de Computación and UMI LAFMIA 3175 CNRS at CINVESTAV-IPN, México D.F., México
e-mail: ccoello@cs.cinvestav.mx

A. Gacek and W. Pedrycz (eds.), *ECG Signal Processing, Classification and Interpretation: A Comprehensive Framework of Computational Intelligence*, DOI 10.1007/978-0-85729-868-3_6, © Springer-Verlag London Limited 2012 medical applications, several important EC techniques have also been applied in this area, as we will see in this chapter. Several EC-based tools have been proposed for medical applications, including those that deal directly with the processing of ECG signals. However, there are also EC-based tools aimed to help other techniques to improve their processing of ECG signals (this could be considered as an indirect way of applying EC approaches in this area). Therefore, the aim of this chapter is to show that EC techniques can be considered as useful tools to be used in this application domain. With that goal in mind, this chapter will review the newest and most relevant proposals on the use of EC techniques for biomedical problems, aiming to provide an appealing perspective of this CI technique and its potential use for medical applications.

The rest of the chapter is organized as follows. Section 6.2 provides the main EC concepts necessary to make this chapter self-contained. This includes a brief description of the most representative EC-based algorithms, seen under a unified perspective. In Sect. 6.3 we give some introductory remarks and definitions on ECG signals. Next, in Sect. 6.4 we present a brief literature review of applications that use EC techniques as either a primary or a secondary tool when dealing with some typical problems related to ECG signals. An additional literature review is given in Sect. 6.5 that describes the application of other bio-inspired metaheuristics such as PSO, AIS, and ACO to ECG signals. The chapter finishes in Sect. 6.6 with some general comments about the state-of-the-art and future research lines in this application domain.

6.2 EC Basics

EC techniques comprise a set of metaheuristics that seek to emulate the mechanism of natural selection described in Charles Darwin's evolutionary theory, with the aim of solving problems. Although the origins of EC can be traced back as far as the early 1930s (Fogel 1995), it was not until the 1960s that the three main techniques based on this notion were developed: genetic algorithms (Holland 1962, 1992), evolution strategies (Schwefel 1965, 1995), and evolutionary programming (Fogel 1966). These approaches, which are now collectively denominated "evolutionary algorithms," constitute the core of the evolutionary computation field.

Nowadays, there exists a large amount of literature devoted to EC techniques and their applications; see for example, Bäck (1996), Bäck et al. (2000), Eiben and Smith (2003), Fogel (1995), and Michalewicz and Fogel (2004). Modern approximations to the theory and practice of EAs can be found in De Jong (2006) as it represents a valuable, comprehensive, and up-to-date source of information about EAs from a unified point of view. Additionally, in Glover and Kochenberger (2003), and in Talbi (2009), one can find good descriptions of EC techniques in the context of modern metaheuristics. These books also describe other bio-inspired algorithms such as Ant Colony Optimization (ACO), Particle Swarm Optimization (PSO), Bee Colony (BC)–based algorithms, and Artificial Immune Systems (AIS).

Considering the most recent perspectives to study EC techniques, we present in the following a general and unified description of EAs that can help readers to better understand their basic operating principles and the ways in which they could be applied in the solution of problems related to the processing of ECG signals.

From a Darwinian perspective (De Jong 2006), the metaphor of adaptation and evolution of a species involves: (a) one or more populations of individuals competing for limited resources, (b) the notion of dynamically changing populations due to the birth and death of individuals, (c) a concept of fitness which reflects the ability of an individual to survive and reproduce, and (d) a concept of variational inheritance (i.e., offsprings closely resemble their parents, but are not identical). An algorithm designed to fulfill the above characteristics implements a *Darwinian evolutionary system* (De Jong 2006). Based on the concept of evolutionary systems, several possibilities arise to design advanced algorithms capable of efficiently exploring complex search spaces for solving complex optimization problems. In this regard, it is necessary to identify the problem components and the way they can be included in the evolutionary system (e.g., a representation of potential solutions, a fitness function to assess the quality of potential solutions, selection mechanisms for mating and reproduction, and evolutionary operators to create offspring from the individuals selected for reproduction). An EA can be considered an advanced expression of an evolutionary system, mainly devoted to solve optimization problems. In the following, we describe the main components (including some examples) of an EA. Next, a general outline of an EA is presented that embodies, in a unified manner, the most representative EAs in current use.

6.2.1 Fundamental Components of an Evolutionary Algorithm

When dealing with a particular problem, a potential user or implementer of an EA must carefully make appropriate design decisions in order to achieve an effective and efficient EA to solve the problem at hand. Those decisions are related to the main components of the EA with regard to the following description:

- *Individuals' Representation*: With no doubt, this is one of the earliest and most important design decisions that must be made. The type of representation adopted will determine the size of the search space (i.e., the set of all possible solutions) as well as the design of the evolutionary operators that will be used for manipulating these solutions. In the jargon of EAs, it is said that an individual[1] encodes (using a particular alphabet) a possible solution for the problem at hand. Many times, the chromosome is an indirect representation of a solution (called genotype) and a decoding process is needed to obtain the solution (called phenotype). However, some other representation encodings directly represent the problem solution, i.e.,

[1]The term *chromosome* is also widely adopted and will be used interchangeably in the following.

the EA search space is a phenotypical one. Thus, we will assume that the search space of an EA can be either genotypical or phenotypical. The binary alphabet is the canonical option in EAs, and the most commonly considered is the set $\{0,1\}$. However, many other encodings are possible as long as we can devise appropriate operators for them. The choice is generally determined by the problem and also by the type of EA that is being implemented. For example, when using Evolution Strategies (Schwefel 1995), the typical representation is a real valued vector. In contrast, the typical representation in Genetic Programming (Koza 1992, 1994) is a tree structure. Another important consideration is about the length of the chromosomes. Their length could be fixed or variable. This depends on the problem we are dealing with. For the sake of a simpler discussion, we will assume in this chapter the use of a fixed length $n \in \mathbb{N}$ for all the individuals in an EA.

- *Population of Individuals:* An EA performs an iterative process that manipulates a population of individuals. Accordingly, a structure $P(t)$ is defined to keep the current population of those individuals at time t (variable t represents the iteration number as described in the following section). Usually, the population size is kept fixed during the evolutionary process; however, the use of variable size populations is also possible.

Definition 6.1. Let $\mathcal{I}$ be the set of all possible encoded solutions, $P(t) \in \mathcal{I}$ a set of the current population at time t, and $m = |P(t)|$ is the population size. The size of $\mathcal{I}$ will depend on n, the length of the chromosome, and the cardinality of the alphabet adopted.

Some examples of possible search spaces regarding the chosen solution representation are the following:

Binary vectors:	$\mathcal{I}_1 = \{(b_1,\ldots,b_n)\vert b_i \in \{0,1\}\}$
Real vectors:	$\mathcal{I}_2 = \{(r_1,\ldots,r_n)\vert r_i \in [a,b] \text{ with } a,b \in \mathbb{R}\}$
Permutations:	$\mathcal{I}_3 = \{(p_1,\ldots,p_n)\vert p_i \in \{1,\ldots,n\}$ and
	$(\text{ if } p_i = p_j, \text{ then } i = j)\}$
Integer vectors:	$\mathcal{I}_4 = \{(a_1,\ldots,a_n)\vert a_i \in \mathbb{N}\}$

- *Fitness Function*: As the emulation of the evolution metaphor implies the survival of the fittest individuals, a measurement mechanism should be defined for assessing the adaptability of the individuals to the environment (i.e., the problem under consideration). The fitness function:

$$F : \mathcal{I} \rightarrow \mathbb{R}^+ \tag{6.1}$$

assigns to each individual a real positive value that is used for the selection mechanism (next item) to guide the search in forthcoming iterations.

- *Selection*: The selection mechanism imposes a bias to the search process toward regions of high-quality solutions. The aim of this mechanism is to preferably select the fittest individuals that will participate in the reproduction phase. The selection mechanism can be seen as the following function:

$$\mathcal{S}el : 2^{\mathcal{I}} \rightarrow 2^{\mathcal{I}} \tag{6.2}$$

- *Reproductive Mechanisms (or Evolutionary Operators)*: This important component is in charge of generating the offspring from the selected set of parents (function $\mathcal{S}el$). Generally speaking, evolutionary operators promote the exploration of the search space by creating offspring which inherit good genetic material from their parents. Thus, these operators are expected to create, on average, individuals with higher quality with respect to their parents. Classical evolutionary operators are crossover (Eq. 6.3) and mutation (Eq. 6.4). The general crossover operator presented in Eq. 6.3 is defined as a binary operator that takes two parents and returns one offspring. However, other domains and ranges are also possible for this operator, e.g., multiple parents, and two or more offspring.

$$\chi_c : \mathcal{I} \times \mathcal{I} \rightarrow \mathcal{I} \tag{6.3}$$

$$\chi_m : \mathcal{I} \rightarrow \mathcal{I} \tag{6.4}$$

A classical example of a crossover operator for binary representation is the so-called 1-point crossover. Its application consists in generating a random number $k \in \{1,\ldots,n-1\}$. The offspring inherits the first k bits from the first parent and the last $n-k$ bits from the second one. For example, given the crossover point $k=3$ and two possible parents $P1$ and $P2$, one of the generated children is the following:

$$\begin{aligned} P1 &= (0\,0\,1\,|0\;\;1\;\;0\,1\;\;1\,1) \\ P2 &= (\mathbf{1\,0\,0}\,|\mathbf{1\;\;1\;\;1\,0\;\;1\,0}) \\ \chi_c(P1,P2) &= (0\,0\,1\;\;\mathbf{1\;\;1\;\;1\,0\;\;1\,0}) \end{aligned}$$

It must be noticed that the original 1-point crossover generates two offspring, by using a very similar procedure to the one described above. In fact, this procedure can be extended to allow the generation of more than two children, to the use of several crossover points and more than two parents.

Following with the binary representation for the individuals, a classical example for the mutation operator is the so-called flip mutation. This simple operator consists of choosing a location $l \in \{1,\ldots,n\}$ that indicates the bit that will undergo mutation. The new value at location l is: $new\_val(l) = 1 - old\_value(l)$. Let $l=4$ be the random location generated and $P1$ the individual that undergoes mutation:

$$\begin{aligned} P1 &= (0\,0\,1\,|0\;\;1\,0\,1\,1\,1) \\ \chi_m(P1) &= (1\,0\,0\,\mathbf{1}\;\;1\,1\,0\,1\,0) \end{aligned}$$

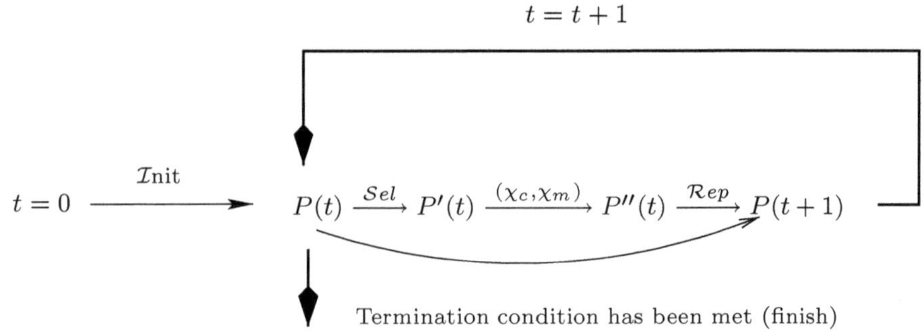

Fig. 6.1 Schematic representation of an EA as a composition of functions: $\mathcal{I}nit$ (applied once), $\mathcal{S}el$, χ_c, χ_m, and $\mathcal{R}ep$

6.2.2 A General Outline of an EA

Having described the main components of an EA, it is now possible to present a general outline of this kind of algorithm. Figure 6.1 displays a schematic representation of an EA's behavior as a composition of the functions $\mathcal{I}nit$ (applied once), $\mathcal{S}el$, χ_c, χ_m, and $\mathcal{R}ep$. Function $\mathcal{I}nit$ is in charge of generating the initial population to be evolved. Several criteria can be used to generate the initial population, but the simpler one is to generate a population completely at random. The last part of the iterative process involves function $\mathcal{R}ep$ which obtains the new population based on the current population ($P(t)$) and the intermediate population ($P''(t)$) generated by applying $\mathcal{S}el$ and operators χ_c and χ_m. In order to have a closer perspective of the implementation of an EA, the corresponding pseudo-code is presented in Algorithm 6.1.

Algorithm 6.1 General outline of an EA

$t = 0$;
$P(t) = \mathcal{I}\text{nit}()$;
while (Termination_Condition **not met**) **do**
  Eval($P(t)$);
  $P'(t) = \mathcal{S}el(P(t))$;
  $P''(t) =$ Apply_Operators($P'(t)$, χ_c, χ_m);
  $P(t+1) = \mathcal{R}\text{ep}(\ P(t)\ ,\ P''(t+1))$;
  $t = t + 1$;
end while

To conclude this section, it is worth mentioning the importance of hybridization in the field of EAs. Several alternatives to design hybrid EAs can be found in the literature. Such examples illustrate the importance of this topic as an alternative to improve the performance of an EA. A recent comprehensive description of hybrid metaheuristics that can be applied to EAs can be found in Talbi (2009). It is also important to highlight that EAs and other related metaheuristics have been widely applied in combination with a large variety of computational intelligence tools as discussed in Sect. 6.4 within the context of ECG signal processing.

6.3 ECG Signals

With the advancements of digital technology in general and the technology used in medical instrumentation, in particular, many different types of medical data are continuously collected from patients for different reasons. Consequently, the hospital and clinical databases are continuously growing as they maintain detailed information from different medical instruments and sources of physiological signals (biosignals) that are usually generated by human beings. For example, magnetic resonance imaging, computerized tomography, electrocardiogram (ECG), electroencephalogram (EEG), and electromyogram (EMG) signals. Although ECG, EEG, and EMG signals are usually associated to the analysis of unimodal signals (i.e., one signal is considered at a time), multimodal signal modeling and processing could be also considered (Laguna and Sörnmo 2009). Particularly, this chapter is devoted to the ECG unimodal signal processing from an evolutionary computation perspective, as an alternative way to deal with some particular problems in this area. In what follows, we first provide the basic concepts and components involved in the processing of ECG signals, and then we discuss the need to use automatic approaches and algorithms for signal processing, as well as the kind of tasks that are more suitable to be solved through the use of EC techniques.

Electrocardiogram (ECG) signal processing conforms one important part of the above-mentioned medical data that are widely available and are also easy to obtain due to the lower costs of medical instruments necessary to collect them among patients under different circumstances. Moreover, heart diseases diagnosis and ECG interpretation is an important noninvasive step in the clinical diagnosis process. The ECG is a valuable indicator of cardiac function, and it represents the electrical activity of the heart over time. In Fig. 6.2, we can observe a normal ECG where the QRS complex and some other waveforms give evidence of mechanical pumping of the heart. Consequently, a correct analysis and interpretation of these waveforms can be extensively used to infer cardiac health as well as cardiac diseases – e.g., arrhythmia, myocardial infarction, and myocardial ischemia; moreover blood and vessels diseases and congenital diseases can also be detected by carefully analyzing the ECG signals. In the next section, we cover some of the main tasks that are usually considered when analyzing the ECG signals in search for patterns that could indicate possible heart diseases or malfunctioning.

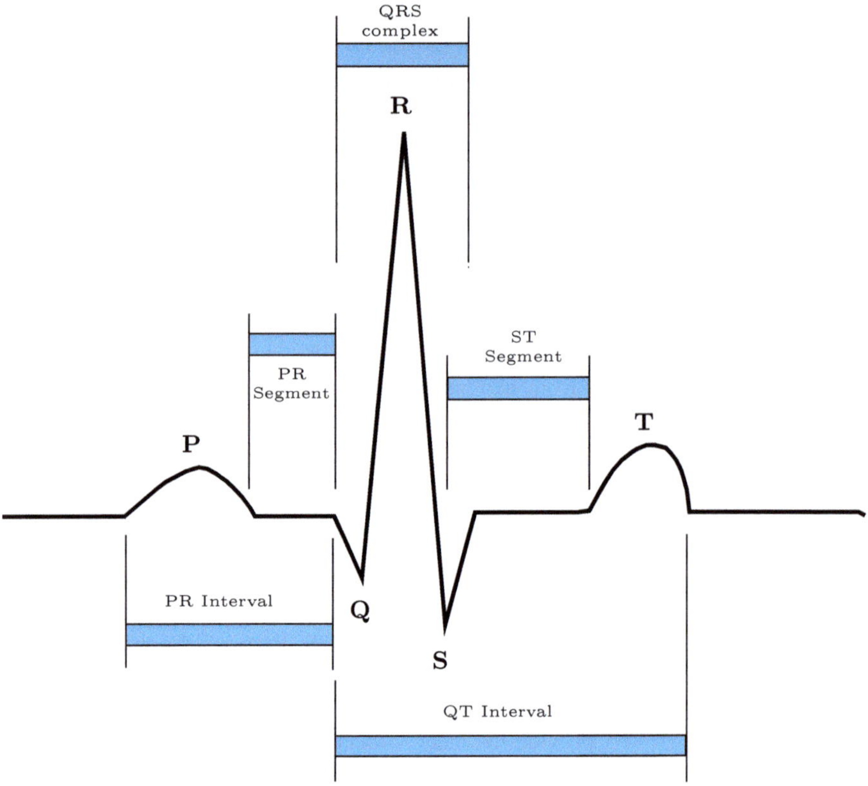

Fig. 6.2 Schematic representation of a normal ECG: QRS complex; PR and ST segments; and PR and QT intervals

6.3.1 ECG Signal Processing

General algorithms for basic ECG signal processing include at least the following components: (a) noise filtering, (b) QRS detection, and (c) wave delineation. In addition to that, (d) a data compression module can be added for further data storage or transmission. Sörnmo and Laguna (2006) describe the interaction among these components which is recreated in this chapter as shown in Fig. 6.3. For further information, an appealing source of introductory information regarding ECG signal processing is precisely the above-mentioned chapter of Sörnmo and Laguna (2006). In the following, we present a short description of the main modules in ECG signal processing which explains their respective functions and scope in the whole processes:

- One important issue when dealing with the interpretation of recorded signals is the presence of noise as indicated in Fig. 6.3 by the respective module in the main sequence of ECG signal processing. In that regard, most of the signal

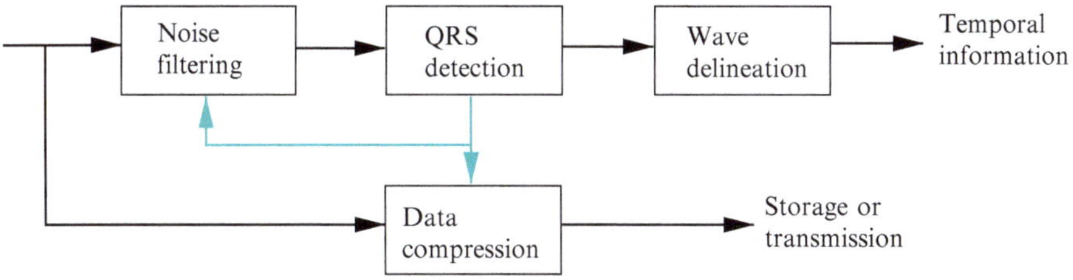

Fig. 6.3 A general scheme of a potential algorithm for basic ECG signal processing. *Light arrows* indicate that the output from QRS complex detection can be used as feedback information in "Data compression" and "Noise filtering" modules to improve their respective performance

processing aims at extracting the expected signal (i.e., uncorrupted) from a noisy one. According to Friesen et al. (1990), there exist several sources of noise that can corrupt in different ways the recorded ECG signal. The following can be considered as the most important sources of noise:

- *Power-Line Interference*: to diminish this kind of noise, filters are designed to suppress ECG components close to the power-line frequency.
- *Electrode Contact Noise*: is a transient interference caused when an electrode loses contact with the skin.
- *Motion Artifacts*: the electrode-skin impedance can produce artifacts with electrode motion.
- *Muscle Contraction*: this causes the generation of millivolt-level potential fields.
- *Baseline Drift*: the beat morphology is suitable for changes that do not have a cardiac origin and can produce important distortions in the collected signal. This type of noise can be generated by the movements of the patient being tested.
- *Instrumentation Noise*: normally generated by electronic devices used in signal processing, e.g., producing a saturation on the input devices that avoid to reach the ECG signals.
- *Electrosurgical Noise*: this type of noise is produced by the instruments that apply electrocauterization and it can completely destroy the ECG signal.

• The QSR wave detection is a very important and determinant step in the ECG signal processing. On one hand, QRS complex detection is directly associated to heartbeat detection. Thus, a poor performance of a potential detector will produce irrecoverable errors in further processing steps, e.g., during the wave delineation. There exists a large number of QRS morphologies that must be detected, and certainly, many different diagnosis tasks that might arise based on the results of the QRS detector. For example, clustering of beat morphologies may be performed for the purpose of characterizing the morphology of a QRS complex, i.e., groups of beats with similar morphology can be assigned to the same cluster.

- Wave delineation is the process through which the boundaries of each wave within the PQRST complex are determined (see Fig. 6.3). This can be done right after the detection of the QRS complex. This process lets us measure the length (or duration) of the waves. From these and other measurements, different characterizations are possible for the waves in the PQRST complex such as amplitude and morphology.
- Data compression implies an efficient use of storage media, transmission under different media; e.g., from the ambulance to the hospital for a rapid diagnostic. Nowadays, the impressive advancements in the creation and improvement of medical instruments to capture huge amounts of data makes necessary to find mechanisms to efficiently transmit, and also store and retrieve the information collected, while avoiding any type of redundancy.

6.3.2 Feature Extraction from ECG Signals

Once the ECG signal processing has finished, a large amount of raw digital data are available for different analysis and interpretation. For undertaking such analysis and interpretation, it is necessary to present such data to the phase of feature extraction which lets us identify the most relevant characteristics that could help us determine possible heart diseases, if any. However, the resulting features from the extraction process can lead us to suboptimal or redundant sets of characteristics. In the suboptimal case, a possible approach to learn and determine heart diseases from some data of a patient will probably fail since there is not enough information available to reach a correct or an acceptable decision. In the second case, the learned prediction model can be very complex and probably inaccurate as well.

The feature extraction problem can be formulated as follows. Let $\mathcal{F}$ be the set of all available features and $n = |\mathcal{F}|$, the number of features. The objective is to select a subset $F \subseteq \mathcal{F}$ with $m = |F| \leq n$ that optimizes a given selection criterion C in regard to $\mathcal{F}$. The feature extraction problem belongs to the class of NP problems. Therefore, computational intelligence (CI) techniques are a suitable alternative for dealing with such problems.

It is also worth noting that from a CI perspective, feature extraction is only one part of the problem, since the main objective is to establish a relationship between the available information (representing the input data) and the corresponding pathology observed in real patients. Here is when EAs or other metaheuristic approaches come to play an important role within ECG signal interpretation as they can be a very useful tools to provide, in a timely manner, high-quality solutions in regard either to the feature extraction task (direct application) or by helping to find more accurate rules in a fuzzy-logic classifier and more efficient neural networks – e.g., optimal weight values or network structure (indirect application). Based on this observation, the next section presents a short review that embodies the most recent research in this area.

6.4 EAs for ECG: A Brief Review

This section presents a short review of the specialized literature that highlights the application of EAs for solving ECG signal processing related problems. This review also includes tasks such as feature extraction, as well as the design of soft computing tools like those found in the field of fuzzy logic and neural networks. It should be noticed, however, that using EAs as either indirect or direct tool to deal with ECG signals, many different solution search spaces are possible. For example, an EA as indirect application could be designed to find a good combination of kernels in a support vector machine or possibly for evolving a neural network structure. Also, EAs are usually applied in the feature selection process before applying another soft computing tool (e.g., for classification). In this case, a binary string is the most widely used representation for the features to select. In the case of direct applications, it is possible to deal with the problem of segmentation of an ECG signal. For that, a real vector can be used as solution representation to approach this particular problem. Accordingly, the reader should be aware that many schemes for solution representation are possible. Certainly, it will depend on the specific problem at hand when dealing with ECG signals and the way that problem is approached. To better characterize the use of EAs in the field of ECG signal processing, we have split the presentation of the review by considering *indirect* and *direct* application of EAs as was explained in the previous section.

6.4.1 *Indirect Application of EAs*

- Wiggins et al. (2006) describe the application of a GA for evolving a Bayesian network devoted to classify patients' ages based on features extracted from ECG signals. The evolutionary process is aimed to produce a high quality network structure for the classification process by evolving a population of chromosomes represented by integer vectors. The GA is compared with K2, a greedy hill-climbing algorithm considering the classification accuracy. The same authors present in (Wiggins et al. 2008) an extended study of Wiggins et al. (2006) in which both the GA and K2 are compared with two naïve Bayesian approaches. The results show that the GA largely outperforms K2 and is also able to achieve an improved performance when compared to the two naïve Bayesian approaches.
- Chua and Tan (2007) use a GA to evolve a non-singleton fuzzy logic system (NSFLS) designed for handling uncertainties in cardiac arrhythmias classification which is a particular pattern classification problem that usually arises when dealing with ECG signals. The NSFLS is supposed to work better than a singleton fuzzy logic system (SFLS) when applied to a noisy environment as it models uncertainty, imprecision, or inaccuracy of the inputs which is a usual situation in ECG signals. In the GA, each possible fuzzy logic system is represented by a binary string (chromosome) which decodes values representing, respectively, three membership functions (for each value, it decodes both the

mean and the standard deviation) and nine possible rules. As the fuzzy logic system is intended to classify three cardiac arrhythmias – i.e., Ventricular Fibrillation (VF), Ventricular Tachycardia (VT), and Normal Sinus Rhythm (NSR), the respective fitness function is calculated as the weighted average on these three correctly classified classes. NSFLS and SFLS are tested and compared on a set of well-known instances of ECG signals (Goldberger et al. 2000). The results show superiority of NSFSL with respect to SFLS regardless of the inputs given.

- Nasiri et al. (2009b) present the Genetic-ESVM, a novel classification system based on a GA, which is designed to improve the generalization performance of the so-called Emphatic Support Vector Machine (ESVM) classifier. The first stage of the Genetic-ESVM is aimed at finding the best subset of features by applying a GA. In order to achieve this goal, each chromosome is represented by a binary vector of length n_f (n_f number of all possible features that can be selected for further classification). The second stage (last) classifies the ECG signals either using a classical SVM (Genetic-SVM) or the proposed ESVM (Genetic-ESVM). The experimental study compares a classical SVM without using the genetic feature extraction and the two genetic-based algorithms: Genetic-SVM and Genetic-ESVM. The dataset MIT-BIH (Goldberger et al. 2000) was considered to assess the algorithms' performance. From the reported results, it can be observed that Genetic-EVSM (with linear kernels) outperformed the other algorithms compared. A related work presented by the same authors (see Nasiri et al. 2009a) compares the performance of a classical SVM, the Genetic-SVM (described above), and PCA-SVM, which is an SVM combined with Principal Component Analysis (PCA). These approaches aim to obtain the subset containing the best possible features for classification. The experimental results show that the feature selection found by the Genetic-SVM greatly improves the quality of classification with respect to the other algorithms studied.
- Jiang et al. (2005) explore the benefit of applying a GA to simultaneously find the internal structure and associated weights of evolvable Block-based Neural Networks (BbNNs). The evolved BbNNs are applied to classify heartbeat patterns from ECG signals. The features of BbNNs make them good candidates to deal with patterns of heartbeats (e.g., these patterns vary for different individuals and, for the same individual, some changes in the pattern can take place at different times of the day as well as in different situations that the individual is experiencing). One of the features of BbNNs is the flexibility of their internal structure which can be adapted as the conditions of the environments change. Additionally, a BbNN can be implemented, for example, through a Field Programmable Gate Array (FPGA) which allows online partial reorganization of its internal structure. Ten records collected from different patients provided by the MIT-BIH Arrhythmia database (see Goldberger et al. 2000) were considered in order to assess the behavior of the evolved BbNN which produced a classification accuracy of more than 90%.
- A novel hybrid method based on the Ant Colony Optimization (ACO) metaheuristic and an evolutionary algorithm is presented by Bursa and Lhotska

(2007). The proposed algorithm, called ACO-DTree is designed to automatically find a classification tree via an evolutionary process which incorporates concepts of the ACO metaheuristic. The main structure of ACO-DTree corresponds to a traditional ACO algorithm. However, the population of solutions found by the colony undergo an evolutionary step (more precisely, the application of a mutation operator) aimed to produce a renewed set of solutions. After that, the usual cycle of the ACO algorithm continues normally by selecting the best solution to proceed with the pheromone evaporation step. The experimental study includes the well-known database MIT-BIH (Goldberger et al. 2000) as well as the Iris data set taken from the UCI repository (Frank and Asuncion 2010). However, the Iris data set is only considered as part of the preliminary parameter estimation of the algorithm. A comparison of results between an EA and ACO-DTree shows a clear benefit of using the hybrid approach (i.e., ACO-DTree) to automatically build high-quality classification trees on the ECG signals, data set considered.

6.4.2 *Direct Application of EAs*

- A genetic segmentation of ECG signals is proposed by Gacek and Pedrycz (2003). The genetic approach is aimed to produce a segmentation of lossy signal compression through evolved geometric constructs (linear functions) which capture the real segments in the ECG signal. The chromosome is represented by a sequence of real numbers which correspond to the respective segments' ending points and the fitness function measures the level on monotonicity of the ECG data analyzed within the segments based on the extreme estimated derivative values (maximum and minimum). In the experimental study, the authors considered three classes of instances of ECG signals taken from the MIT-BIH database (Goldberger et al. 2000) including: normal beats, left bundle branch block beats, and premature ventricular contraction. Although the results are encouraging by using a linear model to approximate the real signal, the authors indicate that more sophisticated approximation models should be considered, e.g., quadratic or polynomials of higher order.
- de Toro et al. (2006) present a methodology consisting in applying either multimodal[2] or multiobjective evolutionary algorithms for the adjustment of medical diagnostic schemes dealing with biosignal analysis and processing. The evolutionary approach is used in two situations: (a) in the process of feature selection and (b) the selection of best parameter setting for different diagnosis schemes as, for example, KNN used in this work. Three different objectives were considered related to the quality of the possible diagnosis

[2]The authors use here the term "multimodal" to refer to single-objective problems that have several optima.

achieved: (a) classification accuracy, (b) sensitivity, and (c) coverage level. In the case of the multimodal EA, the only objective considered out of the three previously mentioned is the classification accuracy. From the multiobjective perspective, SPEA (Zitzler and Thiele 1999) is the algorithm applied and two different objective combinations were considered: (a) classification accuracy and sensitivity, and (b) classification accuracy and coverage level. The proposed methodology was successfully applied on the diagnosis of Paroxysmal Atrial Fibrilation (PAF) on the data set found in PhysioBank (2001). The authors claim that their proposal provides the specialists with a set of different solutions to be used in the diagnostic decision (solutions that include different selected features). Therefore, the specialists have certain freedom to select the parameters for the diagnostic decision process according to the possibilities (e.g., availability of medical instrumentation involved in the features selected).

- Jatoth et al. (2009) present a PSO-based evolutionary tool for extraction of diminished-noise signal from fetal ECGs which allows an effective extraction and further appropriate analysis. The proposed PSO-based tool is intended to optimize the weight vector involved in an adaptive noise cancellation system. This cancellation system aims at minimizing the mean square error between the real and the estimated fetal ECG signal. The estimated signal is referred to as LMS (Least Mean Square) estimation. Although the authors claim that the PSO-based tool outperformed LMS, the experimental study was unfortunately conducted on only one instance of the problem. This makes necessary an extended study of the proposed algorithm to better assess its potential for noise cancellation in fetal ECG.

6.5 Other Nature-Inspired Metaheuristics for ECG

Although EAs are the most extensively used and studied bio-inspired metaheuristics in the current literature, other bio-inspired metaheuristics have also being applied, with different degrees of success, in a variety of real-world problems. The processing, analysis, and interpretation of ECG signals is one of the real-world problems in which an important number of research has been conducted through the use of ACO, PSO, and AISs, just to mention a few. Accordingly, this section is aimed at showing some recent results in this regard, by providing a short review of the literature focused on the aforementioned bio-inspired metaheuristics.

- Bursa and Lhotska (2008b) propose an Ant Colony–inspired clustering algorithm (called Ant Colony Clustering) for arrhythmia diagnosis from the analysis of ECG signals. The authors present a comparative study of their proposal with other clustering algorithms, including: ACO-DTree from the same authors (Bursa and Lhotska 2007), Radial Basis Function Neural Networks (two versions, which are trained by ACO and PSO algorithms, respectively), Kohonen's Self-Organizing Maps (SOMs), Hierarchical Clustering, and *k*-means. Two versions of Ant Colony Clustering were implemented: one using Euclidean Distance (or L2) and another one using the Dynamic Time Warping (DTW) metric. The reported results show a fairly good performance of the Ant Colony Clustering approach with respect to some of the other algorithms studied in the experimental study. A similar proposal from the same authors (see Bursa and Lhotska 2008a) involves the comparison of ACO-DTree, as described in (Begg et al., 2008), but using concepts taken from PSO to improve the solutions and applied at each iteration of the ACO algorithm on the set of solutions previously found. The benefits of the proposed algorithm are demonstrated when compared with a Random Tree Generation method (implemented in the WEKA toolkit). The databases considered include ECG signals instances and also Electroencephalogram (EEG) signals. As a general conclusion, the authors claim that their proposal is suitable for biological data clustering (such as ECG and EEG signals). They also claim that their approach has the advantage of producing readily structures (the decision trees) which have a possible clinical use.

- Korürek and Doĝan (2010) investigate the use of PSO-RBFNN, an algorithm that evolves radial basis function neural networks (RBFNNs) for ECG beat classification. The evolutionary process is based on PSO and is aimed to find a high-quality structure for the neural network. Besides the number of neurons, a RBFNN architecture includes three parameters: (a) center of the neurons (c_i), (b) the respective bandwidth (σ_i), and (c) the weights between the hidden layer and the output layer. In this work, only the center and the respective bandwidth associated to it are considered in the evolutionary process, where each particle in the population is formulated as in Korürek and Doĝan (2010): $net = [(c_1, \sigma_1), \ldots, (c_n, \sigma_n)]$, where n is the number of neurons. The authors present several experiments considering the MIT-BIH arrhythmia database (Goldberger et al. 2000). Preliminary experiments were carried out to determine the most appropriate number of neurons before presenting the main part of the experimental study. The main conclusion of the experimental study indicates a reduction on the network size without compromising the quality of the results expressed in terms of "sensitivity" and "specificity".
- Bereta and Burczynski (2007) designed an Artificial Immune System (AIS) which implements the immune metaphor based on both negative and clonal selection for evolving subsets of features well suited for classification. According to the authors, this proposed algorithm is considered a hybrid AIS as it simultaneously incorporates both selection mechanisms, i.e., negative selection and clonal selection. The hybrid AIS manages binary and real-valued encoding for the subpopulations of detectors (T-lymphocytes). Both versions of the hybrid AIS were compared by using different types of samples taken from the MIT-HIS database (Goldberger et al. 2000), representing normal and pathological ECG signals. The real-coded hybrid AIS showed the best performance regarding computational complexity, while having a lower level of misclassified signals, and a lower number of detectors.
- Korürek and Nizam (2010) investigate an integrated approach based on a combination of wavelets coefficients of the Discrete Wavelet Transform (DWT) and

time domain coefficients for feature selection. In addition, Principal Component Analysis (PCA) is applied on the DWT coefficients in order to decrease the number of features. The resulting subset of features is considered by an ACO algorithm for clustering analysis of ECG arrhythmias instances taken from the MIT-BIH Arrhythmia Database (Goldberger et al. 2000). The design of the ACO algorithm is straightforward, since the number n of elements in the data set determines the number of nodes in the construction graph; m ants are distributed on m nodes to proceed with the search (find the cluster). The ants move from one node to another one by applying rules that depend on the amount of pheromone trails and on information of the nearest neighborhood. An exploration rule is applied to promote exploration by particular ants which are forced to visit the farthest nodes. At each move, an amount of pheromone trail is deposited in the respective connection. The clustering is obtained at the final stage of the algorithm (i.e., when the maximum number of iteration is reached) by considering the final accumulated amount of trail in the whole set of edges in the construction graph. The final step (aimed at improving the clustering) combines small clusters into big ones according to the respective distance from the centroid. The main part of the experimental study includes a comparison of the proposed integrated approach with a similar one except that the clustering is obtained by a Neural Network. As a general conclusion, the authors claim that their proposed approach based on the ACO metaphor slightly outperforms the one based on a Neural Network. In addition, both approaches (ACO and NN-based clustering) can be considered suitable options to accurately classify ECG arrhythmias.

- Poungponsriand and Yu (2009) investigate the use of a hybrid search algorithm for training a Wavelet Neural Network (WNN) for ECG signal modeling and noise reduction. The hybrid algorithm consists of the so-called Adaptive Diversity Learning Particle Swarm Optimization (ADLPSO) (Chen et al. 2006) for global exploration and a gradient descendent algorithm for fine-tuning purposes. The proposed hybrid algorithm can successfully model the ECG signal and remove high-frequency noise.

Finally, a recent publication from Karpagachelvi et al. (2010) presents an interesting survey of different approaches for ECG feature extraction. Such literature review includes an important number of schemes based on Artificial Neural Networks, Genetic Algorithms, Support Vector Machines, and other computational intelligence techniques.

6.6 Conclusions

In this chapter, we have presented some introductory concepts of evolutionary computation techniques, focused on the so-called evolutionary algorithms (EAs). The chapter also provides a short introduction to ECG signal processing which highlights aspects that could be addressed by evolutionary techniques and other related approaches. In addition to that, we also presented a literature review on the use of EAs and other bio-inspired metaheuristics for dealing with ECG signals. This aims to provide an up-to-date perspective of the recent and ongoing research in this area.

As discussed by Begg et al. (2008), we also believe that the oncoming research in this area will focus on the development of tree-breed approaches coming from (a) supervised learning, (b) fuzzy logic, and (c) evolutionary computation. However, the third research area should be extended to include a number of other bio-inspired algorithms as well as local search–based algorithms. The reason for this is that such approaches have shown a lot of potential to deal with complex real-world problems, exhibiting, in many cases, a similar or even better performance than traditional evolutionary computation techniques such as genetic algorithms.

Acknowledgements The second author acknowledges support from CONACyT project no. 103570.

References

Bäck, T.: Evolutionary Algorithms in Theory and Practice: Evolution Strategies, Evolutionary Programming, Genetic Algorithms. Oxford University Press, New York (1996)

Bäck, T., Fogel, D., Michalewicz, Z. (eds.): Evolutionary Computation 1: Basic Algorithms and Operators, vol. 1, 1st edn. Institute of Physics Publishing, Bristol (2000)

Begg, R., Lai, D. T.H., Palaniswami, M.: Computational Intelligence in Biomedical Engineering. CRC Press, Inc., Boca Raton (2008)

Bereta, M., Burczyński, T.: Comparing binary and real-valued coding in hybrid immune algorithm for feature selection and classification of ECG signals. Eng. Appl. Artif. Intell. **20**(5), 571–585 (2007). doi: http://dx.doi.org/10.1016/j.engappai.2006.11.004

Bursa, M., Lhotska, L.: Automated classification tree evolution through hybrid metaheuristics. In: Corchado, E., Corchado, J., Abraham, A. (eds.) Innovations in Hybrid Intelligent Systems. Advances in Soft Computing, vol. 44, pp. 191–198. Springer, Berlin/Heidelberg (2007)

Bursa, M., Lhotska, L.: Ant colony cooperative strategy in electrocardiogram and electroencephalogram data clustering. In: Krasnogor, N., Nicosia, G., Pavone, M., Pelta, D. (eds.) Nature Inspired Cooperative Strategies for Optimization (NICSO 2007). Studies in Computational Intelligence, vol. 129, pp. 323–333. Springer, Berlin/Heidelberg (2008a)

Bursa, M., Lhotska, L.: Nature Inspired Concepts in the Electrocardiogram Interpretation Process. In: Computers in Cardiology, 2008, pp. 241–244. IEEE press, Piscataway, New Jersey, USA (2008b)

Chen, Y., Yang, B., Dong, J.: Time-series prediction using a local linear wavelet neural network. Neurocomput. **69**(4–6), 449–465 (2006). doi: http://dx.doi.org/10.1016/j.neucom.2005.02.006

Chua, T.W., Tan, W.W.: GA optimisation of Non-Singleton Fuzzy logic system for ECG classification. In: IEEE Congress on Evolutionary Computation, 2007 (CEC 2007), pp. 1677–1684. (2007). doi:10.1109/CEC.2007.4424675

De Jong, K.: Evolutionary Computation: A Unified Approach. Complex Adaptive Systems: A Bradford Book. MIT Press, Cambridge, MA (2006)

de Toro, F., Ros, E., Mota, S., Ortega, J.: Evolutionary algorithms for multiobjective and multimodal optimization of diagnostic schemes. IEEE Trans. Biomed. Eng. **53**(2), 178–189 (2006)

Eiben, A.E., Smith, J.E.: Introduction to Evolutionary Computing. Springer, Berlin (2003). ISBN 3-540-40184-9

Fogel, D.B.: Evolutionary Computation. Toward a New Philosophy of Machine Intelligence. The Institute of Electrical and Electronic Engineers, New York (1995)

Fogel, L.J.: Artificial Intelligence through Simulated Evolution. Wiley, New York (1966)

Frank, A., Asuncion, A.: UCI Machine Learning Repository. http://archive.ics.uci.edu/ml (2010). Accessed 1 Sept 2010

Friesen, G., Jannett, T., Jadallah, M., Yates, S., Quint, S., Nagle, H.: A comparison of the noise sensitivity of nine QRS detection algorithms. IEEE Trans. Biomed. Eng. **37**(1), 85–98 (1990). doi:10.1109/10.43620

Gacek, A., Pedrycz, W.: A genetic segmentation of ECG signals. IEEE Trans. Biomed. Eng. **50**(10), 1203–1208 (2003). doi:10.1109/TBME.2003.816074

Glover, F.W., Kochenberger, G.A. (eds.): Handbook of Metaheuristics. Kluwer Academic Publishers, Norwell, Massachusetts, USA (2003)

Goldberger, A.L., Amaral, L.A., Glass, L., Hausdorff, J.M., Ivanov, P.C., Mark, R.G., Mietus, J.E., Moody, G.B., Peng, C.K., Stanley, H.E.: PhysioBank, PhysioToolkit, and PhysioNet: components of a new research resource for complex physiologic signals. Circulation **101**(23), (2000)

Holland, J.H.: Concerning efficient adaptive systems. In: Yovits, M.C., Jacobi, G.T., Goldstein, G.D. (eds.) Self-Organizing Systems – 1962, pp. 215–230. Spartan Books, Washington, D.C. (1962)

Holland, J.H.: Adaptation in Natural and Artificial Systems, 2nd edn. University of Michigan Press/MIT Press, Cambridge, MA (1992)

Jatoth, R., Anoop, S.S.V.K.K., Prabhu, C.M.: Biologically inspired evolutionary computing tools for the extraction of fetal electrocardiogram. WSEAS Trans. Sig. Proc. **5**, 106–115 (2009). http://portal.acm.org/citation.cfm?id=1558867.1558869

Jiang, W., Kong, S.G., Peterson, G.D.: ECG signal classification using block-based neural networks. In: Proceedings of IEEE International Joint Conference on Neural Networks, 2005. IJCNN '05, vol. 1, pp. 326–331. IEEE Operations Center, Piscataway (2005). doi:10.1109/IJCNN.2005.1555851

Karpagachelvi, S., Arthanari, M., Sivakumar, M.: ECG Feature Extraction Techniques – A Survey Approach. Int. J. Comput. Sci. Inf. Secur. **8**(1) (2010)

Korürek, M., Doĝan, B.: ECG beat classification using particle swarm optimization and radial basis function neural network. Expert Syst. Appl. **37**(12), (2010). doi:10.1016/j.eswa.2010.04.087

Korürek, M., Nizam, A.: Clustering MIT-BIH arrhythmias with ant colony optimization using time domain and PCA compressed wavelet coefficients. Digit. Signal Process. **20**(4), 1050–1060 (2010)

Koza, J.R.: Genetic Programming. On the Programming of Computers by Means of Natural Selection. The MIT Press, Cambridge, MA (1992)

Koza, J.R.: Genetic Programming II: Automatic Discovery of Reusable Programs. The MIT Press, Cambridge, MA (1994)

Laguna, P., Sörnmo, L.: Editorial on 'Signal processing in vital rhythms and signs'. Trans. R. Soc. A **367**, 207–211 (2009)

Michalewicz, Z., Fogel, D.: How to Solve It: Modern Heuristics, 2nd Revised and Extended edn. Springer, Berlin (2004). ISBN 3-540-22494-7

Nasiri, J., Naghibzadeh, M., Yazdi, H., Naghibzadeh, B.: ECG arrhythmia classification with support vector machines and genetic algorithm. In: Third UKSim European Symposium on Computer Modeling and Simulation, 2009. EMS '09, pp. 187–192. IEEE Computer Society, Los Alamitos (2009a). doi:10.1109/EMS.2009.39

Nasiri, J.A., Sabzekar, M., Yazdi, H.S., Naghibzadeh, M., Naghibzadeh, B.: Intelligent arrhythmia detection using genetic algorithm and emphatic SVM (ESVM). In: Third UKSim European Symposium on Computer Modeling and Simulation, 2009. EMS '09, pp. 112–117. IEEE Computer Society, Los Alamitos (2009b). doi:10.1109/EMS.2009.116

PhysioBank: CinC challenge 2001 data sets: The PAF prediction challenge database. http://www.physionet.org/physiobank/database/afpdb/ (2001). Accessed 1 Sept 2010

Poungponsriand, S., Yu, X.: Electrocardiogram (ECG) signal modeling and noise reduction using wavelet neural networks. In: IEEE International Conference on Automation and Logistics, 2009. ICAL '09, pp. 394–398. IEEE, Piscataway (2009). doi:10.1109/ICAL.2009.5262892

Schwefel, H.-P.: Kybernetische evolution als strategie der experimentellen forschung in der strömungstechnik. Dipl. -Ing. thesis (1965). (in German)

Schwefel, H.-P.: Evolution and Optimum Seeking. Wiley Interscience, New York (1995)

Sörnmo, L., Laguna, P.: Electrocardiogram (ECG) signal processing. In: Akay, M. (ed.) Wiley Encyclopedia of Biomedical Engineering, vol. 2, pp. 1298–1313. Wiley, Hoboken (2006)

Talbi, E.-G.: Metaheuristics: From Design to Implementation. Wiley, Hoboken (2009)

Wiggins, M., Saad, A., Litt, B., Vachtsevanos, G.: Genetic algorithm-evolved Bayesian network classifier for medical applications. In: Tiwari, A., Roy, R., Knowles, J., Avineri, E., Dahal K. (eds.) Applications of Soft Computing. Advances in Soft Computing, vol. 36, pp. 143–152. Springer, Berlin/Heidelberg (2006). doi: http://dx.doi.org/10.1007/978-3-540-36266-1_14. 10.1007/978-3-540-36266-1_14

Wiggins, M., Saad, A., Litt, B., Vachtsevanos, G.: Evolving a Bayesian classifier for ECG-based age classification in medical applications. Appl. Soft Comput. **8**(1), 599–608 (2008). doi: http://dx.doi.org/10.1016/j.asoc.2007.03.009

Zitzler, E., Thiele, L.: Multiobjective evolutionary algorithms: a comparative case study and the strength pareto approach. IEEE Trans. Evol. Comput. **3**(4), 257–271 (1999)

Chapter 7
Electrocardiogram Application Based on Heart Rate Variability Ontology and Fuzzy Markup Language

Mei-Hui Wang, Chang-Shing Lee, Giovanni Acampora, and Vincenzo Loia

7.1 Introduction

The Electrocardiogram (ECG) trace is highly informative. The most common digital application of the ECG trace is Heart Rate Variability (HRV). Additionally, HRV is widely adopted to measure the heart function, which helps identify patients at risk for a cardiovascular event or death (American Heart Association Inc. and European Society of Cardiology, 1996). The recognition of the beats in ECG is a very significant subject in the intensive care units, where the recognition and classification of the ECG signals in real time is essential for the treatment of patient. In particular, ECG data are normally acquired for clinical diagnosis of cardiac function, and involve the electrical activity of the heart. The state of the cardiac heart is generally reflected in the shape of ECG waveform and heart rate. Heart Rate Variability (HRV) refers to a precise measure in milliseconds in the variation in the intervals between heart beats. HRV analysis is not only a noninvasive tool for assessing cardiovascular system function, but also serves as a useful index for evaluating the function of the autonomic nervous system (ANS) in regulating human organs and muscles (Lin et al. 2010).

In the past decades, many researchers and clinicians have successfully employed HRV analysis for cardiovascular and ANS-related problems and diseases (Lin et al. 2010). However, the HRV analysis is a very specialized domain. Hence, if there is no medical staff nearby, it is very difficult for common people to exactly get the

M.-H. Wang · C.-S. Lee (✉)
Department of Computer Science and Information Engineering, National University of Tainan, Tainan, Taiwan
e-mail: mh.alice.wang@gmail.com; leecs@mail.nutn.edu.tw

G. Acampora · V. Loia
Department of Computer Science, University of Salerno, Fisciano, Italy
e-mail: gacampora@unisa.it; loia@unisa.it

A. Gacek and W. Pedrycz (eds.), *ECG Signal Processing, Classification and Interpretation: A Comprehensive Framework of Computational Intelligence*, DOI 10.1007/978-0-85729-868-3_7, © Springer-Verlag London Limited 2012 information that the results of HRV analysis could provide via the RR interval series, power spectrum density of HRV frequency domain analysis, or the Poincare plots (Pan and Tompkins 1985). Based on such a consideration, it is apparently known that it will make common people easier to understand the results of HRV analysis if they also could be presented in the form of the semantic sentences. However, HRV may be affected by many features, such as exercise, rest, pressure, and disease, so that it is a very specialized medical field. Therefore, building a personal HRV ontology is a good idea for ECG signals processing. However, before presenting them in the form of the semantic sentences, it is a must to construct the HRV ontology based on each person's unique characteristics.

The use of ontologies to provide interoperability among heterogeneous data sources has been applied in many domains, including meeting scheduling (Lee et al. 2006, 2010a), medical information systems (Orgun and Vu 2006), news summarization (Lee et al. 2005), software engineering (Lee et al. 2008; Lee and Wang 2009), health care (Beveridge and Fox 2006; Yan et al. 2006; Lee and Wang 2007, 2008; Lee et al. 2010b; Wang et al. 2010), recruitment (Sanchez et al. 2006), architecture (Liu et al. 2008), and game of Go (Lee et al. 2010c, d). For example, Lee et al. (2010b) proposed a type-2 fuzzy ontology to apply to the knowledge representation in the field of personal diabetic-diet recommendation. Sanchez et al. (2006) designed the ontological model to represent the knowledge of the recruitment domain and developed an intelligent web portal for recruitment. Liu et al. (2008) applied an ontology-based approach to the architecture modeling process and defined the knowledge and semantic units for the ancient Chinese architecture domain. Lee et al. (2005) presented a fuzzy ontology and applied it to news summarization based on the Chinese news of three weather events captured from Chinatimes website from 2002 to 2004. Beveridge and Fox (2006) presented a home monitoring mechanism through an intelligent dialogue system to apply to health care. Lee and Wang (2007, 2008) also presented an ontology-based intelligent healthcare agent for respiratory waveform recognition and ECG application. Yan et al. (2006) proposed a perceptron-based medical decision support system for the diagnosis of heart diseases.

In addition to applying the technologies of ontology to ECG application, another important feature of this chapter is to introduce the fuzzy markup language (FML). Fuzzy Markup Language (FML) is a software technology to create fuzzy-oriented abstraction tools (Acampora and Loia 2005a, b). Additionally, it is also an extensible markup language (XML)-derived technologies and is essentially composed of three layers: (1) XML in order to create a new markup language for fuzzy logic control; (2) document type definition (DTD), initially, and now a XML Schema, in order to define the legal building blocks; and (3) extensible stylesheet language transformations in order to convert a fuzzy controller description into a specific programming language (Acampora and Loia 2005a, b). With the support of the FML, it appears clear that making heterogeneous systems to communicate through standardized, controlled and secured protocols will be able to furnish innovative solutions and satisfy users' needs. FML also provides the way to directly manage fuzzy concepts, fuzzy rules, and fuzzy inference engine

(Acampora and Loia 2005a, b). Since 2008, the Ontology Applications & Software Engineering (OASE) Laboratory, National University of Tainan (NUTN), Taiwan has been cooperated with University of Salerno, Italy together to apply FML to many research fields, including the health care (Wang et al. 2010), game of Go (Lee et al. 2010d), and meeting scheduling (Lee et al. 2010a).

This chapter proposes a fuzzy markup language (FML)-based HRV ontology for ECG application. Based on our previous work (Lee and Wang 2008), an FML-based fuzzy inference mechanism is proposed to infer the nervous level of each involved student according to the collected ECG signals before they took the exams and after they took the exams. The necessary knowledge is stored in the ontology, which consists of some personal ontologies, and is predefined by the domain experts via the developed FML editor. The experimental results show that the proposed approach can work feasibly. The remainder of this chapter is organized as follows. Section 7.2 describes the fuzzy markup language. Section 7.3 introduces the structure of the FML-based HRV ontology. Section 7.4 describes the proposed mechanisms for the ECG application based on the knowledge base and rule base of the FML. The experimental results are shown in Sect. 7.5. Finally, conclusions are drawn in Sect. 7.6.

7.2 Fuzzy Markup Language

Fuzzy Markup Language (FML) is a fuzzy-based markup language that can manage fuzzy concepts, fuzzy rules, and a fuzzy inference engine (Acampora and Loia 2005a, b). Additionally, FML is composed of three layers – eXtensible Markup Language (XML), a XML Schema, and extensible stylesheet language transformations. This section will give an introduction to the FML, including (1) Sect. 7.2.1 gives an FML overview and (2) Sects. 7.2.2 and 7.2.3 introduce the knowledge base and rule base of the FML, respectively (Wang et al. 2010).

7.2.1 Fuzzy Markup Language Overview

Actually, FML can be considered a standalone language used to model the fuzzy controllers from scratch. Now, the FML compiler is based on the integration of different technologies able to instantiate a runtime fuzzy controller without additional work. These technologies are: the *TCP/IP Client/Server application* and the *JAXB XML Binding technology* (Acampora and Loia 2005a). Differently from other similar approaches such as Fuzzy Control Language (FCL) or MATLAB Fuzzy Inference System (FIS) developed by the Matworks, FML exhibits additional benefits in the FLC programming that are related to its XML derivation. Indeed, whereas FCL or FIS code is totally based on a textual representation, FML programs are coded through a collection of correlated semantic tags capable of modeling different controller components by exploiting abstraction benefits offered by XML tools. From the implementation point of view, these benefits allow fuzzy designers (1) to simply code their ideas on heterogeneous hardware without having knowledge about programming details related to the different platforms and (2) to program a fuzzy controller without referring to general purpose computer languages.

In this sub-section, FML is explained starting from a very high-level introduction to fuzzy systems, the most wide-spread application of fuzzy logic. Trivially, a fuzzy control allows the designer to specify the control in terms of sentences rather than equation by replacing a conventional controller, a proportional-integral-derivative (*PID*) controller, with linguistic IF-THEN rules. The use of linguistic variables represents a significant paradigm shift in system analysis: using the linguistic approach, the focus of the attention in the dependencies representations is shifted from differential equations to fuzzy IF–THEN rules in the form *if X is A then Y is B*. The propositions *X is A* and *Y is B* are called fuzzy clauses; *A* and *B* are linguistic variables and *X* and *Y* are their linguistic values (for instance, *if Pressure is high then Volume is low*). The main components of fuzzy controller are (organized in a hierarchical way): (1) fuzzy knowledge base; (2) fuzzy rule base; (3) inference engine; (4) fuzzification subsystem; and (5) defuzzification subsystem.

7.2.2 Fuzzy Markup Language Knowledge Base

An FML implementation is based on the employment of tags able to model different parts of fuzzy controller in a taxonomic way. The root of fuzzy controller taxonomy, the *Controller node*, is represented through the FML tag <FUZZYCONTROL>. Such a tag represents the root tag of FML programs, that is, the opening tag of each FML program. <FUZZYCONTROL> uses two tags: *name* and *ip*. The *name* attribute permits to specify the name of fuzzy controller whereas *ip* is used to define the location of controller in the computer network. The fuzzy knowledge base is defined by means of the tag <KNOWLEDGEBASE> which maintains the set of fuzzy concepts used to model the fuzzy rule base. The <KNOWLEDGEBASE> uses the attribute *ip* that determines the location in the network of whole fuzzy knowledge base of our system. In order to define the fuzzy concept-related controlled system, <KNOWLEDGEBASE> tag uses a set of nested tags: (1) <FUZZYVARIABLE>; (2) <FUZZYTERM>; (3) a set of tags defining a shape of fuzzy sets.

<FUZZYVARIABLE> defines the fuzzy concept, for example () temperature"; <FUZZYTERM> defines a linguistic term describing the fuzzy concept, for example () low temperature"; the set of tags defining the shapes of fuzzy sets are related to fuzzy terms. The attributes of <FUZZYVARIABLE> tags are: *name*, *scale*, *domainLeft*, *domainRight*, *type*, *ip* and, for only an output fuzzy concept, *accumulation*, *defuzzifier*, and *defaultValue*. (1) The *name* attribute defines the name of fuzzy concept, for instance, *temperature*; (2) *scale* is used to define the scale used to measure the fuzzy concept, for instance, *Celsius degree*; (3) *domainLeft* and *domainRight* are used to model the universe of discourse of fuzzy concept, that is,

the set of real values related to fuzzy concept; (4) the position of fuzzy concept into rule (consequent part or antecedent part) is defined by *type* attribute (with value input/output); (5) *ip* defines the position of fuzzy concept in the computer network; (6) *accumulation* attribute defines the method which permits the combination in a final value of fuzzy concept results obtained in each rule; (7) *defuzzifier* attribute defines the method used to execute the conversion from a fuzzy set, obtained after aggregation process, into a numerical value to give in output to system; (8) *defaultValue* attribute defines a real value used only when no rule has fired for the fuzzy concept at issue.

<FUZZYTERM> uses two attributes, *name* used to define the linguistic value associate with fuzzy concept and *complement*, a boolean attribute which denotes, if it is true, it is necessary to consider the complement of membership function defined by given parameters. Some of fuzzy shape tags, used to complete the definition of fuzzy concept, are: <TRIANGULARSHAPE>, <LINEARSHAPE>, <TRAPEZOIDSHAPE>, <SSHAPE>, <ZSHAPE>, and <PISHAPE>. Every shaping tag uses a set of attributes which defines the parameters of corresponding fuzzy set. The number of these attributes depends on the chosen fuzzy set shape. A special tag that can furthermore be used to define a fuzzy shape is <USERSHAPE>. This tag is used to customize fuzzy shape (custom shape).

7.2.3 Fuzzy Markup Language Rule Base

The root of fuzzy rule-base component is modeled by the <RULEBASE> tag which defines a fuzzy rule set. The <RULEBASE> tag six attributes: *name*, *type*, *activationMethod*, *andMethod, orMethod* and *ip*. The former attribute uniquely identifies the rule base. The *type* attribute permits to specify the kind of fuzzy controller (Mamdani or TSK) respect to the rule base at issue. The *activationMethod* attribute defines the method used to implication process; the *andMethod* and *orMethod* attribute define, respectively, the *and* and *or* algorithm to use by default to execute rules. The latter defines the network location of the set of rules used in fuzzy controller. In order to define the single rule, the <RULE> tag is used. The tags used by <RULE> are: *name, connector, operator, weight.* and *ip*. (1) The *name* attribute permits to identify the rule; (2) *connector* is used to define the logical operator used to connect the different clauses in antecedent part (and/or); (3) *operator* defines the algorithm to use for chosen connector; (4) *weight* defines the importance of rule during inference engine time; (5) *ip* defines the location of rule in the computer network. The definition of antecedent and consequent rule part is obtained by using <ANTECEDENT> and < CONSEQUENT > tags. <CLAUSE > tag is used to model the fuzzy clauses in antecedent and consequent part. In order to treat the fuzzy operator "*not*" in clauses, the tag <CLAUSE > uses the Boolean attribute "*not*." To complete the definition of fuzzy clause, the <VARIABLE>, <TERM>, and <TSKPARAM> have to be used. In particular, the pair "<VARIABLE>, <TERM>" is used to define fuzzy clauses in antecedent and consequent part of Mamdani controllers rules as well as in antecedent part of TSK controllers rules. While, the pair "<VARIABLE>, <TSKPARAM>" is used to model the consequent part of TSK controllers rules.

7.3 Structure of FML-Based HRV Ontology

In this section, the structure of the FML-based HRV ontology will be introduced in the following sub-sections. Section 7.3.1 gives an introduction to the basic ECG signal knowledge and the time-domain and frequency-domain parameters about the HRV analysis (Lee and Wang 2008). Section 7.3.2 illustrates the ontology structure (Lee and Wang 2008). Section 7.3.3 describes the HRV ontology based on the knowledge of the HRV analysis (Lee and Wang 2008).

7.3.1 ECG Signal and HRV Knowledge

The electrical activity of the heart can be measured by performing an ECG signal. A typical ECG tracing of the cardiac cycle (heartbeat) consists of a P wave, a QRS complex, and a T wave (American Heart Association Inc. and European Society of Cardiology 1996), shown in Fig. 7.1.

The RR interval (*RRI*) is the time duration between two successive R peaks. HRV refers to the beat-to-beat alterations in heart rate, and the HRV analysis is a well-recognized tool both in the investigation of an autonomic control of the heart and in the prognostic stratification of cardio-logical disease patients. Most studies on HRV have been performed by time-domain and frequency-domain linear methods (American Heart Association Inc. and European Society of Cardiology 1996).

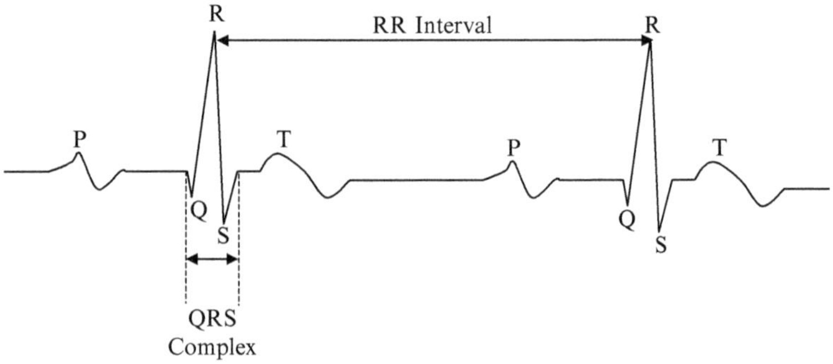

Fig. 7.1 Components of ECG signals (Lee and Wang 2008)

Table 7.1 Time-domain measures of HRV (Lee and Wang 2008)

Variable	Units	Description
meanRRI	ms	The mean of the sequence of the RR interval.
SDNN	ms	Standard deviation of all RR intervals.
RMSSD	ms	The square root of the mean of the sum of the squares of differences between adjacent RR intervals.
NN50	count	Number of pairs of adjacent RR intervals differing by more than 50 ms in the entire recording.
pNN50	%	NN50 count divided by the total number of all RR intervals.

Generally speaking, the average number of the heart beats per minute is about 60–80 for a healthy adult, which means that the mean value of *RRI* is about 600–750 ms for a healthy adult.

For the time-domain analysis, either the heart rate at any point in time or the intervals between successive normal complexes are determined. Simple time-domain variables that can be derived include the mean RR interval (*meanRRI*) and the mean heart rate. The *meanRRI* is normally between 600 and 750 ms. Let us first assume that this person's *meanRRI* is within the normal range. When the *meanRRI* value becomes smaller, it means that the RR interval also becomes smaller. On the other hand, the smaller the *meanRRI* is, the more nervous this person is. Statistical methods include the standard deviation of the RR interval (*SDNN*), the square root of the mean squared differences of successive RR intervals (*RMSSD*), the *NN50*, and the *pNN50* used for time-domain analysis. The *SDNN* represents the level of heart rate variability. The bigger the *SDNN* is, the bigger the HRV is. On the other hand, when the *SDNN* becomes bigger, it means that the person's emotion variability becomes bigger during measuring his ECG signals. The *RMSSD* represents the difference between two consecutive R waves. So, when *RMSSD* tends to be small, it means that this person's heart beat becomes quick. Table 7.1 lists the detailed information about the time-domain measures of HRV.

The frequency-domain analysis involves the spectral analysis of HRV. The HRV spectrum has three components, very low frequency (*VLF*), low frequency (*LF*), and high frequency (*HF*). The physiological effect of the *VLF* ($\leq$0.04 Hz) component is poorly defined. The *LF* (0.04–0.15 Hz) component appears to be mediated by both the vagus and cardiac sympathetic nerves. The *HF* (0.15–0.4 Hz) component is synchronous with respiration, and is identical to respiratory sinus arrhythmia. Additionally, *LF* and *HF* may also be measured in normalized units, which denote the relative value of each power component in proportion to the total power minus the *VLF* component. Table 7.2 lists detailed information about the frequency-domain measures of HRV.

Table 7.2 Frequency-domain measures of HRV (Lee and Wang 2008)

Variable	Units	Description	Frequency range (Hz)
Very Low Frequency (*VLF*)	ms^2	Power in the very low frequency range	≤ 0.04
Low Frequency (*LF*)	ms^2	Power in the low frequency range	0.04–0.15
High Frequency (*HF*)	ms^2	Power in the high frequency range	0.15–0.4
LF norm	n.u.	Low frequency power in normalized units	
HF norm	n.u.	High frequency power in normalized units	
LFHF		Ratio LF/HF	
Total power		The sum of the very low frequency power, low frequency power, and high frequency power	

7.3.2 Ontology Structure

Figure 7.2 shows the domain ontology architecture adopted herein (Lee and Wang 2008), including the *domain layer*, *category layer*, *class layer*, and *instance layer*. The domain ontology adopts two types of inter-conceptual relations, namely the "*association*" and "*instance of*." The "*association*" relation denotes a semantic relationship between concepts in the *concept layer* and the *instance layer*. The relationship between two concepts in the *concept layer* and its corresponding concept in the *instance layer* is "*instance of*." The *domain layer* represents the domain name of an ontology, and comprises various categories defined by domain experts. The *category layer* defines several categories, namely "category 1, category 2, category 3, ..., category *k*." Each concept in the *concept layer*, contains a concept name C_i, an attribute set $\{A_{C_i1},\ldots,A_{C_iq_i}\}$ and an operation set $\{O_{C_i1},\ldots,O_{C_iq_i}\}$ for an application domain. The *instance layer* indicates some instances of the concepts in the *class layer.* The *instance layer* also comprises some instances represented the instances of the domain ontology.

7.3.3 HRV Ontology

The design of the HRV ontology considers all the factors described above. Since the ECG trace expresses cardiac features that are unique to an individual, and ECG data are traditionally acquired for clinical diagnosis of cardiac function (Israel et al. 2005). The HRV ontology is built based on the domain ontology architecture. Figure 7.3 shows the architecture of HRV ontology with some personal HRV ontologies described in the *instance layer* (Lee and Wang 2008).

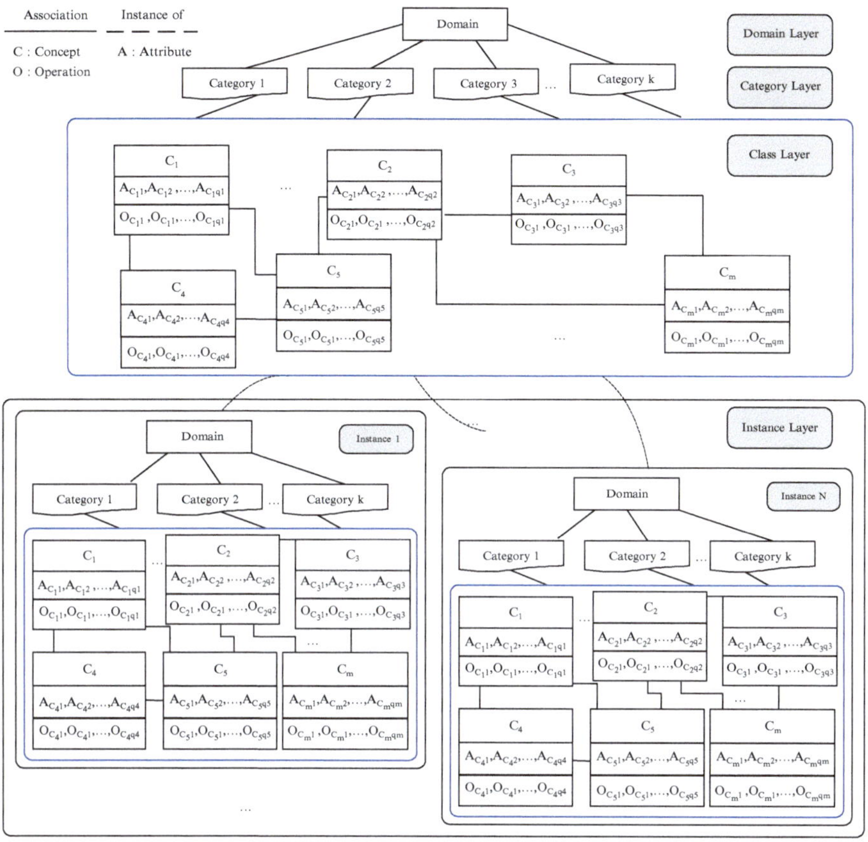

Fig. 7.2 The domain ontology architecture (Lee and Wang 2008)

The process of constructing the HRV ontology follows the description of the (Noy and McGuinness 2001). Take Fig. 7.3, for example, to depict the construction process: (1) Determine the domain and scope of the ontology, that is "Heart Rate Variability." (2) Enumerate important concepts of the constructed ontology such as "Mean RR Interval," "Low Frequency," "Total Power," etc. (3) Define the concepts and the concept hierarchy. Herein, a top-down development process is adopted. (4) Define the properties of the concepts. For example, the parameters of the root of the mean squared difference before examination and after examination are defined. (5) Define the non-hierarchical relations in the ontology. Briefly, the construction of the ontology is built from top to down. The domain name is first decided and then some categories are determined, and next concepts and instances are chosen. Finally, the ontology is formed.

In Fig. 7.3, the domain name of this ontology is "Heart Rate Variability." The categories in the *category layer* include "Time Domain Analysis" and "Frequency

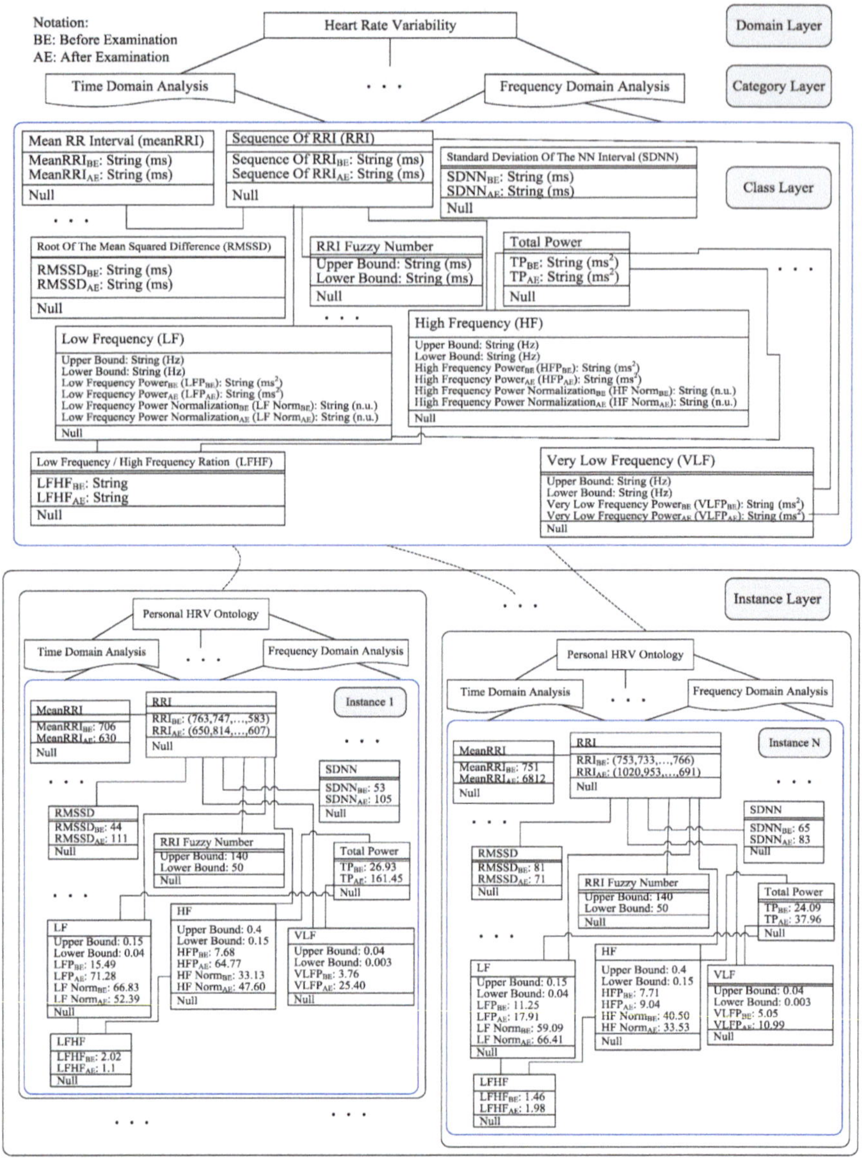

Fig. 7.3 The HRV ontology architecture (Lee and Wang 2008)

Domain Analysis." Each concept in the *concept layer* includes a concept name with an attribute set and an operation set. For example, concept *MeanRRI* has an attribute set $\{MeanRRI_{BE}, MeanRRI_{AE}\}$. The *instance layer* includes some instances representing the personal HRV ontologies. *Instance 1* represents the first personal HRV ontology; *Instance 2* represents the second personal HRV ontology, and *Instance N* represents the *N*th personal HRV ontology. For instance, consider instance 1. The values of the attribute set $\{meanRRI_{BE}, meanRRI_{AE}\}$ are $\{760, 630\}$.

7.4 FML-Based HRV Ontology to Electrocardiogram Application

This section utilizes the predefined HRV ontology to perform the ECG signals applications. The following sub-sections introduce the structure of the FML-based HRV ontology to ECG application, adaptive fuzzy detector, HRV analysis mechanism, and fuzzy inference mechanism.

7.4.1 *Structure*

Figure 7.4 displays the structure of the FML-based HRV ontology to ECG application, including an adaptive fuzzy detector, an HRV ontology repository, and a fuzzy inference mechanism. The structure operates as follows.

- The domain experts construct the FML-based HRV ontology through the provided FML editor, and store the built personal HRV ontology into the FML-based HRV ontology repository.

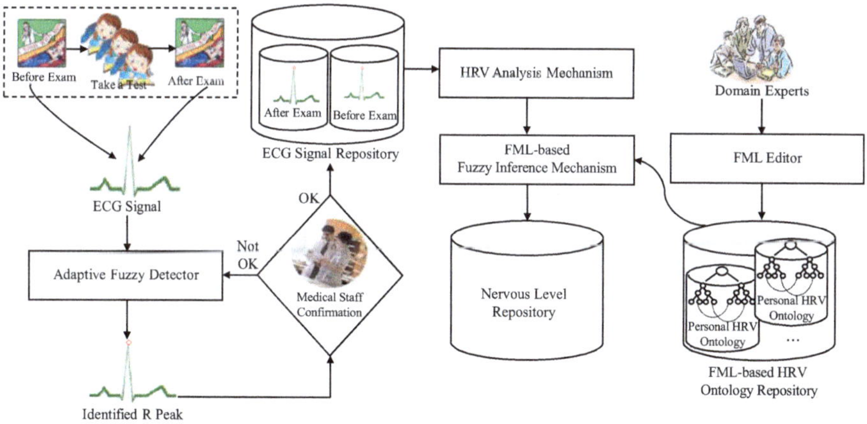

Fig. 7.4 The structure of FML-based HRV ontology to ECG application

- The involved students' ECG signals were measured before their exams and after their exams. After that, an ECG signal is sent to the adaptive fuzzy detector to locate the correct R peak.
- The ECG signal marked with R peaks is then passed to the medical staff to make a confirmation. If the medical staff confirms that the detected R peaks are correct, then the ECG signal is stored into the ECG signal repository.
- The HRV analysis mechanism then performs the HRV by the time-domain and frequency-domain linear methods.
- Based on the pre-defined FML-based HRV ontology, the FML-based inference mechanism infers the nervous level of each involved student via the collected time-domain and frequency-domain parameters, and then stores them into the nervous level repository.

7.4.2 Adaptive Fuzzy Detector

An ECG signal can provide much information on the normal and pathological physiology of the heart activity. Thus, ECG is an important non-invasive clinical tool for the diagnosis of heart diseases (Meau et al. 2006; Israel et al. 2005). The accurate determination of the QRS complex, particularly accurate detection of the R peak, is essential in the computer-based ECG analysis, but is often hard to achieve. Therefore, many different approaches have been developed to enhance the accuracy of QRS detection. For instance, Friesen et al. (1990) developed a comparison of the noise sensitivity of nine QRS detection algorithms and Pan et al. (1985) proposed a real-time algorithm for detecting the QRS complexes of ECG signals. The adaptive fuzzy detector is composed of an adaptive QRS detection mechanism, a double-mean window mechanism, and a sorting mechanism (Lee and Wang 2008). Double-mean window and sorting mechanisms are developed in our previous work (Lee and Wang 2008) to enhance the result of the adaptive QRS detection mechanism presented by (Pan and Tompkins 1985). After executing the adaptive fuzzy detector, the correct R peak is located.

7.4.3 HRV Analysis Mechanism

The HRV analysis mechanism adopts the time series to proceed with the time-domain analysis. Based on the ECG signal with the R peaks marked and the pre-defined FML-based HRV ontology, the HRV analysis mechanism proceeds with the HRV time-domain and frequency-domain analysis to acquire the information such as *meanRRI* and *LF*. Herein, the *meanRRI*, *SDNN*, *RMSSD*, *NN50*, and *pNN50* are calculated as indexes to estimate the state of the heart. Additionally, the nonlinear method, Poincare Plot (Addio et al. 1999), and RRI distribution implemented for different RR intervals. For frequency-domain analysis, the fast

Table 7.3 HRV analysis mechanism algorithm (Lee and Wang 2008)

HRV Analysis Mechanism Algorithm
BEGIN
Input the sequence of the RR interval $T = \{T_1, T_2, \ldots, T_N\}$ after implementing the personal fuzzy filter.
Calculate *meanRRI* by $meanRRI = \frac{\sum_{i=1}^{N} T_i}{N}$
Calculate *SDNN* by $SDNN = \sqrt{\frac{\sum_{i=1}^{N} (Ti - meanRRI)^2}{N}}$
Calculate RMSSD by $RMSSD = \sqrt{\frac{\sum_{i=1}^{N-1} (Ti - T_{i+1})^2}{N-1}}$
Initialize NN50 = 0
DO UNTIL $(i > N)$
  IF $(T_i - T_{i+1}) > 50\text{ms}$ **THEN**
    increment NN50
  END IF
END DO UNTIL
Calculate pNN50 by $pNN50 = \frac{NN50}{N} \times 100\%$
Implement the Berger algorithm to interpolate data points to produce an evenly sampled time series with 4 Hz resampling rate.
Compute an FFT with 1,024 data points.
Integrate the power in very low frequency, low frequency, high frequency range to generate the *VLF*, *LF*, and *HF* power components.
Calculate Total Power by

$$TotalPower = VLF + LF + HF$$

Calculate LFHF ratio by

$$LFHFration = LFP/HFP$$

Calculate HF norm by

$$HF/(TotalPower - VLF) \times 100$$

Calculate LF norm by

$$LF/(TotalPower - VLF) \times 100$$

END

Fourier transform (FFT) is adopted to perform the spectral analysis. To generate an evenly sampled time series prior to FFT-based spectral estimation, the algorithm proposed by Berger et al. (1986) is implemented to resample the RR tachogram to an even time series, HR (beats/minute), at a frequency of 4 Hz. The heart rate power spectra are obtained by computing the magnitude square of the FFT of the 1,024 data points of tachometer signal. The total power is determined by integrating the power spectrum from 0.04 to 0.4 Hz. The algorithm of the HRV analysis mechanism is listed in Table 7.3.

7.4.4 FML-Based Fuzzy Inference Mechanism

In this subsection, the FML-based fuzzy inference mechanism will be introduced. Herein, the trapezoidal membership function $f_A(x:a,b,c,d)$ of fuzzy number A is denoted by Eq. 7.1 and represented as $A = [a,b,c,d]$.

$$f_A(x:a,b,c,d) = \begin{cases} 0, & x < a \\ (x-a)/(x-a) & a \leq x < b \\ 1, & b \leq x < c \\ (d-x)/(d-c), & c \leq x < d \\ 0, & x \geq d \end{cases} \tag{7.1}$$

According to Sect. 7.3.1, three time-domain parameters (*MeanRRI*, *SDNN*, and *RMSSD*) and one frequency-domain parameter (*LFHF*) are chosen as the features to affect the human's nervous level (*NL*). Next, the parameters of membership functions are decided by the domain experts according to the involved students' ECG signals. Figure 7.5a–e show the membership functions for the fuzzy variables *MeanRRI*, *SDNN*, *RMSSD*, *LFHF*, and *NL*, respectively. Based on the FML, an FML editor, developed by the LASA Laboratory, University of Salerno, Italy, is used to construct the knowledge base and rule base of the ECG. Table 7.4 shows part of the FML view of the ECG, including the knowledge base and the rule base. Table 7.5 shows part of the constructed fuzzy rules of the ECG, and the total fuzzy rules is 81.

7.5 Experimental Results

The ontological fuzzy agent for electrocardiogram application described in this chapter is implemented with the Matlab (version 7.0) programming language. The experimental environment is constructed to test the performance of the proposed approach. The experiment involved healthy volunteers, comprising 27 men and 13 women, aged 18–43 years, with average levels of physical activity. The ECG signals are measured in the sitting position before and after an examination. All signals are recorded with a sampling frequency of 1,000 Hz. The duration of experiments under recording ECG signals is 5 min. Table 7.6 lists the time-domain and frequency-domain parameters for the involved 40 students. Table 7.7 shows the mean value, minimum, maximum, and standard deviation (SD) of the parameters listed in Table 7.6.

The first experiment is to observe the variance in time-domain analysis before and after an examination. Figure 7.6a–c display the scattergrams of the *meanRRI*, *SDNN*, and *RMSSD*, respectively. Figure 7.7 shows the statistics results of the number of subjects when the subject's *meanRRI* value before an examination is greater than that after an examination. The same statistics for *SDNN*, *RMSSD*, *NN5*, and *pNN50* are measured similarly as *meanRRI*. Figures 7.6 and 7.7 indicate that

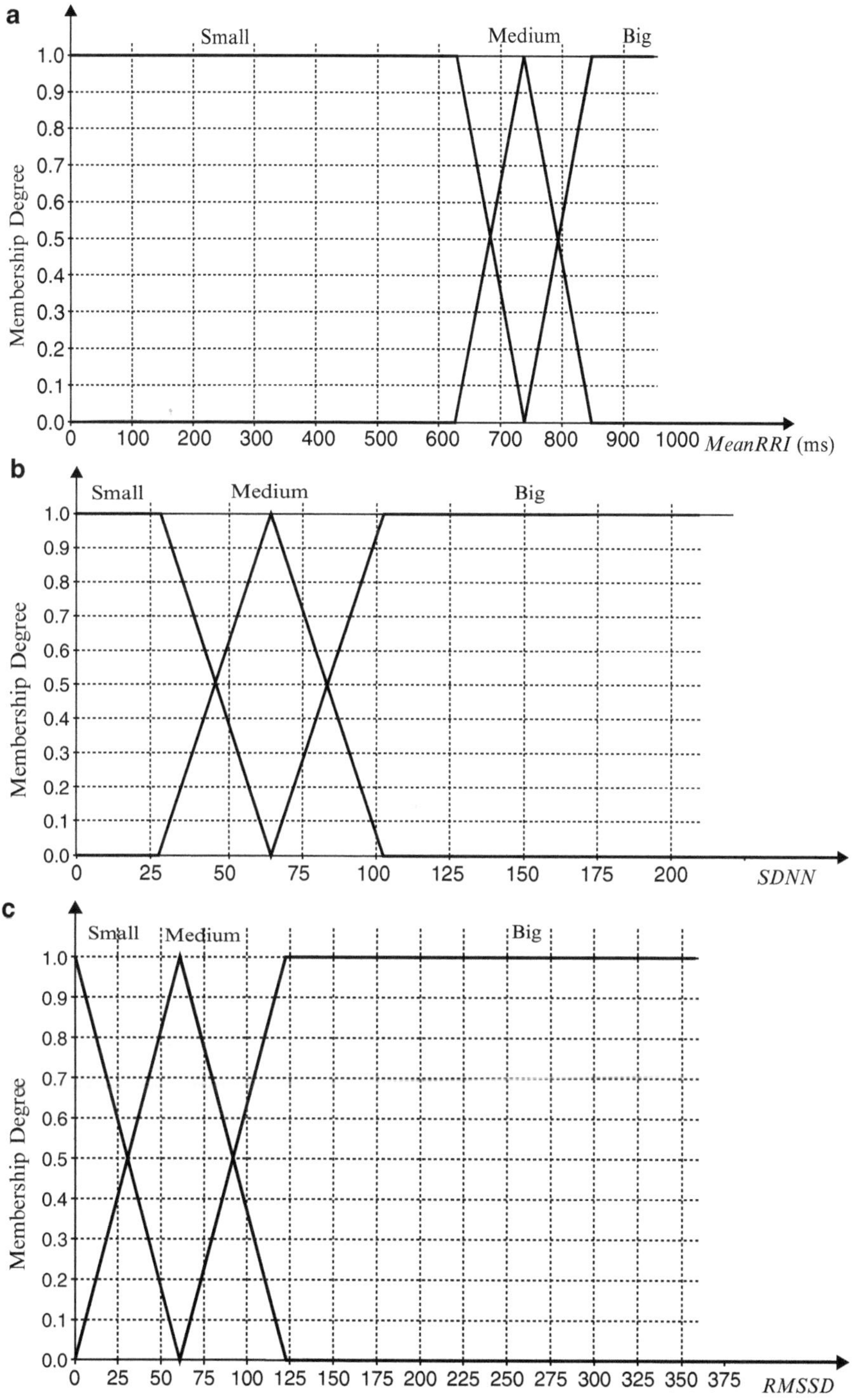

Fig. 7.5 Membership functions for fuzzy variables (**a**) *MeanRRI*, (**b**) *SDNN*, (**c**) *RMSSD*, (**d**) *LFHF*, and (**e**) *NL*

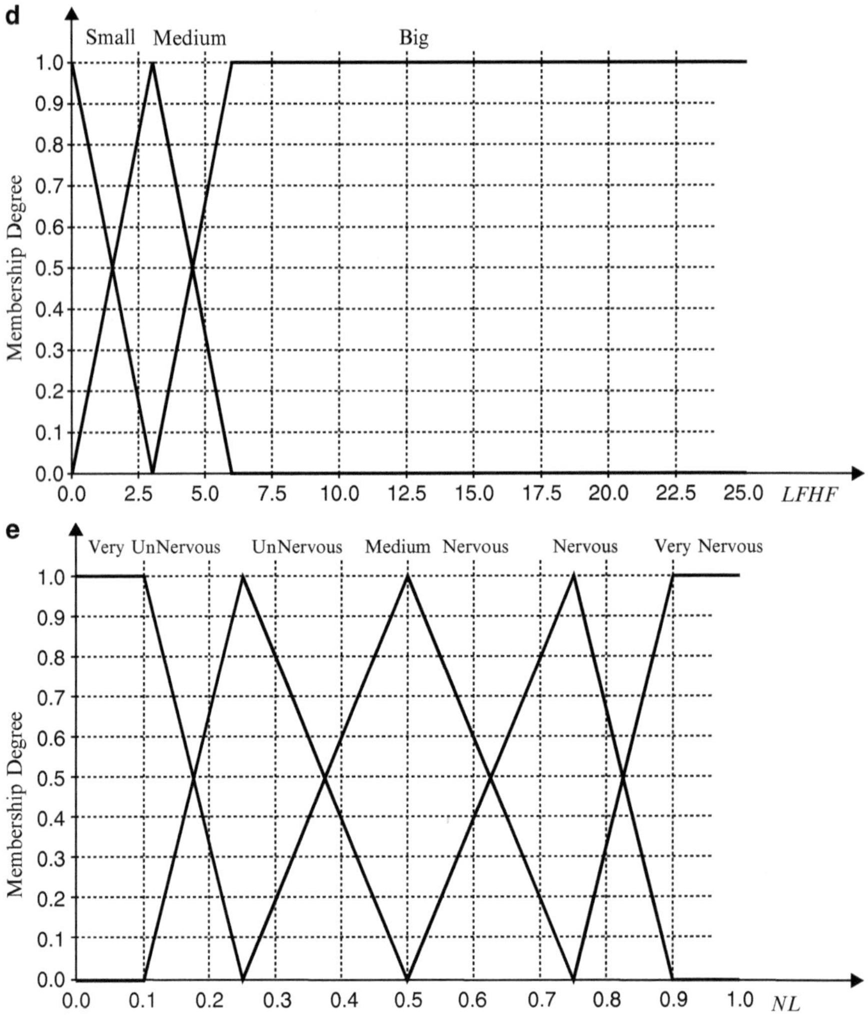

Fig. 7.5 (continued)

for most subjects, the *meanRRI* before an examination is shorter than that after an examination, which means that most subjects feel much more nervous before an examination than after an examination. Experimental results also reveal that the variance of heartbeats is also much lower before an examination than the variance of those after an examination.

The second experiment is to observe the variance in frequency-domain analysis before and after examination. Figure 7.8 shows the scattergrams of the *LFHF* and the pie charts of *LF* and *HF* for all subjects before and after an examination. The results depicted in Fig. 7.8 demonstrate that the percentage of *HF* before an

Table 7.4 Part of the FML view of the ECG knowledge base and rule base

```
<?xml version="1.0" encoding="UTF-8" standalone="no"?>
<FuzzyController ip="140.133.33.2" name="ECG">
  <KnowledgeBase>
<FuzzyVariable domainleft="0.0" domainright="1000.0" name="MeanRRI"
scale="ms" type="input">
  <FuzzyTerm complement="false" name="Big">
    <TrapezoidShape Param1="740.0" Param2="850.0" Param3="1000.0"
Param4="1000.0"/>
  </FuzzyTerm>
  <FuzzyTerm complement="false" name="Medium">
    <TrapezoidShape Param1="630.0" Param2="740.0" Param3="740.0" Param4="850.0"/>
  </FuzzyTerm>
  <FuzzyTerm complement="false" name="Small">
    <TrapezoidShape Param1="461.0" Param2="461.0" Param3="630.0" Param4="740.0"/>
    </FuzzyTerm>
  </FuzzyVariable>
  ...
<FuzzyVariable accumulation="MAX" defaultValue="0.0" defuzzifier="COG"
domainleft="0.0" domainright="1.0" name="NL" scale="" type="output">
  <FuzzyTerm complement="false" name="VeryUnNervous">
    <TrapezoidShape Param1="0.0" Param2="0.0" Param3="0.1" Param4="0.25"/>
  </FuzzyTerm>
  <FuzzyTerm complement="false" name="UnNervous">
    <TrapezoidShape Param1="0.1" Param2="0.25" Param3="0.25" Param4="0.5"/>
  </FuzzyTerm>
  <FuzzyTerm complement="false" name="MediumNervous">
    <TrapezoidShape Param1="0.25" Param2="0.5" Param3="0.5" Param4="0.75"/>
  </FuzzyTerm>
  <FuzzyTerm complement="false" name="Nervous">
    <TrapezoidShape Param1="0.5" Param2="0.75" Param3="0.75" Param4="0.9"/>
  </FuzzyTerm>
  <FuzzyTerm complement="false" name="VeryNervous">
    <TrapezoidShape Param1="0.75" Param2="0.9" Param3="1.0" Param4="1.0"/>
  </FuzzyTerm>
  </FuzzyVariable>
  </KnowledgeBase>
<RuleBase activationMethod="MIN" andMethod="MIN" name="RulcBase1"
orMethod="MAX" type="mamdani">
  <Rule connector="and" name="RULE1" operator="MIN" weight="1.0">
    <Antecedent>
      <Clause>
        <Variable>MeanRRI</Variable>
        <Term>Small</Term>
      </Clause>
      <Clause>
        <Variable>RMSSD</Variable>
        <Term>Small</Term>
```

(continued)

Table 7.4 (continued)

```
    </Clause>
    <Clause>
      <Variable>SDNN</Variable>
      <Term>Small</Term>
    </Clause>
    <Clause>
      <Variable>LFHF</Variable>
      <Term>Small</Term>
    </Clause>
  </Antecedent>
  <Consequent>
    <Clause>
      <Variable>NL</Variable>
      <Term>MediumNervous</Term>
</Clause>
</Consequent>
  </Rule>
...
<Rule connector="and" name="RULE81" operator="MIN" weight="1.0">
    <Antecedent>
      <Clause>
        <Variable>MeanRRI</Variable>
        <Term>Big</Term>
      </Clause>
      <Clause>
        <Variable>RMSSD</Variable>
        <Term>Big</Term>
      </Clause>
      <Clause>
        <Variable>SDNN</Variable>
        <Term>Big</Term>
      </Clause>
      <Clause>
        <Variable>LFHF</Variable>
        <Term>Big</Term>
      </Clause>
    </Antecedent>
    <Consequent>
      <Clause>
        <Variable>NL</Variable>
        <Term>MediumNervous</Term>
      </Clause>
    </Consequent>
      </Rule>
  </RuleBase>
</FuzzyController>
```

Table 7.5 Part of the constructed fuzzy rules of the ECG

	Input Fuzzy variable				Output Fuzzy variable
Rule No	MeanRRI	RMSSD	SDNN	LFHF	NL
1	Small	Small	Small	Small	MediumNervous
2	Small	Small	Small	Medium	Nervous
3	Small	Small	Small	Big	Nervous
4	Small	Small	Medium	Small	Nervous
5	Small	Small	Medium	Medium	Nervous
6	Small	Small	Medium	Big	VeryNervous
7	Small	Small	Big	Small	Nervous
8	Small	Small	Big	Medium	VeryNervous
9	Small	Small	Big	Big	VeryNervous
10	Small	Medium	Small	Small	UnNervous
11	Small	Medium	Small	Medium	MediumNervous
12	Small	Medium	Small	Big	Nervous
13	Small	Medium	Medium	Small	MediumNervous
14	Small	Medium	Medium	Medium	Nervous
15	Small	Medium	Medium	Big	Nervous
16	Small	Medium	Big	Small	Nervous
17	Small	Medium	Big	Medium	Nervous
18	Small	Medium	Big	Big	VeryNervous
19	Small	Big	Small	Small	UnNervous
20	Small	Big	Small	Medium	UnNervous
			...		
71	Big	Medium	Big	Medium	MediumNervous
72	Big	Medium	Big	Big	Nervous
73	Big	Big	Small	Small	VeryUnNervous
74	Big	Big	Small	Medium	VeryUnNervous
75	Big	Big	Small	Big	UnNervous
76	Big	Big	Medium	Small	VeryUnNervous
77	Big	Big	Medium	Medium	UnNervous
78	Big	Big	Medium	Big	UnNervous
79	Big	Big	Big	Small	UnNervous
80	Big	Big	Big	Medium	UnNervous
81	Big	Big	Big	Big	MediumNervous

examination is greater than the percentage of that after an examination, which indicates that the sympathetic nerves are more active before an examination and this situation causes the heart rate of the subjects to be quicker than the ordinary situation.

The final experiment is to evaluate the output of three-dimensional surfaces based on the constructed knowledge base and the rule base. Figure 7.9 represents the surface view for our proposed approach. Major trends can be observed in the following rule descriptions. (1) The *NL* does increase as the *SDNN* increases. (2) The *NL* does increase as the *RMSSD* decreases. (3) The *NL* does increase as the *MeanRRI* approaches about 500–800 ms. (4) The *HDS* does increase as the

Table 7.6 Time-domain and frequency-domain parameters for the involved 40 students

	Before exam				After exam			
No	MeanRRI	SDNN	RMSSD	LFHF	MeanRRI	SDNN	RMSSD	LFHF
1	706.11	53.11	44.28	2.02	652.97	60.12	57.9	2.21
2	905.98	82.8	69.62	1.64	1085.6	155.26	122.15	1.24
3	653.34	49.51	19.35	3.86	645.93	38.88	17.95	5.99
4	586.28	37.84	39.68	1.63	730.5	57.72	79.39	0.77
5	703.64	140.39	221.33	0.28	767.56	49.15	52.84	1.69
6	724.23	120.36	190.34	0.12	795.82	40.25	18.18	5
7	655.42	42.67	22.86	4.96	750.49	58.82	41.18	4.7
8	715.15	89.54	139.18	0.47	721.43	40.28	21.05	2.92
9	616.43	42.94	34.71	1.51	731.8	35.06	23.09	1.02
10	796.25	87.28	70.11	4.09	909.8	67.8	54.16	1.85
11	773.39	70.59	37.12	2.88	753.84	86.87	83.9	1.48
12	856.75	74.12	42.92	3.17	751.62	118.32	97.45	1.09
13	928.41	90.67	64.91	1.23	754.48	80.36	40.09	8.43
14	798.04	65.13	56.89	0.89	823.72	71.78	53.15	2.36
15	590.63	24.76	6.96	9.63	613.76	49.27	12.13	21.03
16	686.04	109.91	129.56	1.5	750.14	209.21	363.85	0.4
17	645.46	41.79	18.39	2.37	740.63	76.55	90.31	0.69
18	653.94	39.25	16.73	9.97	815.7	41.97	37.92	0.92
19	693.71	57.09	45.09	2.01	814.36	76.5	51.95	2.12
20	892.51	66.31	38.3	4.88	875.58	95.71	101.53	2.1
21	676.48	58.08	39.82	1.72	764.45	60.89	58.38	0.4
22	637.57	45.64	24.67	7.67	657.53	88.41	131.17	0.38
23	844.32	215	332.57	0.34	768.73	52.5	31.64	3.24
24	637.58	47.45	17.37	3.57	622.78	41.59	50.81	1.1
25	775.79	135.73	97.54	5.66	831.2	155.71	119.76	4.78
26	654.21	40.21	23.45	4.35	699.37	38.67	22.38	3.52
27	654.77	37.99	19.72	7.95	704.89	34.83	14.79	11.46
28	460.83	14.01	10.86	5.26	512.31	17.85	5.62	10.43
29	723.11	57.9	54.77	1.36	788.19	44.47	39.61	1.52
30	712.54	41.98	45.32	1.51	778.45	43.91	24	6.52
31	744.6	64.75	43.35	3.74	968.14	55.51	65.72	1.27
32	634.89	59.25	66.72	1.68	522.59	18.92	7.91	5.3
33	786.83	57.85	31.93	6.26	833.69	77.81	42.13	2.03
34	654.59	31.7	34.02	1.18	778.99	48.96	36.05	3.02
35	972.71	81.73	99.43	0.24	1032.5	132.82	159.4	1.11
36	759.07	60.84	56.47	0.94	849.06	68.26	68.53	1.65
37	691.92	34.64	24.39	1.68	736.73	42.49	33.74	1.27
38	616.17	33.76	32.28	1.46	708.08	48.65	34.85	2.5
39	625.17	27.28	16.21	3.7	769.2	57.13	42.25	2.1
40	753.1	60.07	63.87	1.57	814.05	80.63	62.14	2.15

Table 7.7 Values of mean, minimum, maximum, and standard deviation (SD) of the parameters

	Values			
Parameters	Mean	Minimum	Maximum	SD
MeanRRI	740.31	460.83	1085.6	110.15
SDNN	66.4	14.01	215	38.01
RMSSD	61.43	0	363.85	61.52
LFHF	3.18	0	21.03	3.24

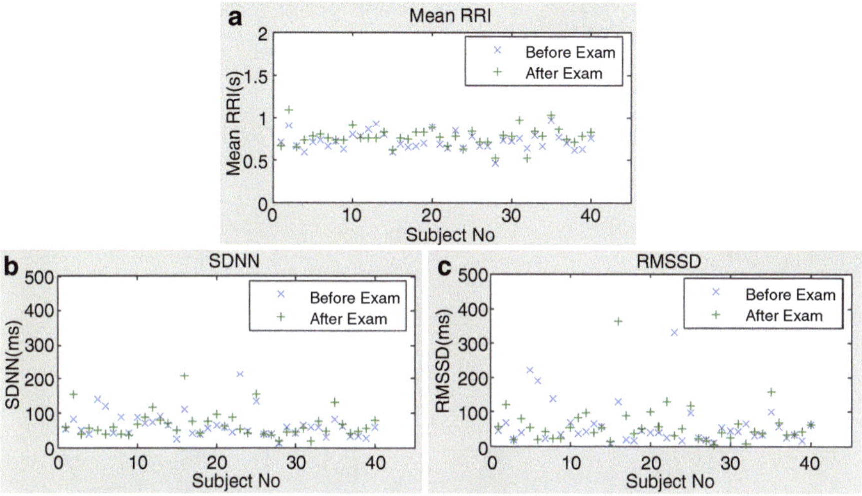

Fig. 7.6 The scattergrams of the (**a**) *meanRRI*, (**b**) *SDNN*, and (**c**) *RMSSD* (Lee and Wang 2008)

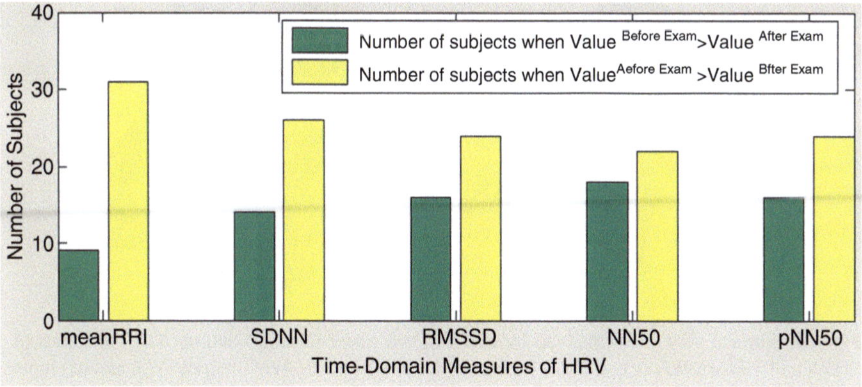

Fig. 7.7 The statistical results of the number of subjects for *meanRRI, SDNN, RMSSD, NN50*, and *pNN50* (Lee and Wang 2008)

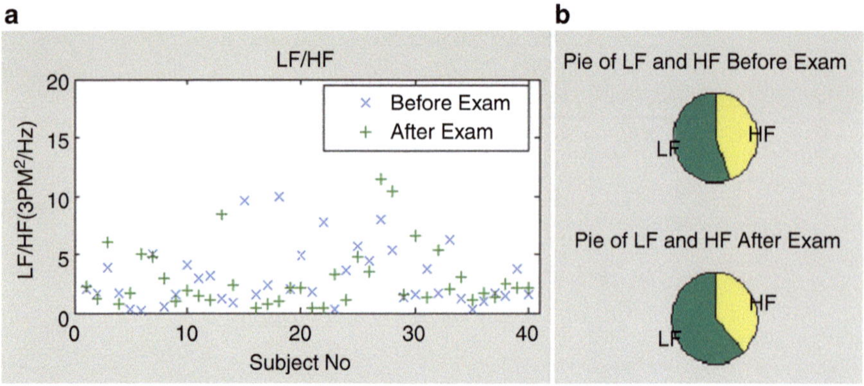

Fig. 7.8 (**a**) The scattergram of *LFHF* and (**b**) the pie charts of *LF* and *HF* for all subjects before and after an examination (Lee and Wang 2008)

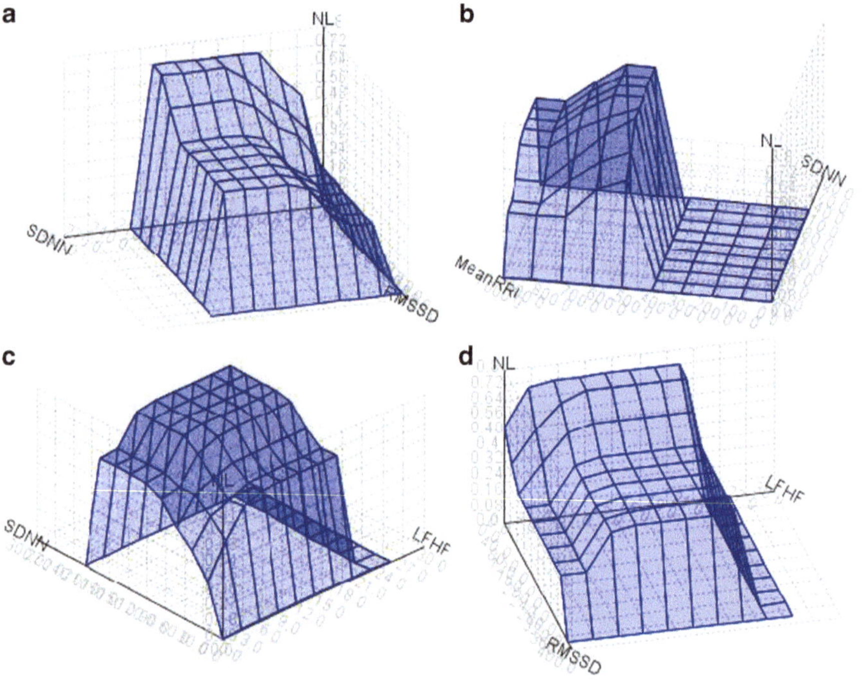

Fig. 7.9 Surface view for *OMAS* (**a**) Inputs (*X-SDNN* and *Y-RMSSD*) output (*NL*), (**b**) Inputs (*X-SDNN* and *Y-MeanRRI*) output (*NL*), (**c**) Inputs (*X-SDNN* and *Y-LFHF*) output (*NL*), and (**d**) Inputs (**X-RMSSD** and *Y-LFHF*) output (*NL*)

LFHF increases. Based on the major trends (Fig. 7.9), the behavior of the proposed approach meets the ECG principles. Hence, the proposed approach is feasible for applying to the ECG domain, which will help people live in a happy life.

7.6 Conclusions

This chapter proposes an FML-based HRV ontology for electrocardiogram application. The needed knowledge is stored in the FML-based HRV ontology. The proposed method comprises an adaptive fuzzy detector, an HRV ontology, and an FML-based fuzzy inference mechanism. Experimental results show that the proposed approach is feasible and can work effectively. Additionally, experimental results also reveal that people are usually more nervous before than after an examination. However, some problems need further to be studied in the future. For example, the proposed approach could be extended to different domain knowledge such as chronic diseases, including asthma and diabetes health care, and a learning algorithm could be applied to learn the membership functions to improve the precision and recall of the ECG signal classification. With these studies, it is hoped to qualify the obtained results in the future.

Acknowledgment The authors would like to thank the National Science Council of Taiwan for financially supporting this research under the grant NSC 98-2221-E-024-009-MY3 and NSC 99-2622-E-024-003-CC3.

References

Acampora, G., Loia, V.: Using FML and fuzzy technology in adaptive ambient intelligence environments. Int. J. Comput. Intell. Res. **1**(2), 171–182 (2005a)

Acampora, G., Loia, V.: Fuzzy control interoperability and scalability for adaptive domotic framework. IEEE Trans. Ind. Inf. **1**(2), 97–111 (2005b)

American Heart Association Inc., European Society of Cardiology.: Guidelines about heart rate variability standards of measurement, physiological interpretation, and clinical use. Eur. Heart J. **17**, 354–381 (1996)

Addio, G.D., Pinna, G.D., Maestri, R., Acanfora, D., Picone, C., Furgi, G., Rengo, F.: Correlation between power-law behavior and poincare plots of heart rate variability in congestive heart failure patients. Comput. Cardiol. **26**, 611–614 (1999)

Beveridge, M., Fox, J.: Automatic generation of spoken dialogue from medical plans and ontologies. J. Biomed. Inf. **39**(5), 482–499 (2006)

Berger, R.D., Akselrod, S., Gordon, D., Cohen, R.J.: An efficient algorithm for spectral analysis of heart rate variability. IEEE Trans. Biomed. Eng. **33**(9), 900–904 (1986)

Friesen, G.M., Jannett, T.C., Jadallah, M.A., Yates, S.L., Quint, S.R., Nagle, H.T.: A comparison of the noise sensitivity of nine QRS detection algorithm. IEEE Trans. Biomed. Eng. **37**(1), 85–98 (1990)

Israel, A.S., Irvine, J.M., Cheng, A., Wiederhold, M.D., Wiederhold, B.K.: ECG to identify individuals. Pattern Recognit. **38**(1), 133–142 (2005)

Lee, C.S., Wang, M.H.: Ontology-based intelligent healthcare agent and its application to respiratory waveform recognition. Expert Syst. Appl. **33**(3), 606–619 (2007)

Lee, C.S., Wang, M.H.: Ontological fuzzy agent for electrocardiogram application. Expert Syst. Appl. **35**(3), 1223–1236 (2008)

Lee, C.S., Wang, M.H.: Ontology-based computational intelligent multi-agent and its application to CMMI assessment. Appl. Intell. **30**(3), 203–219 (2009)

Lee, C.S., Jian, Z.W., Huang, L.K.: A fuzzy ontology and its application to news summarization. IEEE Trans. Syst. Man Cybern. Part B: Cybern. **35**(5), 859–880 (2005)

Lee, C.S., Jiang, C.C., Hsieh, T.C.: A genetic agent using ontology model for meeting scheduling system. Inf. Sci. **176**(9), 1131–1155 (2006)

Lee, C.S., Wang, M.H., Chen, J.J.: Ontology-based intelligent decision support agent for CMMI project monitoring and control. Int. J. Approx. Reason. **48**(1), 62–76 (2008)

Lee, C.S., Wang, M.H., Wu, M.H., Hsu, C.Y., Lin, Y.C., Yen, S.J.: A type-2 fuzzy personal ontology for meeting scheduling system. In: 2010 IEEE World Congress on Computational Intelligence (WCCI 2010), Barcelona, 18–23 July (2010a)

Lee, C.S., Wang, M.H., Hagras, H.: A type-2 fuzzy ontology and its application to personal diabetic-diet recommendation. IEEE Trans. Fuzzy Syst. **18**(2), 374–395 (2010b)

Lee, C.S., Wang, M.H., Yen, S.J., Chen, Y.J., Chou, C.W., Chaslot, G., Hoock, J.B., Rimmel, A., Doghmen, H.: An ontology-based fuzzy inference system for computer Go applications. Int. J. Fuzzy Syst. **12**(2), 103–115 (2010c)

Lee, C.S., Wang, M.H., Yang, Z.R., Chen, Y.J., Doghmen, H., Teytaud, O.: FML-based type-2 fuzzy ontology for computer Go knowledge representation. In: International Conference on System Science and Engineering (ICSSE 2010), Taipei, 1–3 July (2010d)

Lin, C.W., Wang, J.S., Chung, P.C.: Mining physiological conditions from heart rate variability analysis. IEEE Comput. Intell. Mag. **5**(1), 50–58 (2010)

Liu, Y., Xu, C., Zhang, Q., Pan, Y.: The smart architect: scalable ontology-based modeling of ancient Chinese architectures. IEEE Intell. Syst. **23**(1), 49–56 (2008)

Meau, Y.P., Ibrahim, F., Narainasamy, S.A.L., Omar, R.: Intelligent classification of electrocardiogram signal using extended kalman filter based neuro fuzzy system. Comput. Meth. Program Biomed. **82**(2), 157–168 (2006)

Noy, N.F., McGuinness, D.L.: Ontology development 101: a guide to creating your first ontology. Stanford knowledge systems laboratory technical report KSL-01-05 and Stanford medical informatics technical report SMI-2001-0880 (2001)

Orgun, B., Vu, J.: HL7 ontology and mobile agents for interoperability in heterogeneous medical information systems. Comput. Biol. Med. **36**(7–8), 817–836 (2006)

Pan, J., Tompkins, W.: A real-time QRS detection algorithm. IEEE Trans. Biomed. Eng. **32**(3), 230–236 (1985)

Sanchez, F.G., Bejar, R.M., Contreras, L., Bries, J.T.F., Nieves, D.C.: An ontology-based intelligent system for recruitment. Expert Syst. Appl. **31**(2), 248–263 (2006)

Wang, M.H., Lee, C.S., Hsieh, K.L., Hsu, C.Y., Acampora, G., Chang, C.C. Ontology-based multi-agents for intelligent healthcare applications. J. Ambient Intell. Hum. Comput. **1**(2), 111–131 (2010)

Yan, H., Jiang, Y., Zheng, J., Peng, C., Li, Q.: A multiplayer perceptron-based medical decision support system for heart disease diagnosis. Expert Syst. Appl. **30**(3), 272–278 (2006)

Chapter 8
Learning in Artificial Neural Networks

Antônio Pádua Braga

8.1 Introduction

Model induction from data appears in many fields such as Artificial Neural Networks (ANNs), Fuzzy Systems (FS), Dynamic Systems Identification (DSI) and Statistics. Nevertheless, the models that arise from each one of these areas differ from each other by how the problem is represented into their structures. For instance, classical statistical models are naturally generative (Shannon 1948), since they are constructed according to estimations of the data generator density functions. In contrast with such a generative approach, hypersurface approximation by ANN models is accomplished regardless of any hypothesis about the originating distributions. ANN models for classification, for instance, are considered as discriminative (Rosenblatt 1958), since they aim at modeling the separation surface only, not the densities that generated the data.

Although the principles of Fisher Linear Discriminant Analysis (Fisher 1936) were laid down in the literature in the mid-1930s, the notion that ANN-based classifiers could be constructed solely with separation margin data represented a paradigm shift from the classical generative statistical approach in the mid-1980s. The major impact of this new concept was possibly the fact that discriminative models could be built with small samples that were representative of class separation, instead of large samples describing central tendencies. The new approach seemed to break some statistical rules in the beginning, since margin data did not explain the underlying distributions, being inherently located at the distribution tails.

A.P. Braga (✉)
Universidade Federal de Minas Gerais, Departamento de Engenharia Eletrnica,
Avenida Antnio Carlos 6627, 31-270-901, Belo Horizonte, MG, Brazil
e-mail: apbraga@ufmg.br

A. Gacek and W. Pedrycz (eds.), *ECG Signal Processing, Classification and Interpretation: A Comprehensive Framework of Computational Intelligence*,
DOI 10.1007/978-0-85729-868-3_8, © Springer-Verlag London Limited 2012

Nevertheless, the possibility of building models from smaller data sets was promising for many kinds of problems, especially for those that had sampling limitations, which is the case of many real-world applications. However, new ANN users lacked a model that would explain the underlying distributions, what caused a debate in the literature about the pros and cons of "black-box" ANN models (Craven 1996). This long-lasting debate prevailed for many years until it was drifted to more general, non-dichotomic subjects, such as the description of a general theory of learning that would provide a unique framework for both discriminative and generative approaches.

A better understanding of the general Machine Learning (ML) problem was possible after the description of Statistical Learning Theory (SLT) (Vapnik 1995), consolidated in the mid-1990s. Formal descriptions of the margin problem as well as of the upper bounds of risk were important to provide the formal basis of the general *learning from data* problem. The formalism missing in the classical ANN theory provided by SLT and the development of large margin classifiers, like the Support Vector Machine (SVM) (Boser et al. 1992), resulted in a new wave of interest for the area. SLT was later incorporated into the ANN framework and interpreted in the context of current models, like Multi-Layer Perceptron (MLP) and Radial Basis Functions (RBF) (Broomhead and Lowe 1988), resulting in new learning approaches like the Multi-Objective Learning (MOBJ) (Braga et al. 2006; Teixeira et al. 2000). The major contribution of SLT was possibly the description of a general, elegant, and well accepted theory of learning that provided the basis for the understanding of the general learning from data problem in a single framework.

Current trends in ANN design are not anymore the optimization aspects of learning algorithms, convergence, and stochasticity of the results that dominated the area for decades, but more general issues related to approximation theory. Responses to these 1980s–1990s concerns have been well presented in the literature (Hagan and Menhaj 1994) and are less relevant at present. Despite of the non-convexity aspects of learning with ANNs, the universality of function approximation seems to be a more relevant aspect for providing a proper model of learning.

In this chapter, the general problem of ANNs learning is presented in the context of Statistical Learning Theory. It is shown how the ANNs learning problem can be contextualized into this general framework with particular emphasis on its multi-objective aspects. The concepts of multi-objective learning with ANNs are presented and an example of solving an ECG problem is given.

8.2 Statistical Learning Theory

One of the most important contributions of Statistical Learning Theory (Vapnik 1995) was to provide the convergence conditions for the *empirical approximation* of the true risk $R(\mathbf{w})$ of selecting the vector of parameters $\mathbf{w}$ of an approximating function $f(\mathbf{x},\mathbf{w})$. Under ideal conditions, considering that the joint probability density function $p(\mathbf{x}, y)$ is known in advance and that all input-output relations $(\mathbf{x}, y)$ can be assessed, the estimation of the true risk can be represented by Eq. 8.1.

$$R(\mathbf{w}) = \int Q(y, f(\mathbf{x}, \mathbf{w}))p(\mathbf{x}, y)dxdy \tag{8.1}$$

where $Q(y, f(\mathbf{x}, \mathbf{w}))$ is a loss function.

According to Eq. 8.1, the goal of learning is to find the approximating function $f(\mathbf{x}, \mathbf{w}^*)$ with parameters $\mathbf{w}^*$ that minimizes $R(\mathbf{w})$. Of course, this cannot be accomplished, since $p(\mathbf{x}, y)$ is not known in advance, and it is not feasible to cover the full domains of $\mathbf{x}$ and y in order to calcule the integral in Eq. 8.1. Instead of calculating $R(\mathbf{w})$ with the previous equation, *learning from data* models aim at approximating $R(\mathbf{w})$ with an empirical risk function $R_{\text{emp}}(\mathbf{w})$ calculated over a limited set of samples, the *learning set.* Function induction from a limited data set is one of the basic principles of machine learning inductive models; however, this fundamental assumption is only valid under the conditions that the learning set is large enough to provide convergence of $R_{\text{emp}}(\mathbf{w})$. For small samples problems, which is the scenario for most real-world problems, convergence of the empirical risk also depends on model capacity, as will be discussed in the next section.

8.2.1 Model Capacity and Learning

The notion that both error and model capacity should be traded-off in order to reduce approximation error can be well understood from the interpretation of the inequality presented in Expression 8.2, one of the most important formal results of SLT (Vapnik 1995). The interpretation of such expression is that the true risk $R(\mathbf{w})$ is bounded by the empirical risk $R_{\text{emp}}(\mathbf{w})$ plus a square root term that depends both on the sample size N and on the model capacity h.

$$R(\mathbf{w}) \leq R_{\text{emp}}(\mathbf{w}) + \sqrt{\left(\frac{h(log(\frac{2N}{h}) + 1) - log(\frac{\eta}{4})}{N}\right)} \tag{8.2}$$

where N is the sample size, h is the VC dimension (Vapnik 1995), and η is the confidence interval.

It is clear from Expression 8.2 that when the sample size is large, the true risk is bounded by the empirical risk only, since as $N \to \infty \Longrightarrow R(\mathbf{w}) \leq R_{\text{emp}}(\mathbf{w})$. This means that convergence to the true risk in such a situation is yielded by simply minimizing the empirical risk ($R_{\text{emp}}(\mathbf{w}) \approx 0 \Longrightarrow R(\mathbf{w}) \approx 0$ when $N \to \infty$). However, the real challenge of learning is to deal with small samples problems. In such a scenario, $\frac{h}{N}$ is relevant, and a small $R_{\text{emp}}(\mathbf{w})$ does not imply on small $R(\mathbf{w})$. This observation explains why those models based on the empirical risk only do not guarantee good approximation results. Therefore, for small samples, reducing the empirical risk from the data does not guarantee a small approximation error. Since N is fixed for a given problem, the joint minimization of h, which can be achieved by learning, is able to reduce the upper bound of $R(\mathbf{w})$ and assure a better control of the approximation by $R_{\mathrm{emp}}(\mathbf{w})$. In other words, both the empirical risk $R_{\mathrm{emp}}(\mathbf{w})$ and the model capacity h should be reduced in order to reduce the approximation error.

8.3 Bias and Variance Dilemma

The description of the *Bias and Variance Dilemma* (Geman et al. 1992) was also important to understand the factors that affect approximation. Considering that the selected function for the empirical risk is the squared error, as presented in Eq. 8.3, the decomposition of the expected value of the squared error $(y - f(\mathbf{x},\mathbf{w}))^2$ into sampling and approximation error is presented in Eq. 8.4 (Geman et al. 1992)

$$R_{\mathrm{emp}} = \frac{1}{N}\sum_{i=1}^{N}(y - f(\mathbf{x},\mathbf{w}))^2 \tag{8.3}$$

$$E[(y - f(\mathbf{x},\mathbf{w}))^2] = \underbrace{E[(y - E[y|\mathbf{x}])^2]}_{\text{Sampling Error}} + \underbrace{E[(f(\mathbf{x},\mathbf{w}) - E[y|\mathbf{x}])^2]}_{\text{Approximation Error}} \tag{8.4}$$

where $E[y|\mathbf{x}]$ is the expected value of y given the input vector $\mathbf{x}$ yielded by the generator function $f_g(\mathbf{x})$.

The first term $E[(y - E[y|\mathbf{x}])^2]$ of Eq. 8.4 represents the expectation of the sampling error, whereas the second term $E[(f(\mathbf{x},\mathbf{w}) - E[y|\mathbf{x}])^2]$ represents the expectation of the approximation error. The expected value of y for a given $\mathbf{x}$, represented in the equation by $E[y|\mathbf{x}]$, corresponds to the expected value of the target function $f_g(\mathbf{x})$.

As shown in Fig. 8.1, the output data y generated by the system to be modeled corresponds to the outcome of the generator function $f_g(\mathbf{x})$ plus a sampling uncertainty ε. In general, it is assumed that ε exists and that in the particular case when there is no uncertainty, $\varepsilon = 0$. Therefore, the objective of learning from data is to approximate $f_g(\mathbf{x})$ despite of ε. In other words, at the end of learning the approximating function $f(\mathbf{x},\mathbf{w})$ should be as close as possible to $f_g(\mathbf{x})$ and not to $f_g(\mathbf{x}) + \varepsilon$. A proper approximation under the assumption of sampling uncertainty $(\varepsilon \neq 0)$ yields a model with null approximation error and with error residue that is equivalent to system's sampling error. The graph of Fig. 8.2 shows an example of how the residue of a model approximates the uncertainty of the data when $f(\mathbf{x},\mathbf{w}) \approx f_g(\mathbf{x})$.

An important conclusion from Eq. 8.4 is that error minimization can only guarantee control of the approximation error in the no-uncertainty scenario. In such a situation $E[(y - E[y|\mathbf{x}])^2] = 0$ and $E[(y - f(\mathbf{x},\mathbf{w}))^2] = E[(f(\mathbf{x},\mathbf{w}) - E[y|\mathbf{x}])^2]$. Nevertheless, this ideal situation does not happen often in real problems and the

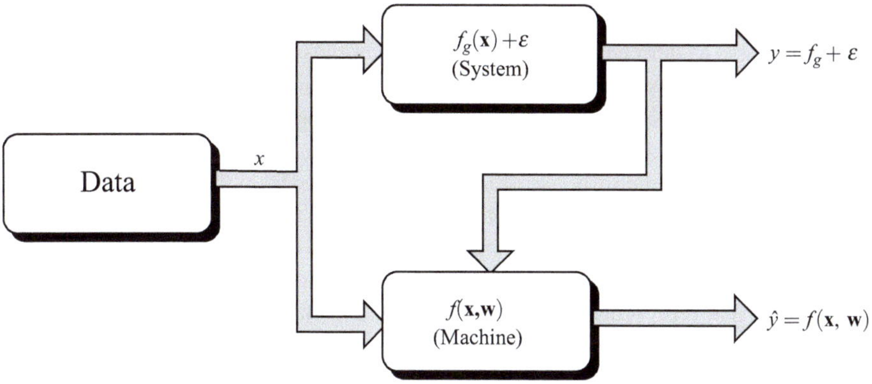

Fig. 8.1 Representation of the uncertainty on learning

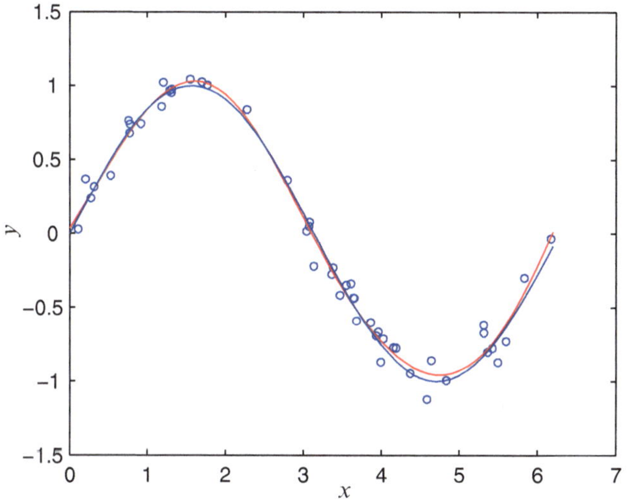

Fig. 8.2 Sine function approximation. Model is close to the generator function resulting in low approximation error and a residue that is equivalent to the sampling error

factors that interfere on the approximation error should be well understood. The bias and variance terms for a family of models are obtained from the decompostion of the second term of Eq. 8.4, as shown in Eq. 8.5.

$$E[(f(\mathbf{x},\mathbf{w})-E[y|\mathbf{x}])^2] = \underbrace{(E[f(\mathbf{x},\mathbf{w})]-E[y|\mathbf{x}])^2]}_{\mu_{\{f(\mathbf{x},\mathbf{w})\}}} + \underbrace{E[(f(\mathbf{x},\mathbf{w})-E[f(\mathbf{x},\mathbf{w})])^2]}_{\sigma^2_{\{f(\mathbf{x},\mathbf{w})\}}} \quad (8.5)$$

From the previous equations, it is possible to conclude that the expectation of the empirical risk, as defined by Eq. 8.3, can be decomposed into the following factors: sampling uncertainty, model bias ($\mu_{\{f(\mathbf{x},\mathbf{w})\}}$), and model variance ($\sigma^2_{\{f(\mathbf{x},\mathbf{w})\}}$). The bias term is the expectation of how far the expected response of the family of models is from the expected response of the target function. Similarly, the variance is a measure of how far the response of a selected model is from the expected response of all models. Since parameter adaptation only affects bias and variance, it can also be affirmed that the objective of learning is to balance these two factors.

According to Statistical Learning Theory, the approximation error, as estimated by the true risk represented in inequality (8.2), depends only on the empirical risk and on the model capacity for fixed N. This important property of learning machines can also be observed in the previous decomposition of the squared error. It is well understood that the larger the model capacity, the larger its ability to adapt to the data set and to the embedded sampling error. It is clear also that models that approximate the uncertainty ($f(\mathbf{x},\mathbf{w}) \approx f_g(\mathbf{x}) + \varepsilon$) are displaced from the target function $f_g(\mathbf{x})$ by ε. Therefore, in order to avoid adaptation to the uncertainty, model capacity should be limited. Nonetheless, capacity control may also affect bias and variance. On one side, if model capacity is less than the required capacity, it may present large bias and small variance. On the other side, if model capacity is larger than required, it may result in small bias and large variance. A low approximation error occurs only if the family of solutions tends to the target function (small bias) with small variability (small variance).

Since $E[y|\mathbf{x}]$ is not known in advance, it is not possible to estimate the bias term of Eq. 8.5 directly. Nevertheless, as discussed previously in this section, the approximation to the target function can be indirectly assessed by how much a model adapts to the uncertainty. A small error model does not imply on small approximation error, since, under the uncertainty assumption ($\varepsilon \neq 0$), it is likely to be far from the target function. Therefore, in order to limit adaptation to the noise, capacity control should be accomplished, what is also consistent with the principles of SLT. Of course, capacity control in the space of parameters affects directly the variance of the model, since this second factor of Eq. 8.5 depends only on the constraints imposed to the parameters of the candidate functions. Therefore, the two terms, bias and variance, that compose the approximation error $E[(f(\mathbf{x},\mathbf{w}) - E[y|\mathbf{x}])^2]$ can be assessed by error ($R_{\text{emp}}(\mathbf{w})$) and capacity ($h$) functions, which present conflicting behavior. This suggests that the general problem of inductive learning should be treated as a bi-objective learning problem, as will be discussed in the next section.

8.4 Multi-Objective Learning

As discussed in the previous section, $R_{\text{emp}}(\mathbf{w})$ and h are conflicting objective functions, since their minima do not coincide. It is clear, therefore, that a single-objective minimization of one of the objective functions may result in the maximization of the other, what paves the way to the Multi-Objective (Chankong and Haimes 1983) treatment of the problem (Liu and Kadirkamanathan 1995; Teixeira et al. 2000). From this perspective, the general problem of model induction (Supervised or Semi-Supervised) can be regarded as the trade-off between $R_{\text{emp}}(\mathbf{w})$ and h.

The different approaches to tackle the supervised learning problem usually include empirical risk (error) minimization and some sort of complexity control, where *complexity* can be *structural* or *apparent*. Structural complexity is associated to the number of network parameters (weights) and apparent complexity is associated to the network response, regardless of its size. Thus, a large structural complexity network may have a small apparent complexity if it behaves like a lower order model. If the network is oversized, it is possible to control its apparent complexity so that it behaves like a lower complexity one.

Structural complexity control can be accomplished by shrinking methods (pruning) (Mozer and Smolensky 1989; LeCun et al. 1990; Karnin 1990) or growing (constructive) methods (Fahlman and Lebiere 1988; Mezard and Nadal 1989), whereas apparent complexity control can be achieved by methods such as smoothing (regularization) (Wahba 1994) and by a restricted search into the set of possible solutions. The latter includes the multi-objective approach that will be described next (Teixeira et al. 2000).

The concepts of flexibility and rigidity are also embodied by the notion of complexity. The larger the network complexity, the higher its flexibility to fit the data. On the other extreme, the lower its complexity, the higher its rigidity to adapt itself to the data set. A model that is too rigid tends to concentrate its responses to a limited region, whereas a flexible one spans its possible solutions into a wider region of the space of solutions. These concepts are also related to the bias-variance dilemma (Geman et al. 1992), since a flexible model has a large variance and a rigid one is biased. The essence of our problem is therefore to obtain a proper balance between error (risk) and complexity (structural or apparent).

8.4.1 Objective Functions for $R_{\text{emp}}(\mathbf{w})$ and h

In order to solve the Multi-Objective problem of trading-off the minimization of $R_{\text{emp}}(\mathbf{w})$ and h, proper objective function representations should be defined for them. The most usual representation for $R_{\text{emp}}(\mathbf{w})$ is the squared error loss function $Q(y_i, f(\mathbf{x}_i, \mathbf{w})) = \sum_{i=1}^{N}(y_i - f(\mathbf{x}_i, \mathbf{w}))^2$, whereas h is usually represented by the L2 norm $||\mathbf{w}||$ of the network weights. Although the squared error representation of $R_{\text{emp}}(\mathbf{w})$ is well accepted, the choice of $||\mathbf{w}||$ may deserve an explanation. The first argument in favor of $||\mathbf{w}||$ is that, for better generalization, it has been shown in the literature that the magnitude of the weights is more important than the number of weights (Bartlett 1997) and, of course, the magnitude of the weights can be directly controlled by $||\mathbf{w}||$. The second argument is that the class separation margin of two classes is inversely proportional to $||\mathbf{w}||$ (Vapnik 1995; Boser et al. 1992), which implies that margin maximization is yielded by $||\mathbf{w}||$ minimization.

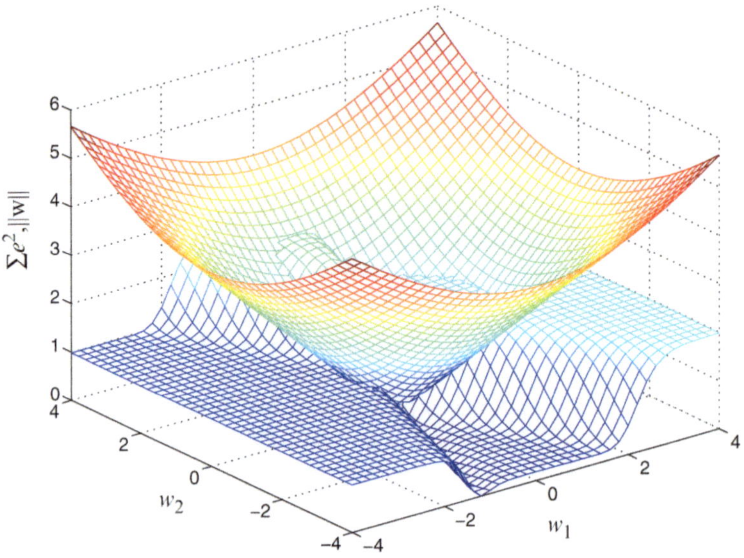

Fig. 8.3 Error and norm surfaces superimposed

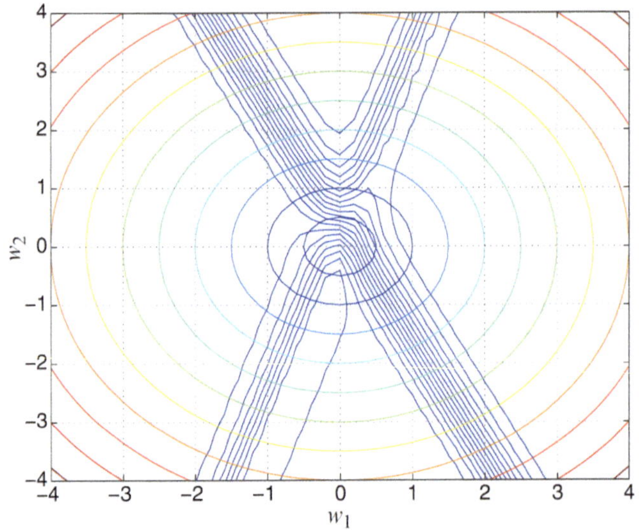

Fig. 8.4 Contour plot of the error and norm surfaces of Fig. 8.3

The role of $||\mathbf{w}||$ in controlling model capacity can be best understood by observing the graphs of Figs. 8.3 and 8.4. Figure 8.3 shows the error and norm functions for a one-variable regression problem approximated by a single logistic neuron with two weights w_1 and w_2. The corresponding contour plots are presented

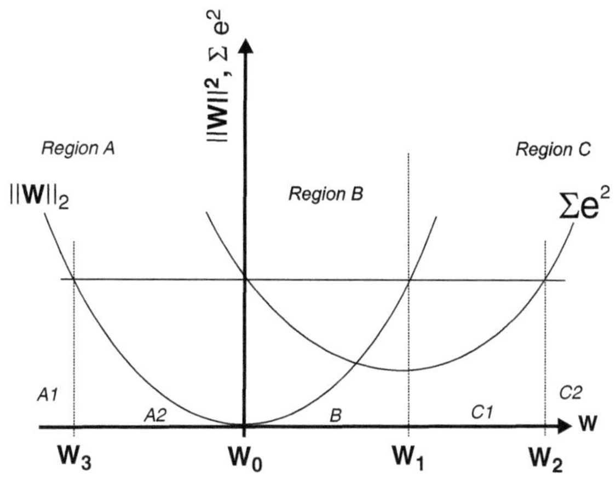

Fig. 8.5 Schematic diagram of the regions of interest of the parameter w

in Fig. 8.4, where it can be seen that the region $||\mathbf{w}|| \leq \delta$ encloses all solutions within a disc, or hypersphere in higher dimensions, with radius δ. Therefore, it is possible to constrain the search space and, consequently, the capacity of a family of functions, by limiting the upper bound of the norm of the weight vector.

8.4.2 *Pareto Set*

The two objective functions $\phi_e(\cdot) = \sum e^2$ and $\phi_c(\cdot) = ||\mathbf{w}||$ are conflicting for the simple reason that error reduction requires weight magnitude increase in order to reach the saturation regions of the sigmoidal activation functions. If they were not conflicting, a trivial solution would be characterized, since a single weight vector would minimize both objectives. The Pareto set (Chankong and Haimes 1983) corresponds to the region of the objective's space where the non-dominated solutions are located. From the optimization point of view, the Pareto set contains *all the optimal solutions* of the formulated optimization problem. From this perspective, any method that is not Pareto-set-based is likely to generate suboptimal solutions that could still be minimized in both objectives. Further discussions and results related to the MOBJ principles were presented in other related works (Teixeira et al. 2000; Braga et al. 2006). Since there is not a single solution in the Pareto set, the learning problem now, after the Pareto set has been generated, becomes the selection of one of them.

In order to represent the solutions, given by individual values of $\mathbf{w}$, in a new space defined by error and norm, the corresponding pair of values $(\sum e^2, ||\mathbf{w}||)$ of Fig. 8.5 are mapped, for every value of $\mathbf{w}$, into a new coordinate system. The new graph obtained is sketched in Fig. 8.6, where the five regions of Fig. 8.5 are also

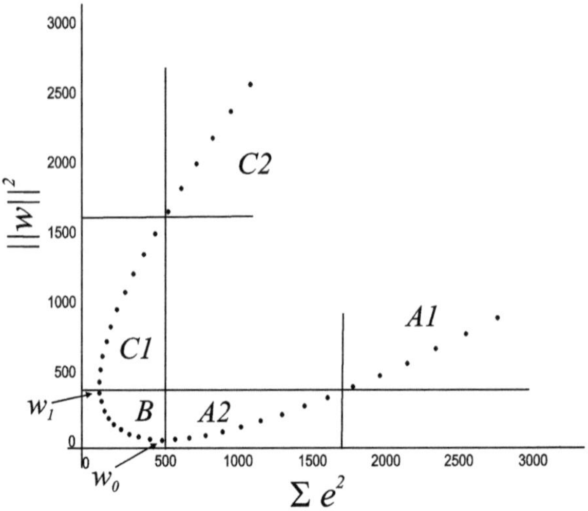

Fig. 8.6 Solutions of Fig. 8.5 mapped onto the space of objectives $||\mathbf{w}||$ and $\sum e^2$

represented. It can be observed in the new graph that regions A1 and C2 are above region B in both coordinates and regions A2 and C1 are above region B in at least one of them. Region B, the Pareto front (Chankong and Haimes 1983), is, therefore, located in the lowest portion of the space of objectives and contains the efficient solutions for the two objective functions.

8.4.3 Multi-Objective Learning Formulation

In order to obtain the Pareto set – efficient solutions for the Multi-Layer Perceptron (MLP) learning problem, the ε-constraint algorithm (Haimes et al. 1971) has been adopted (Teixeira et al. 2000). Basically, the ε-constraint algorithm turns the multi-objective problem into a single objective problem with constraints in order to generate one solution of the Pareto set at a time. From Eq. 8.6, a discrete set of solutions is generated using the ellipsoid algorithm (Bland et al. 1981) for every ε_j constraint value

$$\begin{aligned} &\text{minimize } \textstyle\sum e^2 \\ &\text{subject to } ||\mathbf{w}|| \leq \varepsilon_j \end{aligned} \tag{8.6}$$

for all $j = 1, 2, ..., m$, where $\mathbf{w} \in S$, S is the feasible region and $\varepsilon_j \leq \varepsilon_k$, $\forall j \leq k$.

The analogy between the constraint yielded in the objective's space by limiting the upper bound of $||\mathbf{w}||$ can be best understood by observing Fig. 8.7. Since the error is minimized within the disc with radius $||\mathbf{w}|| \leq \varepsilon_j$, a Pareto set solution is generated for each disc. The optimization problem is then solved for pre-established

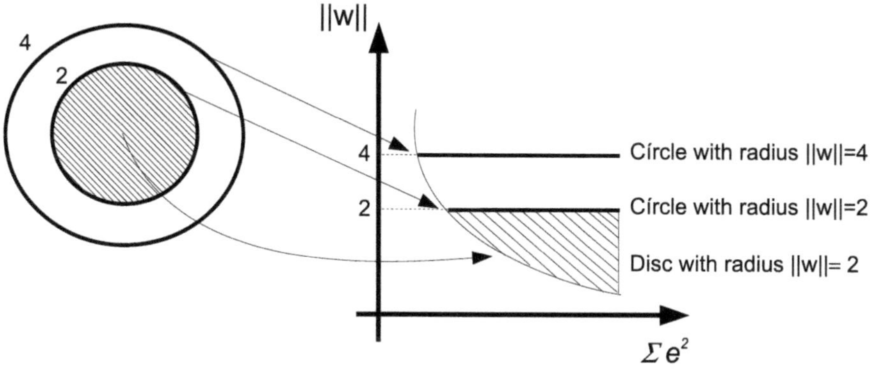

Fig. 8.7 Mapping from parameter's space to objective's space by constraining the solutions to the region $||\mathbf{w}|| \leq \varepsilon$

values of ε_j so that a portion of the Pareto set is generated. Once the set of Pareto set solutions is obtained, a decision-making procedure picks up one of them according to a selection criteria.

8.4.4 Selection Criteria

The Pareto set decider is expected to choose the solution that best fits the generator function $f_g(\mathbf{x})$, without being affected by the additive noise ξ in the data. Consider the supervised learning of a MLP, with the training examples given by the sample points $D_L = \{\mathbf{x}_i, y_i\}_{i=1}^N$: $\{(\mathbf{x}_i, y_i)|y_i = f_g(\mathbf{x}_i) + \xi_i\}_{i=1}^N$. The sampling uncertainty ξ_i is assumed to be an independent and identically distributed (i.i.d.) zero mean random variable, $\mathbf{x}_i$ is a multidimensional input, y_i is a scaled output, N is the sample size, and $f_g(\mathbf{x}_i)$ is the generator function. The training data is also considered to be i.i.d. according to some (unknown) joint probability density function. From a given set of Pareto-optimal solutions, the selection criteria should minimize the distance between the approximating ($f(\mathbf{x}_i, \mathrm{w})$) and generator ($f_g(\mathbf{x}_i)$) functions without any knowledge about $f_g(\mathbf{x}_i)$. Selection is accomplished according to the training data and behavior of the solutions withing the Pareto set.

Although other selection criteria have been developed (Teixeira et al. 2007; Medeiros and Braga 2007), the use of a validation set error seems to be a natural principle. It is based on a validation set $D_v = \{\mathbf{x}_i, d_i\}_{i=1}^{N_v}$ that is presented to every MLP within the Pareto set in the decision phase. The MLP with minimum validation error is chosen as the final solution as can be seen in Eq. 8.7

$$\mathbf{w}^* = \arg \min_{\mathbf{w} \in \mathcal{W}} e_v \tag{8.7}$$

where e_v is represented by

$$e_v = \frac{1}{N_v} \sum_{i=1}^{N_v} [(d_i) - f(\mathrm{x}_i; \mathbf{w})]^2. \tag{8.8}$$

Other strategies for selecting the final solution from the Pareto set have also been developed (Kokshenev and Braga 2008). In the example that follows, the sum of signed errors of the training set was used as a decision strategy.

8.5 ECG Example

In order to provide an example of Neural Networks learning applied to ECG problems, the Arrhythmia dataset available at the UCI website was used (Guvenir et al. 1997). The dataset contains 279 attributes, 206 of which are linear-valued and the rest are nominal. There are 245 examples of normal ECG and 207 of 15 types of arrhythmia, including coronary artery disease, myocardial infarction, sinus tachycardia, sinus bradycardia, right bundle branch block, and atrial fibrillation. In order to treat the problem as a binary classification one, the 207 examples of arrhythmia were joined in a single class.

Due to the high dimensionality of the problem, feature selection based on the F-Score was accomplished in the 279 attributes (Guyon 2003), resulting in a dataset with 18 variables. Since there was also missing data, some records were also eliminated. The final dataset had 428 samples with 18 features, of which 80% were selected for training and 20% for testing.

A multi-layer perceptron trained with the multi-objective learning algorithm was then used to solve the problem. The Pareto set yielded by the training data is presented in Fig. 8.8. The decision-making strategy adopted was based on the sum of signed errors of the training set and yielded solution number 8, as indicated in the graph of Fig. 8.8. The corresponding MLP was then retrieved and applied to the test set, resulting in 77% accuracy. Since the selection criteria adopted are based on the training data only, there was no need for a validation set. Other methods, such as SVMs, would demand an additional validation set which would result in reductions on training/test sets' sizes. Since discrepancies in data set sizes could result in unfair comparisons between models, we have accomplished a grid search on SVM parameters, considering test set data only. Of course, test set performance cannot be used as a performance measure in such a situation, since it was used for model selection. Anyways, it gives us an idea of how good is the MOBJ solution. The SVM parameters obtained with such a procedure were $C = 33$ and $r = 2$, which yielded 79% performance in the test set. This result, of course, cannot be directly compared with the 77% obtained with the MLP, but it shows that the performance of the ANN model obtained with MOBJ training is very close to the best performance that could be obtained if the test set were used for model selection.

Signal representation for practical use of ANNs for ECG classification and prediction is usually accomplished by frequency domain representation and statistical feature extraction. The problem consists basically of representing the ECG data

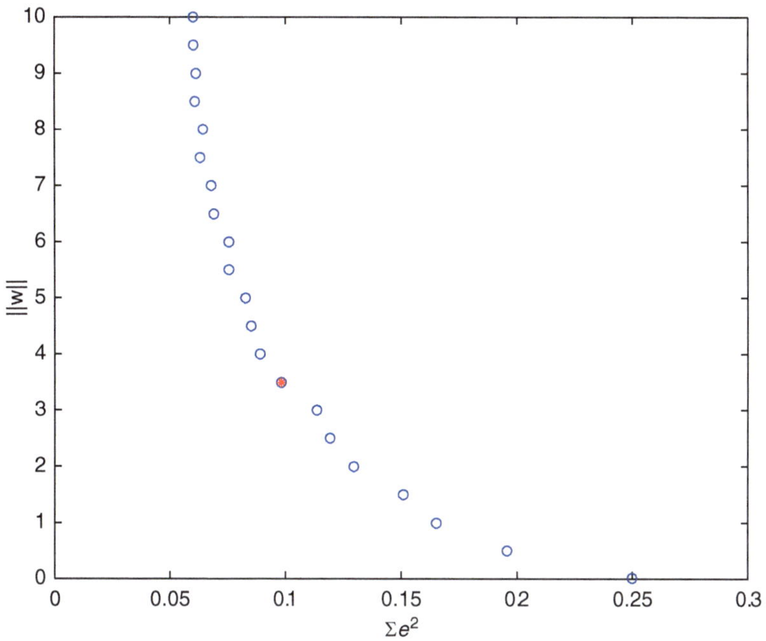

Fig. 8.8 Pareto set obtained (*in circles*) from the ECG dataset and the corresponding solution indicated as a *

points into a few parameters that are representative of the underlying problem. For instance, if a beat classifier is to be developed, parameters representing beat frequency and length should be selected. For this particular problem, Fourier and Wavelet transforms could be applied. There are many other approaches for general feature extraction and selection that are known in the literature (Guyon 2003) which could be used for ANNs applications. The choice for the most appropriate extraction method will depend, however, on the problem itself and on what is aimed to be represented.

8.6 Conclusions

As discussed in this chapter, Neural Networks learning should be accomplished by considering both the empirical risk $R_{\mathrm{emp}}(\mathbf{w})$ and the model capacity h. Convergence to the true risk under the single-objective assumption, considering only $R_{\mathrm{emp}}(\mathbf{w})$, can only be achieved in the large samples scenario. In such a situation, when $N \to \infty$, the approximating function $f(\mathbf{x},\mathbf{w})$ tends to $E[y|\mathbf{x}]$ regardless of model capacity; nevertheless, this situation does not happen very often. In most real problems, the sample size is small and minimization of $R_{\mathrm{emp}}(\mathbf{w})$ does not assure approximation to the generator function. In such situations, model capacity h should also be considered in order to improve convergence to the true risk. Since $R_{\mathrm{emp}}(\mathbf{w})$ and h

do not have coinciding minima, these two objective functions can only be traded-off instead of jointly minimized.

The conflicting behavior of $R_{\text{emp}}(\mathbf{w})$ and h and the need for a trade-off between them suggests that the Neural Networks learning problem is inherently multi-objective and that it should be treated like that. Therefore, from the optimization perspective, the Pareto set solutions are optimal and offer a proper trade-off between $R_{\text{emp}}(\mathbf{w})$ and h. In addition, any other solution, generated by any other method, that is not Pareto-optimal can still be minimized in both objectives.

This chapter presented the general Neural Networks learning problem under the multi-objective learning perspective. A formulation of the problem, based on the ε-constrained optimization method, was presented, so that an approximation of the Pareto-front is achieved. The availability of the Pareto set solutions guarantee that the search is accomplished among the optimal solutions only, and not in the whole parameter's space. Further work in this area should involve the development of new decision-making criteria methods and of improved methods to generate the Pareto set.

References

Bartlett, P.: For valid generalization, the size of the weights is more important than the size of the network. In: Proceedings of NIPS, vol. 9, pp. 134–140. Morgan Kaufmann Publishers, San Mateo (1997)

Bland, R.G., Goldfarb, D., Todd, M.J.: The ellipsoidal method: A survey. Operations Res. **29**, 1039–1091 (1981)

Boser, B., Guyon, I., Vapnik, V.: A training algorithm for optimal margin classfiers. In: Fifth Annual Workshop on Computational Learning Theory, pp. 144–152. ACM, New York (1992)

Braga, A.P., Takahashi, R., Teixeira, R., Costa, M.A.: Multi- objective algorithms for neural networks learning. In: Jin, Y. (ed.) Multiobjective Machine Learning, pp. 151–172. Springer-Verlag, Berlin/Heidelberg (2006)

Broomhead, D.S., Lowe, D.: Multivariable function interpolation and adaptive networks. Complex Syst. **2**, 321–355 (1988)

Chankong, V., Haimes, Y.Y.: Multiobjective Decision Making: Theory and Methodology, vol. 8. North-Holland (Elsevier), New York (1983)

Craven, M.W.: Extracting Comprehensible Models From Trained Neural Network. PhD thesis, University of Wisconsin, Madison (1996)

Fahlman, S.E., Lebiere, C.: The cascade-correlation learning architecture. In: Lippmann, R.P., Moody, J.E., Touretzky, D.S. (eds.) Advances in Neural Information Processing Systems 2. Morgan Kaufmann, San Mateo (1988)

Fisher, R.A.: The use of multiple measurements in taxonomic problems. Ann. Eugenics **7**, 179–188 (1936)

Geman, S., Bienenstock, E., Doursat, R.: Neural networks and the bias-variance dilemma. Neural Comput. **4**, 1–58 (1992)

Guvenir, H.A., Acar, B., Demiroz, G., Cekin, A.: A supervised machine learning algorithm for arrhythmia analysis. In: Computers in Cardiology, pp. 433–436. IEEE, Piscataway (1997)

Guyon, I.: An introduction to variable and feature selection. J. Mach. Learn. Res. **3**, 1157–1182 (2003)

Hagan, M., Menhaj, M.: Training feedforward networks with the Marquardt algorithm. IEEE Trans. Neural Netw. **5**, 989–993 (1994)

Haimes, Y., Lasdon, L., Wismer, D.: On a bicriterion formulation of the problems of integrated system identification and system optimization. IEEE Trans. Syst. Man Cybern. **1**, 296–297 (1971)

Karnin, E.D.: A simple procedure for pruning back-propagation trained neural networks. IEEE Trans. Neural Netw. **1**, 239–242 (1990)

Kokshenev, I., Braga, A.: Complexity bounds and multi- objective learning of radial basis functions. Neurocomput. **71**, 1203–1209 (2008)

LeCun, Y., Denker, J., Solla, S.: Optimal brain damage. In: Touretzky, D. (ed.) Neural Information Processing Systems, vol. 2, pp. 598–605. Morgan Kaufmann, San Mateo/Denver (1990)

Liu, G., Kadirkamanathan, V.: Learning with multi-objective criteria. In: International Conference on Neural Networks (UK), pp. 53–58. IEEE, Perth (1995)

Medeiros, T., Braga, A.P.: A new decision strategy in multi-objective training of artificial neural networks. In: European Symposium on Neural Networks (ESANN07), pp. 555–560. Bruges (2007)

Mezard, M., Nadal, J.: Learning in feedforward neural net- works: The tiling algorithm. J. Phys. A: Math Gen. **22**, 2191–2203 (1989)

Mozer, M.C., Smolensky, P.: Skeletonization: A technique for trimming the fat from a network via relabance assessment. In: Touretzky, D.S. (ed.) Advances in Neural Information Processing Systems, vol. 1, pp. 107–115. Morgan Kaufmann, New York (1989)

Rosenblatt, F.: The perceptron: A probabilistic model for information storage and organization in the brain. Psychol. Rev. **65**, 386–408 (1958)

Shannon, C.: A mathematical theory of communication. Bell. Syst. Tech. J. **27**, 379–423 (1948)

Teixeira, R., Braga, A., Takahashi, R., Rezende, R.: Improving generalization of mlps with multi-objetive optimization. Neurocomput. **35**, 189–194 (2000)

Teixeira, R.A., Braga, A., Saldanha, R.R., Takahashi, R.H.C., Medeiros, T.H.: The usage of golden section in calculating the efficient solution in artificial neural networks training by multi-objective optimization. In: International Conference on Neural Networks (ICANN07). Springer, Berlin/Heidelberg (2007)

Vapnik, V.: The Nature of Statistical Learning Theory. Springer, New York (1995)

Wahba, G.: Generalization and regularization in nonlinear learning systems. Technical Report 921, University of Winsconsin, Madison (1994)

Chapter 9
A Review of Kernel Methods in ECG Signal Classification

José L. Rojo-Álvarez, Gustavo Camps-Valls, Antonio J. Caamaño-Fernández, and Juan F. Guerrero-Martínez

9.1 Introduction

An electrocardiogram (ECG) is the graphical representation of the electrical activity of the heart as it is recorded from the body surface (Kilpatrick and Johnston 1994). Noninvasive electrocardiography has been proven to be a highly useful method for obtaining information about the state of a patient's heart and for detecting cardiac pathologies. The goal of ECG discrimination is to classify the recorded signal into one of a possible number of diagnostic classes, and consequently, to administer the most suitable treatment. The clinical staff can perform this process through visual inspection of the continuous ECG, but this process is time consuming and requires intensive involvement of experts. In addition, the ECG commonly presents high inter- and intra-patient variability both in morphology and timing (Watrous and Towell 1995), and thus even experienced surgeons or cardiologists can misinterpret the data. Actually, although cardiac monitoring has made remarkable progress since the early work of Einthoven (1901), cardiovascular diseases are still a major cause of mortality. It has been demonstrated that rapid treatment leads not only to a reduction in the infarct size, but also to a decrease in the mortality rate. As a consequence, intelligent systems capable of assisting doctors, staff in coronary intensive care units, and pharmacy services in hospitals, are needed. Such systems should be easily implementable, scalable, accurate, robust, and stable. In addition, adaptability to uncommon situations is also desirable. This has led to the appearance

J.L. Rojo-Álvarez (✉) · A.J. Caamaño-Fernández
Universidad Rey Juan Carlos de Madrid, Camino del Molino s/n, Fuenlabrada, Madrid, Spain
e-mail: joseluis.rojo@urjc.es; antonio.caamano@urjc.es

G. Camps-Valls · J.F. Guerrero-Martínez
Universitat de València, C/ Dr. Moliner, 50. Burjassot (València), Spain
e-mail: gustavo.camps@uv.es; juan.guerrero@uv.es

A. Gacek and W. Pedrycz (eds.), *ECG Signal Processing, Classification and Interpretation: A Comprehensive Framework of Computational Intelligence*,
DOI 10.1007/978-0-85729-868-3_9,

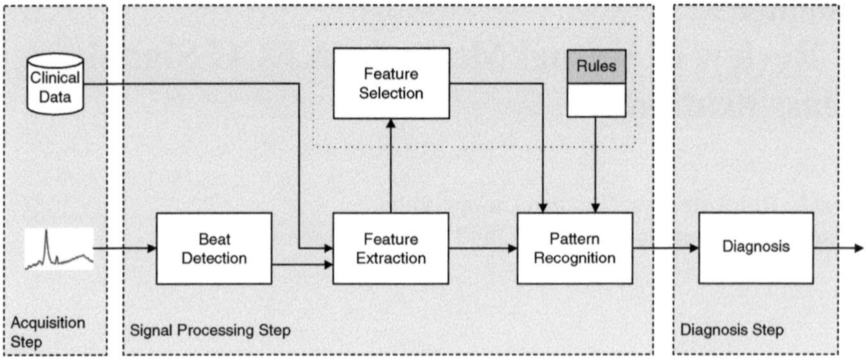

Fig. 9.1 Schematic representation of a usual learning scheme for electrocardiogram (ECG) pattern recognition

of computer-based classification approaches and their implementation in the daily clinical routine to yield more consistent and faster detection.

Intelligent supervision systems (Mora et al. 1993) appeared in the 1990s aiming to overcome the drawbacks of first-generation monitors (Le Blanc 1986). Their purpose was to integrate several sources of observation and several types of medical knowledge, and to build interactive and helpful supervision systems. Their main objectives today are: (1) to detect abnormal situations by analyzing the signals, (2) to predict the occurrence of abnormal events, (3) to give therapeutic advice, and (4) to explain the underlying mechanism generating the disorder.

In these approaches, three main tasks are identified: (1) the acquisition step, in which acquired ECGs and data from patients' follow-up are gathered; (2) the signal-processing step, which processes the acquired signals and data to produce a relevant description of the signals; and (3) the diagnosis step, which has to detect potential pathologies as early as possible, and to characterize the situation on the basis of the previous processing steps. Figure 9.1 illustrates this general learning scheme for ECG pathology discrimination. In this chapter, we will focus on the second step, which has been previously formalized by some authors (Carrault et al. 2003; Nugent et al. 1999). Various methodologies of automated ECG classification for simultaneous (or posterior) diagnosis are found in the literature. The entire process can be generally subdivided into a number of processing modules: (1) beat detection, (2) feature extraction/selection, and (3) classification or diagnosis.

The first preprocessing block of beat detection aims to locate each cardiac cycle QRS in each of the recording leads, for subsequent insertion of reference markers indicating the beginning and end of each inter-wave component (Nugent et al. 1999). The accuracy of detection of each cardiac cycle is of great importance since it contributes significantly to the overall classification result. The markers are subsequently processed during the feature extraction step, where measurements are generated for wave amplitudes, frequencies, and durations.

In the majority of cases, detection of abnormal waves requires a preliminary feature extraction step, in which characteristics from the signal in time (duration, slope, or amplitude of waves), frequency (energy in bands), or time-frequency domains (time and energy simultaneous feature scales), are extracted. An optional feature selection can be included in this process, by which the dimensionality of feature vectors is reduced, including only the most relevant features necessary for discrimination and sometimes assisted by a priori knowledge or rules.

The pattern recognition step involves development of intelligent systems dealing with the extracted and selected information in the previous step. A large number of machine learning approaches have been used to identify different types of cardiac pathology. The diagnosis step consists of identifying pathological conditions. It is worth noting that the diagnosis step can either directly exploit the classification provided by the signal-processing step (relevant features and classifier) or translate the information provided by the signal-processing step into the most accurate diagnosis according to a predetermined protocol. In the first case, the classifier is trained to provide an explicitly defined diagnosis class. In the second case, the clinical diagnosis is provided by means of a determined inductive principle from the signal-processing step. Abduction reasoning is generally associated to model-based diagnosis. However, these techniques are computationally demanding and useless for real-time monitoring. As a consequence, models closer to classification/recognition are usually preferred for diagnosis.

In the literature, there are excellent reviews of applications of machine learning algorithms in medicine in general, and cardiology in particular (Dybowski 2000; Miller et al. 1992; Kumaravel et al. 1997; Abreu-Lima and de Sa 1998; Itchhaporia et al. 1996; Watrous and Towell 1995; Abboud et al. 2002; Lisboa et al. 2002; Camps-Valls and Guerrero-Martínez 2006). It is worth to note that the use of nonparametric classification tools, such as decision trees (Exarchos et al. 2007), neural networks (Camps-Valls and Guerrero-Martínez 2006), or Support Vector Machines (SVMs), has yielded promising results for the discrimination of different types of cardiac pathology. The use of such methods is commonly encouraged by their theoretical and practical advantages, given that it is not strictly necessary to assume a specific relationship between variables. They provide nonlinear flexible mappings, and they have proven to be effective techniques in a wide range of applications.

In the task of ECG classification, the classical feedforward neural network trained with the back-propagation learning algorithm is usually employed. However, further improvement can be obtained when using more elaborate neural or kernel methods. After a thorough revision of the literature, researchers and medical staff often use sophisticated approaches in easy problems and vice versa. Sometimes the authors notice poor performance and lack of interpretability of neural networks compared to simpler models. Other problems have been also identified. For instance, the risk of falling in local minima or the need for regularization should be considered (Lisboa et al. 2002). This chapter concentrates on the recent spread of SVMs for pathology discrimination, which alleviates some of the previous problems. SVM is a well-known regularized kernel-based method which can handle large input spaces efficiently, and can effectively work with reduced datasets, alleviate overfitting by controlling the margin, and automatically identify the most critical informative examples in the training set, namely, support vectors. In fact, an important issue in model development, previously highlighted in Lisboa et al. (2002), is model regularization, which allows us to obtain smooth and robust solutions, combating, in a certain way, the overfitting problem. There are some works aimed at obtaining fast and regularized neural-network solutions, but using heuristics (Mahalingam and Kumar 1997). However, kernel methods provide more elegant formulations for the regularization task, which is drawn naturally from the minimizing function. The SVM classifier has been widely used in the ECG data processing community in the recent years. However, SVMs are only one particular kernel method. In this chapter we aim at reviewing the theory of generic kernel machines and revising the main applications in ECG data processing. However, noting that most of the applications deal with the use of SVM, we provide with a systematic revision of other kernel methods that could be eventually used in this application field.

The rest of this chapter is outlined as follows. Section 9.2 presents a brief introduction to kernel methods, fixes notation of SVM classifiers, and reviews the basic properties. Section 9.3 is devoted to review the main applications of SVM in the field of ECG data classification. Section 9.4 reviews the recent developments and foresees the future trends in kernel machines for ECG data analysis. Section 9.5 concludes the chapter with some final remarks.

9.2 Introduction to Kernel Classification Methods

This section includes a brief introduction to kernel methods. After setting the scenario and fixing the most common notation, we give the main properties of kernel methods. We also pay attention to the development of kernel methods by means of particular properties drawn from linear algebra and functional analysis (Golub and Van Loan 1996; Reed and Simon 1980).

9.2.1 Measuring Similarity with Kernels

Kernel methods rely on the notion of similarity between examples. Let us define a set of empirical data $(\mathbf{x}_1, y_1), \ldots, (\mathbf{x}_n, y_n) \in \mathcal{X} \times \mathcal{Y}$, where $\mathbf{x}_i$ are the *inputs* taken from $\mathcal{X}$ and $y_i \in \mathcal{Y}$ are called the *outputs*. Learning means using these data pairs to predict well on test examples $\mathbf{x} \in \mathcal{X}$. To develop machines that generalize well, kernel methods try to exploit the structure of the data and thus define a similarity between pairs of samples.

Since $\mathcal{X}$ may not have a proper notion of similarity, examples are mapped to a (dot product) space $\mathcal{H}$, by using a mapping $\phi : \mathcal{X} \to \mathcal{H}, \mathbf{x} \mapsto \phi(\mathbf{x})$. The similarity between the elements in $\mathcal{H}$ can now be measured using its associated dot product

$\langle\cdot,\cdot\rangle_{\mathcal{H}}$. Here, we define a function that computes that similarity, $K:\mathcal{X}\times\mathcal{X}\rightarrow\mathbb{R}$, such that $(\mathbf{x},\mathbf{x}')\mapsto K(\mathbf{x},\mathbf{x}')$. This function, called *kernel*, is required to satisfy:

$$K(\mathbf{x},\mathbf{x}')=\langle\phi(\mathbf{x}),\phi(\mathbf{x}')\rangle_{\mathcal{H}}. \tag{9.1}$$

The mapping ϕ is its *feature map*, and the space $\mathcal{H}$ is its *feature space*.

9.2.2 Positive Definite Kernels

The class of kernels that can be written in the form of (9.1) coincides with the class of positive definite kernels.

Definition 9.1. A function $K:\mathcal{X}\times\mathcal{X}\rightarrow\mathbb{R}$ is a positive definite kernel *if and only if* there exists a Hilbert space $\mathcal{H}$ and a feature map $\phi:\mathcal{X}\rightarrow\mathcal{H}$ such that for all $\mathbf{x},\mathbf{x}'\in\mathcal{X}$ we have $K(\mathbf{x},\mathbf{x}')=\langle\phi(\mathbf{x}),\phi(\mathbf{x}')\rangle_{\mathcal{H}}$.

In practice, a real symmetric $n\times n$ matrix $\mathbf{K}$, whose entries are $K(\mathbf{x}_i,\mathbf{x}_j)$ or simply K_{ij}, is called *positive definite* if for all $c_1,\ldots,c_n\in\mathbb{R}$, $\sum_{i,j=1}^{n}c_ic_jK_{ij}\geq 0$. Note that a positive definite kernel is equivalent to a positive definite Gram matrix in the *feature space*.

Therefore, algorithms operating on the data only in terms of dot products can be used with any positive definite kernel by simply replacing $\langle\phi(\mathbf{x}),\phi(\mathbf{x}')\rangle_{\mathcal{H}}$ with kernel evaluations $K(\mathbf{x},\mathbf{x}')$, a technique also known as the *kernel trick* (Schölkopf and Smola 2002). Another direct consequence is that, for a positive definite kernel, one does not need to know the explicit form of the feature map since it is implicitly defined through the kernel.

9.2.3 Standard Kernels

The bottleneck for any kernel method is the definition of a kernel mapping function ϕ that accurately reflects the similarity among samples. However, not all kernel similarity functions are permitted. In fact, valid kernels are only those fulfilling Mercer's Theorem (roughly speaking, corresponding to positive definite similarity matrices) and the most common ones are the linear $K(\mathbf{x},\mathbf{z})=\langle\mathbf{x},\mathbf{z}\rangle$, the polynomial $K(\mathbf{x},\mathbf{z})=(\langle\mathbf{x},\mathbf{z}\rangle+1)^d$, $d\in\mathbb{Z}^+$, and the radial basis function (RBF), $K(\mathbf{x},\mathbf{z})=\exp\left(-\|\mathbf{x}-\mathbf{z}\|^2/2\sigma^2\right)$, $\sigma\in\mathbb{R}^+$. Note that, by Taylor series expansion, the RBF kernel is a polynomial kernel with infinite degree. Thus the corresponding Hilbert space is infinite dimensional, which corresponds to a mapping into the space of smooth functions $\mathcal{C}^\infty$. The RBF kernel is also of practical convenience – stability and only one parameter to be tuned –, and it is the preferred kernel measure in standard applications (Schölkopf and Smola 2002).

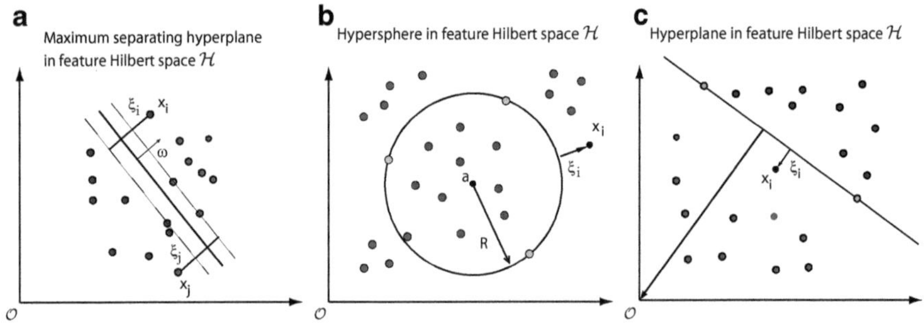

Fig. 9.2 Illustration of kernel classifiers. (**a**) SVM: Linear decision hyperplanes in a nonlinearly transformed, feature space, where *slack* variables ξ_i are included to deal with errors. (**b**) SVDD: The hypersphere containing the target data is described by center **a** and radius R. Samples in the boundary and outside the ball are unbounded and bounded support vectors, respectively. (**c**) OC-SVM: Another way of solving the data description problem, where all samples from the target class are mapped with maximum distance to the origin

9.2.4 SVM Equations

The SVM is defined as follows. Notationally, given a labeled training data set $\{\mathbf{x}_i, y_i\}_{i=1}^n$, where $\mathbf{x}_i \in \mathbb{R}^N$ and $y_i \in \{-1, +1\}$, and given a nonlinear mapping $\phi(\cdot)$, the SVM method solves:

$$\min_{\mathbf{w},\xi_i,b} \left\{ \frac{1}{2}\|\mathbf{w}\|^2 + C\sum_{i=1}^{n} \xi_i \right\} \tag{9.2}$$

constrained to:

$$y_i(\langle \phi(\mathbf{x}_i), \mathbf{w} \rangle + b) \geq 1 - \xi_i \quad \forall i = 1, \ldots, n \tag{9.3}$$

$$\xi_i \geq 0 \qquad \forall i = 1, \ldots, n \tag{9.4}$$

where **w** and b define a linear classifier in the feature space, and ξ_i are positive slack variables enabling to deal with permitted errors (Fig. 9.2a). Note that the functional to be minimized in (9.2) has two terms: a regularization term $\|w\|^2$, whose minimization is equivalent to the maximization of the margin (the separation between classes), and the loss function, which in the case of SVMs is a linear function of the committed errors. Appropriate choice of nonlinear mapping ϕ guarantees that the transformed samples are more likely to be linearly separable in the (higher dimension) feature space. The regularization parameter C controls the generalization capability of the classifier, and it must be selected by the user. Primal problem (9.2) is solved using its dual problem counterpart (Schölkopf and Smola 2002), and the decision function for any test vector $\mathbf{x}_*$ is finally given by

$$f(\mathbf{x}_*) = sgn\left(\sum_{i=1}^{n} y_i \alpha_i K(\mathbf{x}_i, \mathbf{x}_*) + b\right) \tag{9.5}$$

where α_i are Lagrange multipliers corresponding to constraints in (9.3), being the support vectors (SVs) those training samples $\mathbf{x}_i$ with nonzero Lagrange multipliers $\alpha_i \neq 0$; $K(\mathbf{x}_i, \mathbf{x}_*)$ is an element of a kernel matrix $\mathbf{K}$ defined as in (9.1); and bias term b is calculated by using the *unbounded* Lagrange multipliers as $b = 1/k \sum_{i=1}^{k} (y_i - \langle \phi(\mathbf{x}_i), \mathbf{w} \rangle)$, where k is the number of *unbounded* Lagrange multipliers ($0 \leqslant \alpha_i < C$); and $\mathbf{w} = \sum_{i=1}^{n} y_i \alpha_i \phi(\mathbf{x}_i)$ (Schölkopf and Smola 2002).

9.2.5 *ν*-Support Vector Machine

One interesting variation of the SVM is the ν-SVM introduced by Schölkopf et al. (2000). In the SVM formulation, the soft margin is controlled by parameter C, which may take any positive value. This makes difficult to adjust it when training the classifier. The idea of the ν-SVM is forcing the soft margin to lie in the range $[0, 1]$. This is carried out by redefining the problem as

$$\min_{\mathbf{w}, \xi_i, b, \rho} \left\{ \frac{1}{2} \|\mathbf{w}\|^2 + \nu\rho + \frac{1}{n} \sum_{i=1}^{n} \xi_i \right\} \tag{9.6}$$

subject to:

$$y_i(\langle \phi(\mathbf{x}_i), \mathbf{w} \rangle + b) \geq \rho - \xi_i \quad \forall i = 1, \ldots, n \tag{9.7}$$

$$\rho \geq 0,\ \xi_i \geq 0 \qquad \forall i = 1, \ldots, n \tag{9.8}$$

In this new formulation, parameter C has been removed and a new variable ρ with coefficient ν has been introduced. This new variable ρ adds another degree of freedom to the margin, the size of the margin increasing linearly with ρ. The old parameter C controlled the trade-off between the training error and the generalization error. In the ν-SVM formulation, this is done adjusting ν in the range $[0, 1]$, which acts as an upper bound on the fraction of margin errors, and it is also a lower bound on the fraction of support vectors.

9.2.6 Support Vector Data Description

A different problem statement for classification is given by the support vector domain description (SVDD) (Tax and Duin 1999). The SVDD is a method to solve one-class problems, where one tries to describe one class of objects, distinguishing them from all other possible objects.

The problem is defined as follows. Let $\{\mathbf{x}_i\}_{i=1}^n$ be a dataset belonging to a given *class of interest*. The purpose is to find a minimum volume *hypersphere* in a high-dimensional feature space $\mathcal{H}$, with radius $R > 0$ and center $\mathbf{a} \in \mathcal{H}$, which contains most of these data objects (Fig. 9.2b). Since the training set may contain outliers, a set of *slack variables* $\xi_i \geq 0$ is introduced, and the problem becomes

$$\min_{R,\mathbf{a}} \left\{ R^2 + C \sum_{i=1}^{n} \xi_i \right\} \tag{9.9}$$

constrained to

$$\|\phi(\mathbf{x}_i) - \mathbf{a}\|^2 \leq R^2 + \xi_i \quad \forall i = 1, \ldots, n \tag{9.10}$$

$$\xi_i \geq 0 \qquad \forall i = 1, \ldots, n \tag{9.11}$$

where parameter C controls the trade-off between the volume of the hypersphere and the permitted errors. Parameter ν, defined as $\nu = 1/nC$, can be used as a rejection fraction parameter to be tuned as noted in Schölkopf et al. (1999).

The dual functional is a quadratic programming problem that yields a set of Lagrange multipliers (α_i) corresponding to constraints in Eq. 9.10. When the free parameter C is adjusted properly, most of the α_i are zero, giving a sparse solution. The Lagrange multipliers are also used to calculate the distance from a test point to the center $R(\mathbf{x}_*)$:

$$R(\mathbf{x}_*) = K(\mathbf{x}_*, \mathbf{x}_*) - 2 \sum_{i=1}^{n} K(\mathbf{x}_i, \mathbf{x}_*) + \sum_{i,j=1}^{n} K(\mathbf{x}_i, \mathbf{x}_j) \tag{9.12}$$

which is compared with ratio R. Unbounded support vectors are those samples $\mathbf{x}_i$ satisfying $0 \leqslant \alpha_i < C$, while bounded SVs are samples whose associated $\alpha_i = C$, which are considered outliers.

9.2.7 One-Class Support Vector Machine

In the One-Class SVM (OC-SVM), instead of defining a hypersphere containing all examples, a hyperplane that separates the data objects from the origin with maximum margin is defined (Fig. 9.2c). It can be shown that when working with normalized data and the RBF Gaussian kernel, both methods yield the same solutions (Schölkopf et al. 1999).

In the OC-SVM, we want to find a hyperplane $\mathbf{w}$ which separates samples $\mathbf{x}_i$ from the origin with margin ρ. The problem thus becomes

$$\min_{\mathbf{w},\rho,\xi} \left\{ \frac{1}{2}\|\mathbf{w}\|^2 - \rho + \frac{1}{\nu n}\sum_{i=1}^{n} \xi_i \right\} \tag{9.13}$$

constrained to

$$\langle \phi(\mathbf{x}_i), \mathbf{w} \rangle \geq \rho - \xi_i \quad \forall i = 1, \ldots, n \tag{9.14}$$

$$\xi_i \geq 0 \quad \forall i = 1, \ldots, n \tag{9.15}$$

The problem is solved through its Langrangian dual introducing a set of Lagrange multipliers α_i. The margin ρ can be computed as $\rho = \langle \mathbf{w}, \phi(\mathbf{x}_i) \rangle = \sum_j \alpha_j K(\mathbf{x}_i, \mathbf{x}_j)$.

9.3 Applications of Kernel Methods in ECG Data Classification

In this section, we review the vast field of ECG signal classification with kernels in a categorized taxonomy based on the most relevant fields of application. When considered as relevant, the analysis of other cardiac signals, such as intracardiac electrograms (EGMs) recorded in implantable devices, is also included in the review. It is noteworthy to say that during the last years, almost all the usual processing stages of ECG have been revisited from SVM or kernel methods problem statements.

9.3.1 Beat Detection and Arrhythmia Discrimination

As we have seen in the previous sections, an important step for ECG classification is beat detection, which represents the basis for all the subsequent systems. Beat detection usually consists of the estimation of fiducial points allowing to segment the signal into beats, and it is different from the classification of the segmented beat into a number of categories. We next summarize a set of relevant applications of kernel methods to the early stages of ECG processing, namely, wave delineation, abnormal beat detection, and arrhythmia discrimination.

9.3.1.1 Wave Delineation

The wave delineation stage consists not only of the determination of the R wave for a beat-by-beat segmentation (which is the basis for virtually all the subsequent analysis), but also of the automatic identification of the beginning and end of the most relevant waves in the ECG. Accordingly, R wave detection, and time segments for P wave, QRS complex, and T wave, have to be correctly identified in this stage. The usual approach is to use semisupervised systems, so that an expert can then review the annotations of a given algorithm and correct them. However, in today's systems, the correction time can range from some few minutes to more than one hour (for a typical 24-h Holter recording), and hence, algorithms with improved performance are required in order to reduce as much as possible the expensive time of the specialist in this task.

In Mehta and Lingayat (2008a), a system for QRS complexes recognition in ECG is delivered. After preprocessing (low-band and high-band noise removal), an SVM classifier is used to delineate QRS and non-QRS region, achieving 99% of detection rate. In Mehta and Lingayat (2008b), combined entropy criterion is used to enhance the QRS complexes in the same system. In Mehta and Lingayat (2007), a method for detection of T waves in 12-lead ECG is presented. After digital filtering of low-band and high-band noise, an SVM is used as a classifier for T-wave detection on a sliding-window basis. In the CSE Database, the system is capable of reaching 91% detection. In Mehta and Lingayat (2008c), the method is presented for delineation of T wave, QRS complex, and T wave. These works consider an input space given by the amplitudes of the 12-lead ECG gradients, and a desired output given by the ECG samples labeled as inside or outside the delineated intervals. Hence, they can be considered as instantaneous nonlinear envelopment detectors, and comparison to conventional classifiers (such as trees or neural networks) with the same input and output spaces would be informative about the actual superiority of the kernel method. Interestingly, this is one of the few SVM works in which the sigmoid kernel (not always a Mercer's kernel) is chosen as the best performing kernel.

9.3.1.2 Beat Classification

After ECG segmentation based on the previous stage of wave delineation, each segmented beat has to be assigned into a given category. Simplest algorithms just make a distinction between normal and premature ventricular complexes (PVCs), whereas the most advanced algorithms are designed to be able to distinguish among a family of possible kinds of beats (see Fig. 9.3).

In Ribeiro et al. (2007), the detection of PVC is addressed, by means of a system with three stages: feature extraction (amplitudes, durations, and areas), eigen-decomposition of data, and finally an SVM classifier trained for PVC with examples. After using a feature extraction system (recursive feature elimination, RFE), a reduced set of features is combined with spectral clustering to increase the performance of the detection process. In Ribeiro et al. (2008), a system for PVC detection and data visualization is delivered, which exploits the intrinsic

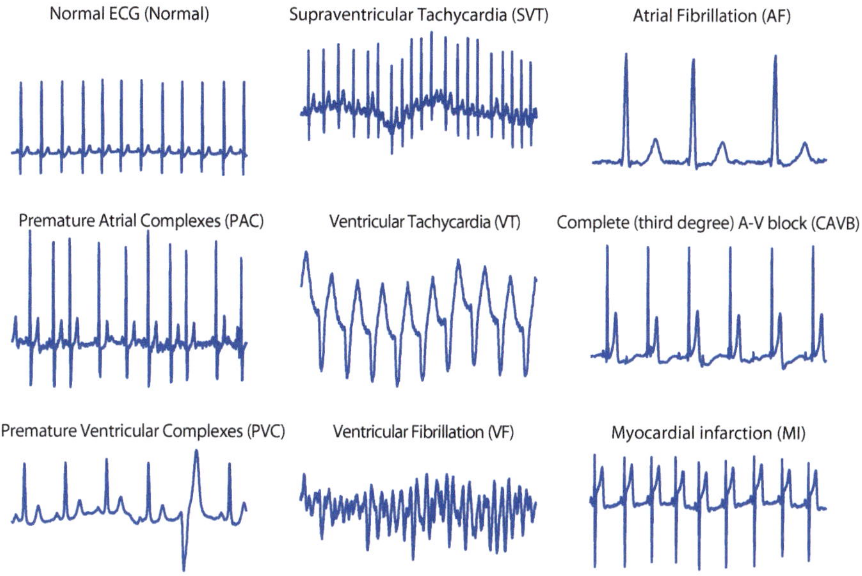

Fig. 9.3 ECG acquisitions for different pathologies and arrhythmias (source: Physionet, http://www.physionet.org/)

geometry of the high-dimensional data using manifold learning and SVM. In brief, a neighborhood-preserving projection is built, which allows to uncover the low-dimensional manifold and can be used for preprocessing and subsequent labeling.

In Zhao and Zhang (2005), the feature extraction of ECG and subsequent classification is addressed by using the wavelet transform and an SVM classifier. Not only the wavelet coefficients are used as features, but also autoregressive modeling is used to obtain the temporal structures of ECG waveform in the considered time segments. Recognition of six different heart rhythm types (normal, left and right bundle branch block, pace, PVC, and atrial premature complex) reaches in this work up to 99% in overall accuracy in the MIT-BIH Arrhythmia Database. In Zellmer et al. (2009), an ECG-based beat classification system is presented, which uses wavelet transform and time domain morphology analysis to form three separate feature vectors from each beat. These vectors are fed separately to three different SVM independent classifiers, and with the result of each, a voting strategy is used to yield the multiclassifier. Up to 99% accuracy is obtained in six different rhythms from MIT-BIH Arrhythmia Database (see precedent work). In Melgani and Bazi (2008), a detailed experimental study is presented to show the capabilities of the SVM for automatic classification of ECG beats. Additionally, authors improve the generalization performance of the SVM classifier by including a particle swarm optimization system, by searching for the best values of the free parameters, and for the best subset of input features. On the MIT-BIH Arrhythmia Database, up to overall 89% accuracy was obtained. In Ubeyli (2007), a multiclass SVM with correcting output codes is presented for classification of four ECG kinds of beats (normal, congestive heart failure, ventricular tachyarrhythmia, atrial fibrillation), from the Physiobank database.

9.3.1.3 Arrhythmia Discrimination

After each segmented beat is assigned a label, the detection of arrhythmias is usually based on joint considerations of time cycle (in average and/or in scatter terms) and the kind of consecutive beats. However, the separation between beat labeling and arrhythmia detection is not always the same across different ECG systems. Also, specific arrhythmias have been paid special attention in terms of their discrimination, deserving devoted schemes. The most relevant arrhythmia discrimination problems are probably the following: (1) the supraventricular tachycardia (SVT) versus the ventricular tachycardia (VT) discrimination, as far as the former does not require an immediate therapy in implantable devices, whereas the latter does require it; (2) the ventricular fibrillation (VF) detection, as far as this is the most life-threatening arrhythmia and the main cause of sudden cardiac death; and (3) the atrial fibrillation (AF) detection, as this is the most prevalent arrhythmia, specially in the elderly people nowadays.

Among the high number of arrhythmias, the discrimination of wide QRS tachycardias in VT and SVT has become a complex area in electrocardiography. Also, detection of VF at an early stage is crucial in order to reduce the risk of sudden death and allow the specialist to have longer reaction time to give the patient appropriate therapy. Consequently, some relevant attempts have been made to develop classifiers and establish criteria for this differentiation (Brugada et al. 1991). More arrhythmia-oriented schemes are described next.

Arrhythmia classification is addressed in Uyar and Gurgen (2007) by using serial fusion of SVM classifiers and logistic regression in ECG signals. The two-stages serial fusion system is based on SVM rejection option. The SVM distance outputs are related to confidence measure, and ambiguous samples with first SVM level are rejected to classify. The rejected samples are forwarded to the logistic regression stage, and finally, both decisions are combined. In Joshi et al. (2009), a hybrid SVM is used for multiclass arrhythmia classification, capable of reducing the patients falsely classified as normal, and validated in the MIT-BIH arrhythmia database for seven different arrhythmias. In Osowski et al. (2004), a committee of experts formed by several SVMs was proposed for the recognition of 13 heart rhythm types including VF, and confirmed the reliability of the proposed approach. An updated comparison among neural networks and SVM in this setting can be found in Ubeyli (2007).

In Rojo-Alvarez et al. (2002a), the discrimination between SVT and VT is addressed in Implantable Cardioverter Defibrillator (ICD) stored electrograms (EGM). The system analyzes the waveform and different transformations. Furthermore, in Rojo-Alvarez et al. (2002b), the electrophysiological meaning of the support vector is scrutinized. In Kamousi et al. (2009), again SVM classifiers are used for the same application, this time using the covariance feature description for accounting with three simultaneously recorded waveforms.

The automatic recognition of VF from any other rhythms has been also addressed from kernel methods problem statements. In Alonso-Atienza et al. (2008), a system for learning the relevant features from temporal and spectral domain description is presented, together with a nonparametric bootstrap resampling procedure for selecting the relevant features. This approach considers the automatic classification into VF vs non-VF of every 1-second segment, which is usually the basis for subsequent rhythm discrimination schemes. The validation is presented in ECG data from the MIT-BIH Arrhythmia Database and the AHA Database.

The automatic recognition of AF has also been improved with SVM classifiers. In Kostka and Tkacz (2008), time and frequency domain features, together with wavelet transform coefficients, yielded the input features for an SVM classifier. AF episodes in the MIT-BIH Arrhythmia Database were classified with higher performance when using a feature-selection strategy (88% sensitivity, 85% specificity for Gaussian kernel SVM).

In the comparative analysis presented in these works, it can be seen that the classification rates given by the SVM are often similar to those given by other learning schemes. However, some of the main advantages in these applications are the flexibility and the ease of free-parameter search compared to other techniques, which are often desirable features in this field.

9.3.2 Myocardial Ischemia and Infarction

Myocardial ischemia is caused by a lack of oxygen and nutrients to the contractile cells of cardiac muscle and may lead to myocardial infarction with severe consequences of heart failure and arrhythmia.

Many studies have used kernel methods for the characterization of myocardial infarction (MI), which is one of the leading causes of death in Europe and the United States. Detection of MI has been extensively treated by means of retrospective studies in which some clinical variables are used to train the models. Early diagnosis of acute myocardial infarction (AMI) in patients with severe chest pain presenting at emergency units has attracted considerable interest for the application of SVMs.

In Konttila et al. (2005), the SVM classifier forms the basis for a system capable of identifying acute myocardial ischemia with a reduced set of body surface potential map electrodes. In Sepúlveda-Sanchis et al. (2002), a system for detecting patients with unstable angina is presented. An SVM classifier is used to discriminate those patients with mortality or readmission within 6 months after the onset of unstable angina for any of the following reasons: acute myocardialinfarction, unstable angina, congestive heart failure, SVT, or VF. A previous feature selection step was performed using genetic algorithms, before using the final set of features with the SVM classifier (66% sensitivity, 79% specificity).

9.3.3 Other Applications

Some brief examples of other applications are summarized here.

9.3.3.1 Heart Rate Variability

Heart rate variability analysis addresses the estimation of the autonomic nervous balance (sympathetic versus vagal branch), the estimation of the stress or relaxation condition, and the evaluation of physiological or mental workload. In Kampouraki et al. (2009), binary SVM classifiers are used to analyze two databases. First, long-term ECG recordings with young and elderly screened healthy subjects (Fantasia Database) were considered. Second, long ECG recordings from subjects suffering from coronary artery disease were compared to the recordings coming from healthy subjects. The SVM outperformed standard classification techniques (such as k Nearest Neighbors and Neural Networks with Radial Basis Functions) in terms of recall and precision.

9.3.3.2 Automated Diagnostic Systems

A variety of automated diagnostic system can be used in other applications, by taking advantage of SVM classifier schemes. In Ji et al. (2009), a system for early detection of hemorrhagic injuries is presented. The system uses discrete wavelet transform coefficients from physiological signals (ECG, together with arterial blood pressure, and thoracic impedance). The data were collected from healthy subjects conducting a hemorrhage model protocol. SVM yielded the highest accuracy (82%) among classification methods.

9.3.3.3 Sleep Apnea

In Khandoker et al. (2009b), SVMs are used for automated recognition of obstructive sleep apnea syndrome using ECG information from nocturnal recordings in normal subjects and apnea patients. The features were extracted from wavelet coefficient levels of heart rate variability signals and ECG-derived respiration. This system reached a 92% accuracy in an independent test set. In Patangay et al. (2007), a system to monitor obstructive sleep apnea in heart failurepatients is delivered. Heart sounds and ECG features are used to build an SVM classifier yielded 85% sensitivity and 92% specificity in the apnea epochs detection on a database from 17 patients with 2 min epochs.

9.3.3.4 Fetal Analysis

In Khandoker et al. (2009a), the recognition of abnormal fetus is addressed by considering simultaneously ECG signals and simultaneously recorded Doppler ultrasound signals. Multiresolution wavelet was used to link the frequency contents of the Doppler signals with the opening and closing of the aortic and mitral valves. An SVM with polynomial kernel yielded 100% accuracy (8 abnormal vs 29 normal fetuses).

9.3.3.5 Risk Stratification

A number of applications for SVM in risk stratification have been presented, in a variety of different stratification contexts. In Graja and Boucher (2005), the classification of patients prone to atrial fibrillation is addressed with an SVM scheme from ECG parameters (P-wave delineation and subsequent parameter extraction). Up to 90% sensitivity and 85% specificity were reached.

9.3.3.6 Intelligent Garment

Intelligent garment is embedded with electrical vital sign recording and analysis, and it can be used for personal health monitoring systems. In Yi-Zhi et al. (2008), a fuzzy SVM-based classifier is used for diagnostic of chronic fatigue syndrome. The architecture and design for intelligent garment embedded in an online chronic fatigue syndrome evaluation system is improved by decreasing the input feature space with principal component analysis, and the diagnostic is addressed with a fuzzy multiclass SVM classifier, reaching 99% sensitivity.

In Miyaji et al. (2009), a system for driver cognitive distraction detection is presented, which uses physiological features, not only from ECG (R–R interval series), but also stereo camera (for eyes tracking, head movements, or pupil diameter). An SVM classifier and a faster detection from adaboost are discussed in the cited work.

9.4 Future Trends in ECG Kernel Learning

As we have noted in the reviewed literature throughout the chapter, the vast majority of applications and ECG data processing problems made use of the standard SVM. Interestingly, other kernel methods have not been used in the field. We review in the following sections, other approaches that we think should be explored in the near future, given the special peculiarities of the data.

9.4.1 Other Kernel Machines and Learning Paradigms

It is not surprising that the field has not explored other kernel methods than classification, as far as most of the problems in ECG data processing are concerned with annotation and pathology discrimination. What it is surprising though is the fact that the SVM is the only kernel method used. Other classifiers have been obviated, such as the SVDD and the ν-SVM (see Sects. 9.2.5, 9.2.6, and 9.2.7).

Another field that should be paid attention is that of regression, function approximation, and time series prediction with kernels. This is a quite advanced field in which state of the art results in terms of accuracy are obtained. ECG data processing is sometimes confronted with problems in which noise in the acquired must canceled out by approximation, prediction models of HRV, or the particular shape of waves using ARMA models. There are kernel methods for tackling these problems with improved accuracy and robustness. Another related field is that of *causal learning*. Estimation of dependences between random variables is a common problem in science, and is the key in many ECG processing problems. The goal may be diverse but mainly tries to discern if sensed variables or ECG signals are related, to measure the strength of these relations, and to eventually identify cause–effect relations. Kernel methods can be used to find confounders and causal relations in ECG databases as well.

Kernel methods for feature extraction have been extensively used in other communities, such in speech or image processing, whereas they have not been explored for analyzing the structure of ECG data manifolds. This chapter has presented an updated literature review on kernel classification, since it is apparently the predominant approach. However, new kernel-based learning methodologies are being constantly introduced in the machine learning community and they could be exploited for ECG data processing too.

The special peculiarities of the ECG data lead to develop new methods. And vice versa, the new learning paradigms available offer new ways of looking at old, yet unsolved, problems in ECG signal processing. In what follows, we review recent research directions in the context of ECG data kernel-based learning.

9.4.2 Other Kernel Functions

To our knowledge, in all SVM applications, the standard kernel functions have been used, namely, linear, polynomial, or RBF kernel functions. However, by taking advantage of some algebra and functional analysis properties (Golub and Van Loan 1996; Reed and Simon 1980), one can derive very useful properties of kernels. Be K_1

and K_2 two positive definite kernels on $\mathcal{X} \times \mathcal{X}$, $\mathbf{A}$ a symmetric positive semidefinite matrix, $d(\cdot,\cdot)$ a metric fulfilling distance properties, f any function, and $\mu > 0$. Then, the following kernels are valid (Schölkopf and Smola 2002):

$$K(\mathbf{x},\mathbf{x}') = K_1(\mathbf{x},\mathbf{x}') + K_2(\mathbf{x},\mathbf{x}') \tag{9.16}$$

$$K(\mathbf{x},\mathbf{x}') = \mu K_1(\mathbf{x},\mathbf{x}') \tag{9.17}$$

$$K(\mathbf{x},\mathbf{x}') = K_1(\mathbf{x},\mathbf{x}') \cdot K_2(\mathbf{x},\mathbf{x}') \tag{9.18}$$

$$K(\mathbf{x},\mathbf{x}') = \mathbf{x}^\top \mathbf{A}\mathbf{x}' \tag{9.19}$$

$$K(\mathbf{x},\mathbf{x}') = \exp(-d(\mathbf{x},\mathbf{x}')) \tag{9.20}$$

$$K(\mathbf{x},\mathbf{x}') = K(f(\mathbf{x}), f(\mathbf{x}')) \tag{9.21}$$

These basic properties give rise to the construction of refined similarity measures better fitted to the data characteristics. In ECG data processing, one can sum dedicated kernels to different features (spectral, temporal, etc) through Eq. 9.16. A scaling factor to each kernel can also be added (Eq. 9.17).

Another common problem in the field is the following. ECG signals are typically processed by extracting a potentially high number of features of different nature and their efficient combination is a key problem. Composite kernels can provide a valid and consistent framework for the combination of different features. Essentially, the methodology uses some properties of kernel methods (such as the direct sum of Hilbert spaces, see Sect. A.1) to combine kernels dedicated to different signal sources, e.g., the sum of a kernel on spectral feature vectors can be summed up to a kernel defined over spatially extracted feature vectors. More advanced methodologies of kernel combination, such as Multiple Kernel Learning (MKL), are continuously developed in the machine learning domain. Here, different weights and scales are learned jointly from the data. This corresponds to developing *convex combinations* of kernels by exploiting Eqs. 9.16 and 9.17 to define (and optimize) linear combinations of kernels working on feature subsets:

$$K(\mathbf{x},\mathbf{x}') = \sum_{m=1}^{M} d_m K_m(\mathbf{x},\mathbf{x}')$$

Note that this kernel offers some insight in the problem, since relevant features receive higher values of d_m, and the corresponding kernel parameters θ_m yield information about pairwise similarity scales.

9.4.3 Adaptive Kernel Machines

While most of the problems in ECG signal processing are *supervised*, they are typically confronted with the problems of scarce labeled data points or over-representativity of some classes in the problem. This is related to the field of *semisupervised learning* in which unlabeled data (wealth and relatively cheap to obtain) are used to improve the decision function. Many kernel machines exist in this context, and some recent advances include the following.

Deforming kernels. The field of semisupervised kernel learning deals with techniques to modify the values of the training kernel including the information from the whole data distribution, hence K is either deformed through a graph distance matrix built with both labeled and unlabeled samples, or by means of kernels built from clustering solutions.

Generative kernels. By exploiting (9.21), one can construct kernels from probability distributions by defining $K(\mathbf{x},\mathbf{x}') = K(\mathbf{p},\mathbf{p}')$, where $\mathbf{p}$, $\mathbf{p}'$ are defined on the space $\mathcal{X}$. This kind of kernels is known as *probability product kernels between distributions* and is defined as

$$K(\mathbf{p},\mathbf{p}') = \langle \mathbf{p},\mathbf{p}' \rangle = \int_{\mathcal{X}} \mathbf{p}(\mathbf{x})\mathbf{p}'(\mathbf{x})\mathrm{d}\mathbf{x}.$$

Joint input–output mappings. Typically, kernels are built on the input samples. Lately the framework of *structured output learning* deals with the definition of joint input–output kernels, $K((\mathbf{x},y),(\mathbf{x}',y'))$.

Another interesting and common problem in ECG data processing is the lack of adaptation to new circumstances. This is known as transfer learning or domain adaptation. This setting implies that unlabeled test examples and training examples are drawn from different domains or distributions. A related problem is also that of classifying data using labeled samples from other problems, which induces the sample selection bias problem, also known as covariate shift. Here, unlabeled test data are drawn from the same training domain, but the estimated distribution does not correctly model the true underlying distribution since the number (or the quality) of available training samples is not sufficient.

9.4.4 Structured-Output Kernel Machines

Most of the techniques revised so far assume a simple set of outputs. However, more complex output spaces can be imagined, e.g., predicting multiple labels, multi-temporal sequences, or in multicenter (yet related) data. Such complex output spaces are the topic of structured learning, one of the most recent developments in machine learning. Certainly this field of learning joint input–output mappings will receive attention in the future.

9.4.5 *Active Sample Selection with Kernels*

Finally, we would like to spot the relatively new field of active learning. When designing a supervised classifier, the performance of the model strongly depends on the quality of the labeled information available. This constraint makes the generation of an appropriate training set a difficult and expensive task requiring extensive manual human-signal interaction. Therefore, in order to make the models as efficient as possible, the training set should be kept as small as possible and focused on the examples that really help to improve the performance of the model. Active learning aims at responding to this need, by constructing effective training sets.

9.5 Conclusions

Kernel methods allow us to transform almost any linear method into a nonlinear one, while still operating with linear algebra. The methods essentially rely on embedding the examples into a high-dimensional space where a linear method is designed and applied. Access to the mapped samples is done implicitly through kernel functions. This chapter reviewed the field of kernel machines in ECG signal processing.

We adverted the fact that only the SVM has been paid attention in the field. Even if successful in many important applications, SVM with the RBF kernel is just the baseline classifier nowadays in the field of machine learning, though more powerful SVM formulations and specific kernel functions can be used for data classification. Also, other kernel methods are currently available for regression, density estimation, anomaly detection, system identification, measure dependence and discover causal relations between variables. We believe this becomes an opportunity to practitioners in the field of ECG data processing.

This chapter merely aimed to note this fact and to provide some ideas for future exploitation of kernel machines in ECG signal processing. We foresee some other future research lines in the development of specific kernel methods to deal with the data peculiarities. New developments are expected in the near future to encompass both ECG data complexity and new problem settings.

A.1 Operations with Kernels

We now review some basic properties with kernels. Note that, although the space $\mathcal{H}$ can be very high dimensional, some basic operations can still be performed.

Translation. A translation in feature space can be written as the modified feature map $\tilde{\phi}(\mathbf{x}) = \phi(\mathbf{x}) + \Gamma$ with $\Gamma \in \mathcal{H}$. Then, the translated dot product for $\langle \tilde{\phi}(\mathbf{x}), \tilde{\phi}(\mathbf{x}') \rangle_{\mathcal{H}}$ can be computed if we restrict Γ to lie in the span of the functions $\{\phi(\mathbf{x}_1), \ldots, \phi(\mathbf{x}_n)\} \in \mathcal{H}$.

Centering. The previous translation allows us to center data $\{\mathbf{x}_i\}_{i=1}^n \in \mathcal{X}$ in the *feature space*. The mean of the data in $\mathcal{H}$ is $\phi_\mu = \frac{1}{n} \sum_{i=1}^n \phi(\mathbf{x}_i)$ which is a linear combination of the span of functions and thus fulfills the requirement for Γ. One can center data in $\mathcal{H}$ by computing $\mathbf{K} \leftarrow \mathbf{HKH}$ where entries of $\mathbf{H}$ are $H_{ij} = \delta_{ij} - \frac{1}{n}$ and the Kronecker symbol $\delta_{i,j} = 1$ if $i = j$ and zero otherwise.

Subspace Projections. Given two points Ψ and Γ in the feature space, the projection of Ψ onto the subspace spanned by Γ is $\Psi' = \frac{\langle \Gamma, \Psi \rangle_{\mathcal{H}}}{\|\Gamma\|_{\mathcal{H}}^2} \Gamma$. Therefore one can compute the projection Ψ' expressed solely in terms of kernel evaluations.

Computing Distances. The kernel corresponds to a dot product in a Hilbert space $\mathcal{H}$, and thus one can compute distances between mapped samples entirely in terms of kernel evaluations:

$$d(\mathbf{x}, \mathbf{x}') = \|\phi(\mathbf{x}) - \phi(\mathbf{x}')\|_{\mathcal{H}} = \sqrt{K(\mathbf{x}, \mathbf{x}) + K(\mathbf{x}', \mathbf{x}') - 2K(\mathbf{x}, \mathbf{x}')}$$

Normalization. Exploiting the previous property, one can also normalize data in feature spaces:

$$K(\mathbf{x}, \mathbf{x}') \leftarrow \left\langle \frac{\phi(\mathbf{x})}{\|\phi(\mathbf{x})\|}, \frac{\phi(\mathbf{x}')}{\|\phi(\mathbf{x}')\|} \right\rangle = \frac{K(\mathbf{x}, \mathbf{x}')}{\sqrt{K(\mathbf{x}, \mathbf{x}) K(\mathbf{x}', \mathbf{x}')}}$$

Acknowledgements This work was partially supported by projects CICYT-FEDER TEC2009-13696, AYA2008-05965-C04-03, CSD2007-00018, TEC2009-12098, and TEC2010-19263.

References

Abboud, M.F., Linkens, D.A., Mahfouf, M., Dounias, G.: Survey on the use of smart and adaptive engineering systems in medicine. Artif. Intell. Med. **26**, 179–209 (2002)

Abreu-Lima, C., de Sa, J.P.: Automatic classifiers for the interpretation of electrocardiograms. Rev. Port. Cardiol. **17**, 415–28 (1998)

Alonso-Atienza, F., Rosado-Muñoz, A., Rojo-Álvarez, J.L., Camps-Valls, G.: Learning the relevant features of ventricular fibrillation from automatic detection algorithms. In: Hines, E., Martínez-Ramón, M., Pardo, M., Llobet, E., Leeson, M., Iliescu, D., J.Y. (eds.) Intelligent Systems: Techniques and Applications, pp. 505–534. Shaker Publishing, Maastrich, Netherlands (2008)

Brugada, P., Brugada, J., Mont, L., Smeets, J., Andries, E.W.: A new approach to the differential diagnosis of a regular tachycardia with a wide QRS complex. Circulation **83**, 1649–59 (1991)

Camps-Valls, G., Guerrero-Martínez, J.F.: Neural networks in ECG classification: what is next in adaptive systems? In: Kamruzzaman, J., Begg, R.K., Sarker, R.A., (eds.) Neural Networks in Healthcare: Potential and Challenges, pp. 81–104. http://www.idea-group.com/books/details.asp?ID=5529. Idea Group Publishing, Hershey (2006). ISBN: 1-59140-848-2

Carrault, G., Cordier, M.O., Quiniou, R., Wang, F.: Temporal abstraction and inductive logic programming for arrhythmia recognition from electrocardiograms. Artif. Intell. Med. **28**, 231–63 (2003)

Dybowski, R.: Neural computation in medicine: perspectives and prospects. In: Proceedings of the Artificial Neural Networks in Medicine and Biology Conference, pp. 26–36. Springer, Göteborg, Sweden (2000)

Einthoven: Un Nouveau galvanométre. Arch Néerland Sci exactes naturelles, Serie 2, **6**, 625–633 (1901)

Exarchos, T., Tsipouras, M., Exarchos, C., Papaloukas, C., Fotiadis, D., Michalis, L.: A methodology for the automated creation of fuzzy expert systems for ischaemic and arrhythmic beat classification based on a set of rules obtained by a decision tree. Artif. Intell. Med. **40**, 187–200 (2007)

Golub, G.H., Van Loan, C.F.: Matrix Computations (Johns Hopkins Studies in Mathematical Sciences). The Johns Hopkins University Press, Baltimore (1996)

Graja, S., Boucher, J.: SVM classification of patients prone to atrial fibrillation. In: IEEE International Workshop on Intelligent Signal Processing, pp. 370–374. Faro (2005)

Itchhaporia, D., Snow, P.B., Almassy, R.J., Oetgen, W.J.: Artificial neural networks: current status in cardiovascular medicine. J. Am. Coll. Cardiol. **28**, 515–21 (1996)

Ji, S.Y., Chen, W., Ward, K., Rickards, C., Ryan, K., Convertino, V., Najarian, K.: Wavelet based analysis of physiological signals for prediction of severity of hemorrhagic shock. In: International Conference on Complex Medical Engineering, pp. 1–6. ICME, IEEE press Tempe, AZ, USA (2009)

Joshi, A., Chandran, S., Jayaraman, V., Kulkarni, B.: Hybrid SVM for multiclass arrhythmia classification. In: IEEE International Conference on Bioinformatics and Biomedicine, pp.287–290. IEEE Computer Society, Piscataway (2009)

Kamousi, B., Tewfik, A., Lin, B., Al-Ahmad, A., Hsia, H., Zei, P., Wang, P.: A new approach for icd rhythm classification based on support vector machines. In: International Conference of the IEEE Engineering in Medicine and Biology Society, pp. 2478–2481. IEEE Computer Society, Minneapolis (2009)

Kampouraki, A., Manis, G., Nikou, C.: Heartbeat time series classification with support vector machines. IEEE Trans. Inf. Technol. Biomed. **13**, 512–518 (2009)

Khandoker, A., Kimura, Y., Palaniswami, M.: Automated identification of abnormal fetuses using fetal ECG and Doppler ultrasound signals. In: Computers in Cardiology, pp. 709–712. IEEE, Piscataway (2009a)

Khandoker, A., Palaniswami, M., Karmakar, C.: Support vector machines for automated recognition of obstructive sleep apnea syndrome from ECG recordings. IEEE Trans. Inf. Technol. Biomed. **13**, 37–48 (2009b)

Kilpatrick, D., Johnston, P.: Origin of the electrocardiogram. IEEE Eng. Med. Biol. Mag. **13**, 479–486 (1994)

Konttila, T., Stenroos, M., Vaananen, H., Hanninen, H., Lindholm, M., Tierala, I., Katila, T.: Support vector classification of acute myocardial ischemia with reduced sets of body surface potential map electrodes. In: Computers in Cardiology, pp. 869–872. IEEE, Piscataway (2005)

Kostka, P., Tkacz, E.: Feature extraction for improving the support vector machine biomedical data classifier performance. In: Information Technology and Applications in Biomedicine, 2008. International Conference on ITAB 2008. 362–365. Shenzhen (2008)

Kumaravel, N., Rajesh, J., Nithiyanandam, N.: Equivalent tree representation of electrocardiogram using genetic algorithm. Biomed. Sci. Instrum. **33**, 573–578 (1997)

Le Blanc, R.: Quantitative analysis of cardiac arrhythmias. crc: Critical review in biomedical engineeering. In: MIT-BIH Database Distribution. 2003. http://ecg.mit.edu/ Mitchell, T.M., Machine Learning. pp. 14–1 (1986)

Lisboa, P.J., Vellido, A., Wong, H.: Bias reduction in skewed binary classification with Bayesian neural networks. Neural Netw. **13**, 407–410 (2000)

Mahalingam, N., Kumar, D.: Neural networks for signal processing applications: ECG classification. Austral. Phys. Eng. Sci. Med. **20**, 147–151 (1997)

Mehta, S., Lingayat, N.: Detection of T-waves in 12-lead electrocardiogram. In: International Conference on Computational Intelligence and Multimedia Applications, 2007, vol. 2. 512–516. IEEE Computer Society, Washington (2007)

Mehta, S., Lingayat, N.: SVM-based algorithm for recognition of QRS complexes in electrocardiogram. IRBM **29**, 310–317 (2008a)

Mehta, S., Lingayat, N.: Combined entropy based method for detection of QRS complexes in 12-lead electrocardiogram using SVM. Comput. Biol. Med. **38**, 138–145 (2008b)

Mehta, S., Lingayat, N.: Development of SVM based classification techniques for the delineation of wave components in 12-lead electrocardiogram. Biomed. Signal Process. Control **3**, 341–349 (2008c)

Melgani, F., Bazi, Y.: Classification of electrocardiogram signals with support vector machines and particle swarm optimization. IEEE Trans. Inf. Technol. Biomed. **12**, 667–677 (2008)

Miller, A.S., Blott, B.H., Hames, T.K.: Review of neural network applications in medical imaging and signal processing. Med. Biol. Eng. Comput. **30**, 449–464 (1992)

Miyaji, M., Kawanaka, H., Oguri, K.: Driver's cognitive distraction detection using physiological features by the adaboost. In: International IEEE Conference on Intelligent Transportation Systems, pp. 1–6. IEEE, St. Louis (2009)

Mora, F., Passariello, G., Carrault, G., Le Pichon, J.P.: Intelligent patient monitoring and management systems: a review. IEEE Eng. Med. Biol. Mag. **12**, 23–33 (1993)

Nugent, C.D., Webb, J.A.C., Black, N.D., Wright, G.T.H., McIntyre, M.: An intelligent framework for the classification of the 12-lead ECG. Artif. Intell. Med. **16**, 205–222 (1999)

Osowski, S., Hoai, L.T., Markiewicz, T.: Support vector machine-based expert system for reliable heartbeat recognition. IEEE Trans. Biomed. Eng. **51**, 582–589 (2004)

Patangay, A., Vemuri, P., Tewfik, A.: Monitoring of obstructive sleep apnea in heart failure patients. In: Annual International Conference of the IEEE Engineering in Medicine and Biology Society, pp. 1043–1046. IEEE, Lyon (2007)

Reed, M.C., Simon, B.: Functional Analysis. Volume I of Methods of Modern Mathematical Physics. Academic, New York (1980)

Ribeiro, B., Marques, A., Henriques, J., Antunes, M.: Premature ventricular beat detection by using spectral clustering methods. In: Computers in Cardiology, 2007, pp. 149–152. IEEE, Piscataway (2007)

Ribeiro, B., Henirques, J., Marques, A., Antunes, M.: Manifold learning for premature ventricular contraction detection. In: Computers in Cardiology, pp. 917–920. IEEE, Piscataway (2008)

Rojo-Alvarez, J.L., Arenal-Maiz, A., Artes-Rodriguez, A.: Discriminating between supraventricular and ventricular tachycardias from egm onset analysis. IEEE Eng. Med. Biol. Mag. **21**, 16–26 (2002a)

Rojo-Alvarez, J.L., Arenal-Maiz, A., Artes-Rodriguez, A.: Support vector black-box interpretation in ventricular arrhythmia discrimination. IEEE Eng. Med. Biol. Mag. **21**, 27–35 (2002b)

Schölkopf, B., Smola, A.: Learning with Kernels – Support Vector Machines, Regularization, Optimization and Beyond. MIT Press, Cambridge, MA (2002)

Schölkopf, B., Williamson, R.C., Smola, A., Shawe-Taylor, J.: Support vector method for novelty detection. In: Advances in Neural Information Processing Systems (NIPS), Vol. 12. MIT Press, Cambridge, MA, (1999)

Schölkopf, B., Smola, A.J., Williamson, R.C., Bartlett, P.L.: New support vector algorithms. J. Neural Comput. **2**, 1207–1245 (2000)

Sepúlveda-Sanchis, J., Camps-Valls, G., Soria-Olivas, E., Salcedo-Sanz, S., Bousoño-Calzón, C., Sanz-Romero, G., Marrugat de la Iglesia, J.: Support vector machines and genetic algorithms for detecting unstable angina. In: Computers in Cardiology, Vol. 29, pp. 261–265. IEEE, Piscataway (2002)

Tax, D., Duin, R.P.: Support vector domain description. Pattern Recognit. Lett. **20**, 1191–1199 (1999)

Ubeyli, E.D.: ECG beats classification using multiclass support vector machines with error correcting output codes. Digit. Signal Process. **17**, 675–684 (2007)

Uyar, A., Gurgen, F.: Arrhythmia classification using serial fusion of support vector machines and logistic regression. In: IEEE Workshop on Intelligent Data Acquisition and Advanced Computing Systems, Technology and Applications, pp. 560–565. IEEE, Piscataway (2007)

Watrous, R., Towell, G.: A patient-adaptive neural network ECG patient monitoring algorithm. In: Computers in Cardiology 1995. pp. 229–232. IEEE Computer Society, Long Beach (1995)

Yi-Zhi, W., Hong-An, X., Yong-Sheng, D., Jin-Lan, S., Bo-Hui, Z.: SVM based chronic fatigue syndrome evaluation for intelligent garment. In: International Conference on Bioinformatics and Biomedical Engineering. pp. 1947–1950. IEEE Xplore, Piscataway (2008)

Zellmer, E., Shang, F., Zhang, A.: Highly accurate ECG beat classification based on continuous wavelet transformation and multiple support vector machine classifiers. In: International Conference on Biomedical Engineering and Informatics. pp. 1–5. IEEE, Piscataway (2009)

Zhao, Q., Zhang, L.: ECG feature extraction and classification using wavelet transform and support vector machines. In: International Conference on Neural Networks and Brain, Vol. 2, pp. 1089–1092. IEEE, Piscataway (2005)

Chapter 10
Hyperellipsoidal Classifier for Beat Classification in ECG Signals

G. Bortolan, I. Christov, and W. Pedrycz

10.1 Introduction

Electrocardiogram (ECG) signal analysis is a useful and widely accepted way to study and diagnose cardiac dysfunctions.

In the last few years, a significant effort in ECG signal processing, classification, and interpretation has been witnessed.

Detection and classification of ECG beats is of considerable importance in critical care units and during patient monitoring. In heart conduction disorders, ventricular excitation may not originate as it is normal from the sinus node, but from other ectopic centres in the myocardium. Thus premature contractions are generated, called also extrasystoles or ectopic beats. The premature beat itself does not cause symptoms but the occurrence of multiple single premature beats is considered clinically important, since it becomes a sign for disturbance in the depolarization process preceding in many cases the appearance of malignant cardiac arrhythmias. Pattern recognition algorithms have emerged as a meaningful and useful algorithmic tool in the computerized classification techniques.

In ECG signal analysis and classification, a variety of different descriptors have been analyzed: morphological parameters coming from both the ECG and the derived vectorcardiogram (VCG) (Christov and Bortolan 2004; Christov et al. 2005; Jekova et al. 2004), time–frequency features, Karhunen-Loève transform, and

G. Bortolan (✉)
Institute of Biomedical Engineering, ISIB-CNR, Padova, Italy
e-mail: bortolan@isib.cnr.it

I. Christov
Institute of Biophysics and Biomedical Engineering, BAS, Sofia, Bulgaria
e-mail: christov@clbme.bas.bg

W. Pedrycz
Department of Electrical & Computer Engineering, University of Alberta, Edmonton, Canada and Systems Research Institute Polish Academy of Sciences, Warsaw, Poland
e-mail: pedrycz@ece.ualberta.ca

A. Gacek and W. Pedrycz (eds.), *ECG Signal Processing, Classification and Interpretation: A Comprehensive Framework of Computational Intelligence*,
DOI 10.1007/978-0-85729-868-3_10,

Independent Component Analysis (Christov et al. 2006; Gómez-Herrero et al. 2005, 2006). Various clustering methods for classification have been studied, analyzed, and applied: neural networks, K-nearest neighbor classifiers (K-NNs), discriminant analysis, hyperbox classifiers, fuzzy logic, and fuzzy clustering (Bortolan et al. 2007, 2005; Bortolan and Pedrycz 2007; Christov and Bortolan 2004; Christov et al. 2005; Jekova et al. 2004). Attention has been paid to the formation of learning sets. Acknowledged was their great importance in achieving classification accuracy: global (with application of the "leave one out rule"), basic (without the application of the "leave one out rule"), and local (consisting of heartbeats coming only from the tested patient) (Jekova et al. 2008).

Interesting studies are also present in the framework of ECG beat classification and interpretation, ranging from the use of neural networks to self-organized maps (Bortolan et al. 1996; Bortolan and Pedrycz 2002a, b; Bortolan and Willems 1994; Silipo et al. 1999).

There is an increasing interest in studying and examining specific classification techniques in which the induced feature space possess a simple geometry, which becomes beneficial mainly in the process of interpreting the results. The family of hyperbox classifiers exhibits these characteristics to a significant extent (Gabrys and Bargiela 2001; Simpson 1992). In fact, they form a useful tool for achieving a high level of interpretability of the classification rules, providing a simple structure of the overall classifier and a visualization of the obtained results. In general the hyperboxes do not possess differentiable boundaries, and for that reason the learning process is not directly suitable for gradient-based optimization techniques. Consequently, the learning process is developed by hybrid learning strategy, for example with fuzzy clustering and genetic algorithms.

The aim of this research, realized in the framework of ECG signal processing and beat classification, is to study families of hyperbox or hyperellipsoid classification techniques, characterized by simple geometry and coming with interpretation clarity.

10.2 Hyperboxes and Hyperellipsoids

The geometry of pattern classifiers reveals great importance in the determination, defining, and quantification of the resulting performance of the proposed classifier. There are a very large number of topologies of classifiers and associated learning mechanisms. Neural networks, fuzzy rule-based systems, and k-nearest neighbor classifiers are just the more commonly used categories of pattern classifiers. The shapes of the classes are not of immediate visual interpretation.

The geometry of the feature space imposed (restrained) by the classifier is connected with the ability to interpret the classification process as well as classification results and to understand the decision boundaries produced by the classifiers. In general, the boundaries are linear, piecewise linear, or nonlinear. From the interpretation point of view, the most intuitive classifiers are those in which the regions are intuitive by a visual inspection, at least in the low dimensional spaces. One category of "intuitive" geometry is represented by the family of hyperboxes and hyper-ellipsoids.

The hyperboxes (HB) located in an n-dimensional feature spaces are regions described in the following form:

$$\{x_i \in [x_{iA}, x_{iB}]\} \quad i = 1, \ldots.., N$$

Given this description, one can directly translate them into the following well-known format of rule-based classification rules:

> "IF feature X_1 assume values in $[X_{1A}, X_{1B}]$ and feature X_2 assume values in $[X_{2A}, X_{2B}] \ldots$ and feature X_N assume values in $[X_{NA}, X_{NB}]$, THEN class W_i,"

where the interval limits are the respective edges of the corresponding hyperbox.

An example of hyperbox-based classifier formed in a two-dimensional feature space is shown in Fig. 10.1, where two hyperboxes HB_1 and HB_2 cover data of class W1, whereas the patterns belonging to class W2 are excluded:

$$\begin{aligned} HB_1 &= \{x \in [X_1, X_2]; \quad y \in [Y_1, Y_2]\} \\ HB_2 &= \{x \in [X_3, X_4]; \quad y \in [Y_3, Y_4]\}, \end{aligned}$$

which can be interpreted as:

$$\text{IF feature } x \in [X_1, X_2] \text{ and feature y} \in [Y_1, Y_2], \text{THEN class } W_1$$

The hyperboxes exhibit some important characteristics:

- The underlying geometry of the hyperboxes is simple and comes with a visual interpretation, at least in the low dimensional feature space
- The resulting hyperboxes can be easily interpreted as a set of IF–THEN rules
- The hyperboxes explicitly localize (and describe) the region in the feature space that are pertinent to the given class of patterns

An interesting and intuitively appealing generalization of hyperboxes comes in the form of hyper-ellipsoids, a family of geometric constructs formed as the spherical product of the two superquadratic curves. This family can be used to model a wide variety of shapes including sphere, ellipsoids, and parallelepipeds, as well as all shapes positioned in-between (Jaklic et al. 2000).

For example, in the case of a three-dimensional space, a hyperellipsoid is described by the following equation:

$$\left(\frac{x}{x_r}\right)^m + \left(\frac{y}{y_r}\right)^m + \left(\frac{z}{z_r}\right)^m = 1,$$

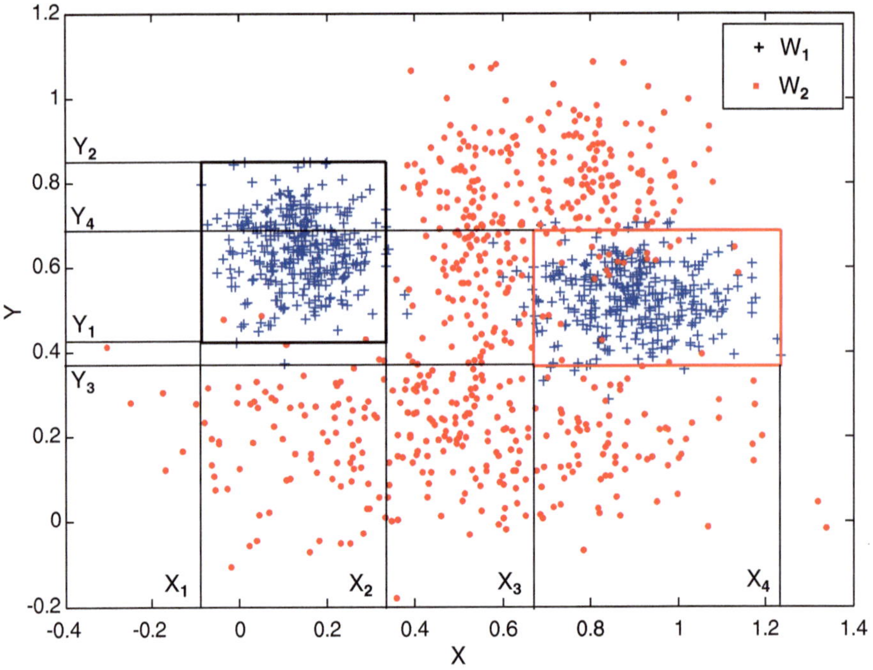

Fig. 10.1 Classification of class W_1 with two hyperboxes in two-dimensional feature spaces

where x_r, y_r, and z_r are the equatorial and polar radii, and the parameter m determines the form or the shape of the object. In particular, we encounter the following geometric constructs:

$m = 1$	diamond
$m = 2$	sphere ($x_r = y_r = z_r$)
$m = 2$	ellipsoid
$m = 4$	hyperellipsoid
$m = \inf$	hyperbox

In Fig. 10.2 we visualize the shape of hyperellipsoids in the three-dimensional space, considering various values of the parameter m. For $m = 1$ we have a diamond shape. For $m = 2$ one has a sphere or an ellipsoid. With the increasing values of "m" the shape of the geometric constructs changes starting resembling hyperboxes (which happens when the value of "m" is around 20).

In other words, we can note that hyperboxes form a particular case of hyperellipsoids.

Figure 10.3 refers to the same examples as shown in Fig. 10.1 in the two dimension, where the two ellipsoids have been optimized for classification purposes. Figure 10.4 pertains to the same data but here we are concerned with hyperellipsoids

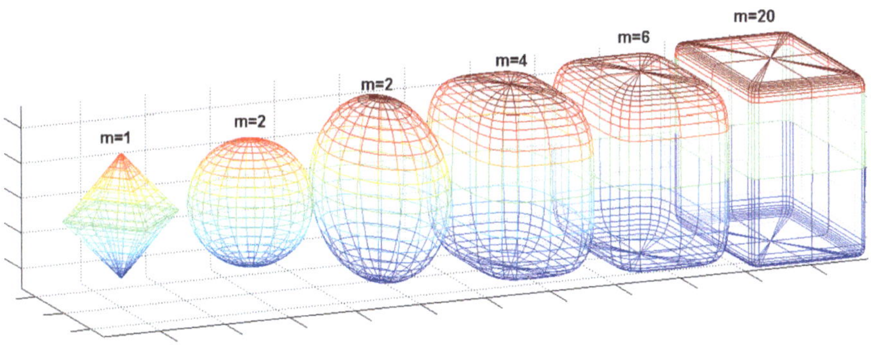

Fig. 10.2 Examples of members of the family of hyperellipsoid

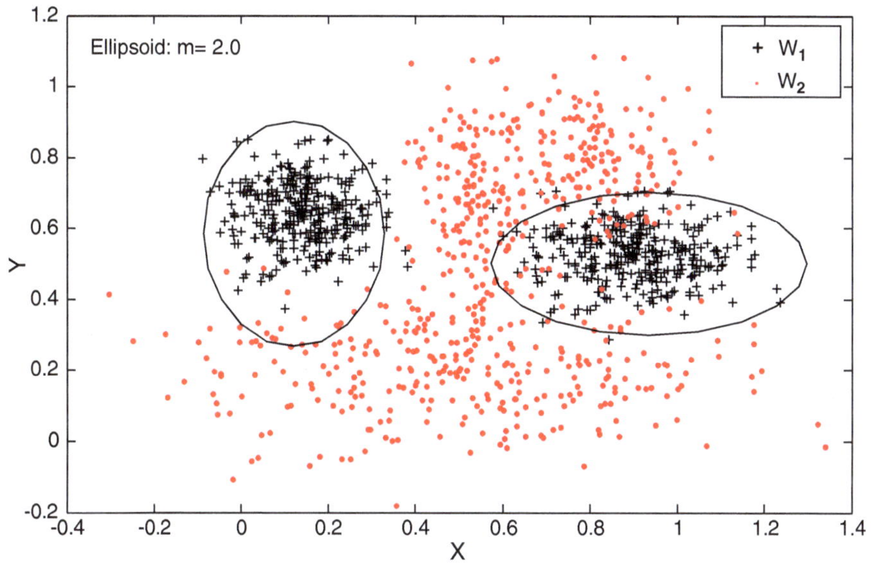

Fig. 10.3 Delineation of class W_1 with the use of two ellipsoids $(m = 2)$ realized in a two-dimensional feature space

with $m = 4$. It becomes quite apparent that the shape of the geometric constructs is effectively controlled by choosing a suitable value of "m". It is also worth noting that the use of the family of hyperellipsoids comes with well-defined analytical expressions of the ensuing classifiers; however in comparison with hyperboxes (where $m = \infty$) we loose some interpretation capabilities of "if–then" rules associated with these geometric constructs.

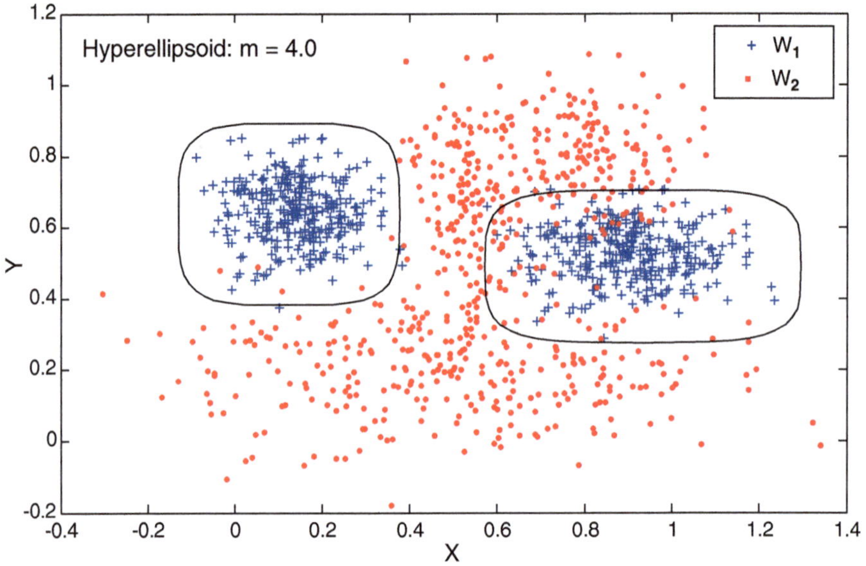

Fig. 10.4 Determination of class W_1 with the aid of two ellipsoids (with $m = 4$)

10.3 The Learning Process

To identify "optimal" hyperboxes or hyperellipsoids in the feature space, viz. regions that capture objects belonging to a certain class, the learning process is developed using two approaches of pattern recognition, namely the fuzzy c-means algorithm and the genetic algorithms. In what follows, we briefly recall the essential conceptual and algorithmic aspects of the FCM algorithm and genetic optimization.

10.3.1 Fuzzy C-Means

The Fuzzy C-means (FCM) algorithm (Bezdek 1981) realizes clustering of data located in a certain feature space. This is accomplished by the minimization of the following objective function:

$$Q = \sum_{i=1}^{c} \sum_{k=1}^{N} u_{ik}^2 \left\| x_k - v_i \right\|^2,$$

where $x_1, \ldots, x_N$ represents the n-dimensional patterns defined in the space $x_k \in R^n$, $U = [u_{ik}]$ represents the partition matrix, $\|.\|$ stands for the distance function, c is the number of clusters, and $v_1, \ldots, v_c$ are the centers of the clusters (prototypes).

The minimization is carried out under the following constraints imposed on the partition matrix U:

$$0 \leq \sum_{k=1}^{N} u_{ik} \leq N \quad \text{for } i = 1,2,\ldots,\mathbf{c}$$

$$\sum_{k=1}^{c} u_{ik} = 1 \quad \text{for } k = 1,2,\ldots,N$$

The number of clusters **c** is provided in advance. The FCM algorithm starts with a random distribution of the **c** prototypes, and iteratively modifies the prototypes and the partition matrix U in order to minimize the objective function Q. This constrained optimization locates iteratively the prototypes in regions where we encounter the highest density of homogeneous data (viz. the data belonging to the same class). The FCM phase is introduced in order to orient the search process of the Genetic Algorithm mechanism to explore only those areas around the selected prototypes.

10.3.2 Genetic Algorithms

The genetic optimization of the organization of the learning process uses a real coded Genetic Algorithm where the chromosomes are represented by real valued vectors. The genetic algorithm has the objective to optimize the location and dimension of hyperboxes built around the **c** prototypes determined by the previously described FCM algorithm. In addition this approach has been tested and validated for determining **c** hyperboxes or hyperellipsoids with no location or dimension constraints. In both cases, the chromosomes represent the parameters that characterize the hyperboxes or the hyperellipsiods. The genetic Algorithm repeatedly modifies a population of individual solutions.

At each step, the algorithm selects in a random way individuals from the current population to be parents and uses them to produce the children for the next generation. The population evolves toward an optimal solution over successive generations.

The genetic algorithms use three main types of rules in every step of the learning process, in order to create the next generation from the current generation of individuals:

- Selection rules: select the individuals (parents) that contribute to the population of the next generation
- Crossover rules: combine two parents to form children for the next generation
- Mutation rules: apply random changes to individual parents to form children

The fitness function of the Genetic Algorithm represents the function to be optimized and minimized.

The Genetic Algorithm uses the Augmented Lagrangian Genetic Algorithm to solve nonlinear constraint problem (Conn et al. 1991).

In the present study the chromosomes represent the characteristic features of the classifiers. Considering "*c*" hyperboxes and "*n*" variables, the length of the chromosomes is given by 2^*n^*c. In particular in the case of hyperboxes, the minimum and maximum values of the hyperboxes, while in the case of hyperellypsiod, the central value and the radius in every dimension are codified.

In the problem of ECG classification, the fitness function has to navigate the genetic algorithm to find the optimal solutions and the more "readable" ones, and this purpose can be reached by the optimization of the following criteria:

- Maximize the accuracy of the resulting classifier
- Maximize the accuracy and minimize the area/volume of the resulting classifier.

which corresponds to the following fitness functions:

$$\mathrm{FT}_1 = 1 - \mathrm{accuracy} = 1 - (\mathrm{TP} + \mathrm{TN})/\mathrm{N}$$

$$\mathrm{FT}_2 = 1 - \mathrm{accuracy} + \mathbf{K}^*\mathrm{area\_HB},$$

where TP + TN (True Positive and True Negative classification) represents the total number of right classification, N is the number of considered records, **K** is an appropriate weight factor, and area_HB is the area/volume of the considered hyperbox/hyperellipsoid.

Consequently, at each step, the genetic algorithm usually selects individuals that have better fitness values as parents, and create the children for the next generation considering three groups of individuals:

- Individuals with the best fitness function
- New individuals (crossover children) by combining the vectors of pair of parents
- New individuals (crossover children) crated by introducing random changes or mutations to single parents.

Once we reach a stopping condition for the algorithm (time limit, fitness function limit, or function tolerance), the GA produces the optimal hyperbox configuration.

10.3.3 Learning Strategies

In order to characterize and to search in the feature space the optimal Hyperbox/Hyperellipsoid that better characterize the considered class, different learning processes have been developed with the use and the combination of fuzzy clustering and genetic algorithms. In particular, the following three methods have been considered and tested:

1. (FCM-GA) The learning process is developed with a hybrid architecture in two phases. The fuzzy clustering (Fuzzy C-Means) represents the first step, in which the clusters are localized and characterized by the corresponding prototypes. In the second step, hyperboxes will be defined around the prototypes, and optimized with the use of genetic algorithm, which are very suitable for problems with high dimensions (Bortolan and Pedrycz 2007).
2. (GA-HB) The learning process is developed using only the genetic algorithm, and the optimal hyperboxes will be characterized by the ability of the GA to find the optimal solution of the HB.
3. (GA-HE) The GA has been used for determining the optimal generalized hyperbox that better represents and discriminate the analyzed classes. For this purpose, a family of hyperellipsoids was sought. For this experiment, in order to have a visual interpretability of the results, the case of 3D was considered.

Two sets of features were taken into account in the experiments:

(A) All the 26 features were considered in the FCM-GA learning strategy for testing the global capacity of the classifier,
(B) A limited number of features was considered in the GA-HB and GA-HE learning strategies.

In (B) selection we are at position to better study the aspects of geometrical interpretability of the classifier. In particular, maximal positive and negative peaks, and the area of QRS complex in lead 1 were selected.

10.3.4 The Validation Process

The sensitivity, the specificity, the total accuracy, the positive predictive values, and the negative predictive values have been used as validation indices. Considering a general classification task, the following indices can be defined for every record under consideration:

TP (true positive): correctly predicted positive
TN (true negative): correctly predicted negative
FP: (false positive): incorrectly predicted positive
FN: (false negative): incorrectly predicted negative
Accuracy: $(\mathrm{TP}+\mathrm{TN})/\mathrm{N}$
Sensitivity: $\mathrm{TP}/(\mathrm{TP}+\mathrm{FN})$
Specificity: $\mathrm{TN}/(\mathrm{TN}+\mathrm{FP})$
Positive predictive value: $\mathrm{TP}/(\mathrm{TP}+\mathrm{FP})$
Negative Predictive value: $\mathrm{TN}/(\mathrm{TN}+\mathrm{FN})$

Due to the fact that the total accuracy or classification rate depends on the composition of the different records (the percentage of positive/negative events), the mean values of sensitivity, specificity, positive and negative predictive values and accuracy have been reported and used for the validation process.

10.4 The ECG Database

The MIT-BIH Arrhythmia Database was used for testing and validating the proposed methods. This database contains 48 half-hour excerpts of two-channel ambulatory ECG recordings, obtained from 47 subjects studied by Boston's Beth Israel Hospital (BIH) Arrhythmia Laboratory between 1975 and 1979. Each record consists of two leads sampled at 360 Hz for a period of 30 min (Mark and Moody 1988). Forty-two of the MIT-BIH arrhythmia database recordings are of leads II and V1. The remaining are of leads II and V5 (recordings: 100, 114, 123), V2 and V5 (recordings: 102, 104), II and V4 (recording: 124).

Two or more cardiologists have been annotated all beats in the database. Approximately 70% of the beats have been annotated as Normal (N).

No selection based on the quality of the signal was performed, thus the analysis was applied even in the presence of artifact or noise in the ECG signal.

Since we focused only on the N/PVC classification, we followed the AHA records equivalent annotation, including some of the abnormal beats (left bundle branch block, right bundle branch block, aberrantly conducted beat, nodal premature beat, atrial premature beat, nodal or atrial premature beat, nodal escape beat, left or right bundle branch block, atrial ectopic beat, and nodal ectopic beat) in the 'normal' group. In addition, fusion premature ventricular contractions, ventricular flutter waves, ventricular escape beats, blocked atrial premature beats, paced beats, missed beats and questionable beats were excluded from the study.

Preprocessing filtration, taken from the work of Christov and Bortolan (2004), is having the advantage for future real-time implementation. The following procedures were realized:

- A notch filter for elimination of the power-line interference, implemented by moving averaging of samples in one period of the interference;
- A low-pass filter for suppression of the tremor noise, realized by moving averaging of samples in 30-ms time interval, thus having a first zero at about 35 Hz;
- A high-pass recursive filter for drift suppression (Daskalov et al. 1998) with cut-off frequency of 2.2 Hz.

The method for calculation of the large collection of morphological descriptors was applied to all QRS complexes annotated as N, PVC, LBBB, RBBB, or PB in the MIT-BIH arrhythmia database. The QRS pattern recognition technique (Daskalov and Christov 1999) identified the onset and the offset of the QRS complex by simultaneous analysis of the two ECG leads with relatively easy computation procedures. Then a number of 26 morphological descriptors representing information of the amplitude, the area, specific interval durations, and measurements of the QRS vector in the vectorcardiographic (VCG) plane were calculated as follows: (1) 11 descriptors were extracted by individual assessment of each lead (their total number is 22 considering the two leads); (2) one descriptor was derived by the simultaneous leads analysis; and (3) three descriptors were calculated from the VCG signal in the

Table 10.1 Morphological descriptors derived from the two ECG leads: (L1 + L2) – simultaneous analysis of Lead1 and Lead2; (L1), (L2) – individual analysis of Lead1 and Lead2

Label	Description	Leads
Width	QRS complex width – the time-interval between the onset and the offset of the identified pattern	(L1 + L2)
Pp	Maximal amplitude of the positive peak	(L1),(L2)
Pn	Maximal amplitude of the negative peak	(L1),(L2)
ArP	Area of the positive samples in the identified pattern	(L1),(L2)
ArN	Area of the negative samples in the identified pattern	(L1),(L2)
Ar	Area of the QRS complex – the sum of the absolute values of the ECG samples in the identified pattern; (Ar = ArP + ArN)	(L1),(L2)
Av1	Sum of the absolute values of the velocities in the pattern interval	(L1),(L2)
No	Number of samples crossing a threshold of 70% of the highest peak amplitude	(L1),(L2)
Ima	Time-interval from the QRS complex onset to the maximal positive peak	(L1),(L2)
Imi	Time-interval from the QRS complex onset to the maximal negative peak	(L1),(L2)
S1	QRS slope velocity calculated for the time-interval between the QRS complex onset and the first peak;	(L1),(L2)
S2	QRS slope velocity calculated for the time-interval between the first peak and the second peak;	(L1),(L2)
VCGamp	Maximal amplitude of the VCG vector	(L1 + L2)
VCGsin	Sine component of the angle of the maximal amplitude vector	(L1 + L2)
VCGcos	Cosine component of the angle of the maximal amplitude vector	(L1 + L2)

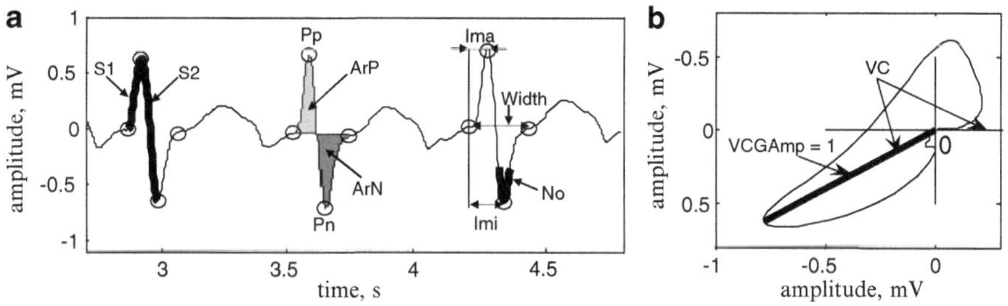

Fig. 10.5 Morphological descriptors

single-plane formed by the two leads. The 26 morphological descriptors are shown in Table. 10.1 and Fig. 10.5 (The Table and the Figure are taken from the work of Jekova, Bortolan and Christov (Jekova et al. 2008) with the kind permission of all the authors).

All the 26 parameters have been used for the testing and validation of the proposed methods, except in same particular cases to better visualize the classifier, where the three most significative parameters (maximal positive peak, maximal negative peak, and area of negative values in the QRS interval in lead I) were selected (Christov and Bortolan 2004, Christov et al. 2005, Jekova et al. 2008).

Four ECG records (102, 104, 107, and 217) were excluded from this study for the presence of paced heartbeats, considering the AAMI recommendations (AAMI 2008). All the remaining 44 ECG records present in the MIT-BIH ECG arrhythmia database has been tested, for a total of 92,855 Normal beats and 6,901 Premature Ventricular Contraction (PVC). Some ECG records (101, 103, 112, 113, 115, 117, 122) have no PVC, and some others (100, 102, 104, 111, 121, 123, 209, 230, 231, 234) have only a limited number (<5) of them. The ECG beats of each record were randomly divided in learning set (66.7%) and test set (33.3%). One particular experiment (FCM-GA) completed two scenarios, performing the characterization of the feature space of (1) Normal beats and (2) PVC complexes. In this case, ECG records with at least 20 PVC were selected, with the consequence that 22 ECG records have been effectively used in the testing and validation process.

10.5 Results

The study of the classification techniques based on hyperbox and hyperellipsoid, characterized by simple geometry and by interpretation clarity, have been performed considering the following three learning process:

1. The Fuzzy clustering and Genetic algorithm (FCM-GA) for the optimization of hyperboxes
2. Hyperbox with the use of genetic algorithm (GA-HB)
3. Hyperellipsoid with the use of genetic algorithm (GA-HE)

The following two fitness functions, previously described, have been considered:

$$\mathrm{FT}_1 = 1 - \text{accuracy}$$
$$\mathrm{FT}_2 = 1 - \text{accuracy} + \mathbf{K}^* \text{ area of the hyperellypsoid}$$

The specificity, the sensitivity, the positive predictive value, the negative predictive value, and the accuracy are the indices reported in order to test and validate the capacity of the proposed techniques, and for the characterization of the classifiers. The mean values of sensitivity, specificity, positive predictive values, negative predictive value, and accuracy on the examined 44 ECG records from the MIT-BIH database were reported.

FCM-GA procedure with fitness function $\mathbf{FT_1}$. The first experiment considers a two-phase learning strategy (FCM-GA). The first step of fuzzy clustering was useful for the determination of the prototypes and consequently to delimit the search region when running the genetic algorithm. All the 26 parameters were used for testing the potential of the proposed method, and 22 ECG records with at least 20 PVC were

Table 10.2 Classification of N class and PVC class with FCM-GA (22 ECG records and 26 features)

# of HB	Classification	Se	Sp	P+	P−	Accuracy
1	N	97.6%	97.9%	99.8%	78.0%	97.7%
2	N	97.7%	98.9%	99.8%	79.3%	97.9%
3	N	98.0%	99.2%	99.9%	81.9%	98.2%
7	N	98.0%	98.4%	99.8%	80.0%	98.1%
1	PVC	75.3%	99.9%	99.6%	97.3%	97.6%
2	PVC	75.5%	99.9%	99.6%	97.5%	97.8%
3	PVC	74.7%	99.9%	99.6%	97.3%	97.6%
7	PVC	73.4%	99.9%	99.8%	97.2%	97.6%

Mean values of sensitivity (*Se*), specificity (*Sp*), positive predictive values (*P*+), negative predictive values (*P*−), and accuracy are reported for 1, 2, 3, and 7 Hyperboxes

selected. Different number of hyperboxes (1, 2, 3, and 7) was considered. The mean values of the validation indices are reported in Table. 10.2 for the classification of N beats (upper part) and for the classification of PVC beats (lower part).

With one hyperbox the mean sensitivity and specificity were 97.6% and 97.9% for N and 75.3% and 99.9% for PVC, whereas two hyperboxes produced 97.7% and 98.9% for N and 75.5% and 99.9% for PVC. The use of seven hyperboxes improved partially the results, but not significantly, and with the drawback of limiting the interpretability and increasing of the complexity of the classifier. These findings indicate that a low number or hyperboxes are quite sufficient to describe the feature space of N or PVC classes.

Figure 10.6 reports an example (ECG #223) with two Hyperboxes for the classification of Normal (N) beats. Only three features are visualized. The discriminant capacity of the two hyperboxes is visible only partially due to the imposed reduction of the feature space.

GA-HB technique with fitness function FT_1. In the second experiment, the learning procedure used only the Genetic Algorithm (GA-HB) to provide optimal hyperboxes. In this case three parameters (maximal positive peak, maximal negative peak, and area as a sum of negative values in the QRS interval reported for lead I) were used for a more direct way to evaluate the geometrical interpretability of the results, and the validation process was performed on 44 ECG records. The results are reported in Table 10.3 (upper part) for the classification of N beats, considering 1, 2, and 3 HB. Two HB produces a sensitivity of 99.7% and a specificity of 87.7% and a mean accuracy of 99.4%. Figure 10.7 reports the same ECG example, and in this case the discriminant ability of the two HB is more evident.

GA-HE technique with fitness function FT_1. The third experiment considers the use of GA for searching the optimal hyperellipsoid (GA-HE), with the use of three features, the same as in GA-HB. As in the previous experiment, 3 ECG parameters were used in 44 ECG records. Table 10.3 (lower part) reports the results with two hyperellipsoid and the value of the parameter m is 2, with no constraints for the

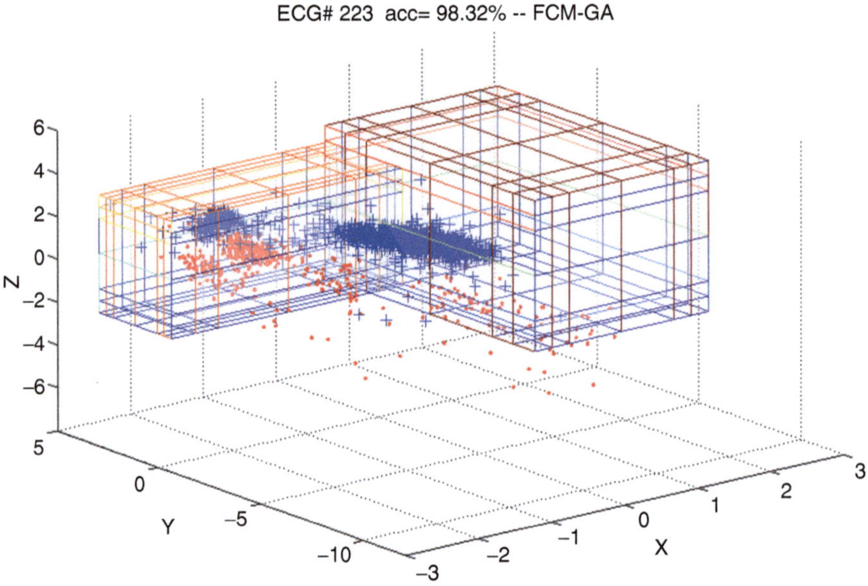

Fig. 10.6 Example of classification of N class with FCM-GA method with two hyperboxes (*PVC*: • marks, *N*: + marks)

Table 10.3 Classification of N class with GA-HB and GA-HE ($m = 2$) methods, considering the entire MIT-BIH database

# of HB	Method	Se	Sp	P+	P−	Accuracy
1	GA-HB	99.6%	82.0%	99.4%	82.9%	99.2%
2	GA-HB	99.7%	87.7%	99.7%	86.4%	99.4%
3	GA-HB	99.7%	90.6%	99.7%	83.9%	99.4%
1	GA-HE(m = 2)	99.7%	86.2%	99.7%	82.5%	99.5%
2	GA-HE(m = 2)	99.7%	92.1%	99.8%	90.0%	99.5%
3	GA-HE(m = 2)	99.7%	93.2%	99.8%	87.4%	99.5%

Mean values of sensitivity (*Se*), specificity (*Sp*), positive predictive values (*P*+), negative predictive values (*P*−), and accuracy are reported for 1, 2, and 3 Hyperboxes

equatorial and polar radii. For example, the use of two HB produce an improvement in the specificity (92.1%) and a light improvement in the accuracy (99.5%), and the visual inspection of the example reported in Fig. 10.8 shows clearly the ability and the geometrical interpretability of the classifier.

GA-HB, GA-HE techniques with fitness function FT_2 (minimization of the area). A further improvement in the classification transparency consists in minimizing the number and the size of hyperboxes/hyperellipsoids in order to simplify the visual interpretation. This task can be done in two steps: first including the

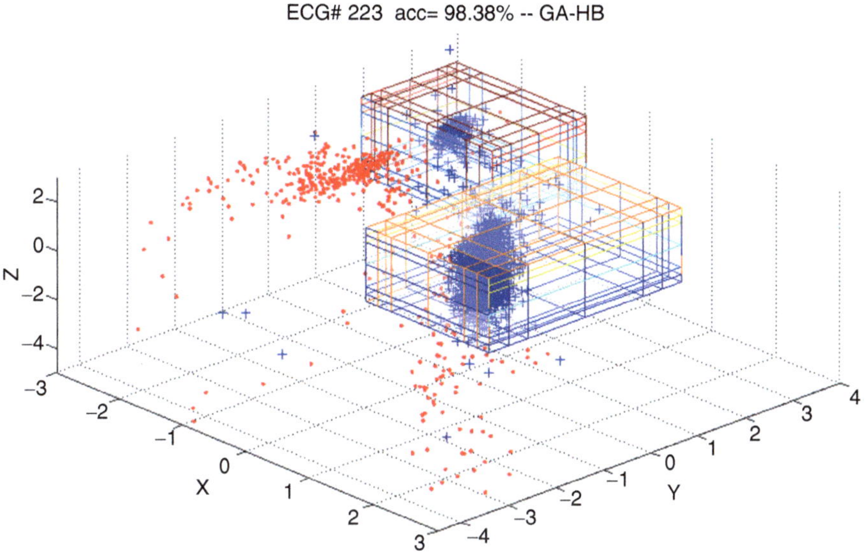

Fig. 10.7 Example of classification of N class with GA-HB method with two hyperboxes (*PVC*: · marks, *N*: + marks)

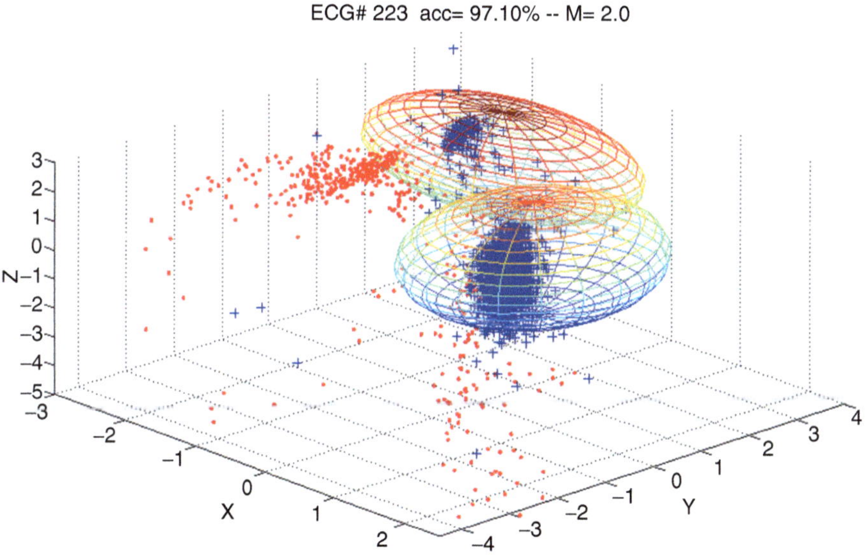

Fig. 10.8 Example of classification of N class with GA-HE method with two hyperellipsoid ($m = 2$) (*PVC*: · marks, *N*: + marks)

Table 10.4 Classification of N class with GA-HB and GA-HE without (−) and with (+) the optimization of the area, considering the entire MIT-BIH database

	Mean # of HB(−)	Acc(−)	Mean # of HB (+)	Size reduction (+)	Acc(+)
GA-HB	1	99.2%	1.00	89.0%	98.1%
GA-HB	2	99.4%	1.50	90.5%	98.1%
GA-HB	3	99.4%	1.80	90.7%	98.2%
GA-HE(m = 2)	1	99.5%	1.00	90.3%	96.1%
GA-HE(m = 2)	2	99.5%	1.82	92.8%	97.7%
GA-HE(m = 2)	3	99.5%	2.27	91.9%	98.0%

Mean number of Hyperboxes, mean size reduction, and mean accuracy are reported

area/volume in the fitness function of the Genetic algorithm and then a subsequent optimization of the number of hyperboxes deleting the meaningless ones. The first step is obtained by considering the following fitness function:

$$FT_2 = 1 - \text{accuracy} + \mathbf{K}^* \text{area\_HB} = 1 - (TP + TN)/N + \mathbf{K}^* \text{area\_HB}$$

where **K** is an appropriate constant in order to equilibrate the values of the accuracy and the area of the hyperboxes.

The second step concerns a suitable optimization algorithm for reducing the number of hyperboxes, eliminating those with very few samples.

In this experiment the same three parameters previously described were selected, and the validation process was performed for all 44 ECG records.

Table 10.4 reports a comparison of the GA-HB and GA-HE algorithms with and without the described optimization. The mean number of hyperellipsoids and the mean value of the total accuracy with and without the optimization of the area and the percentage of size reduction are reported. Considering one HB, only the first part of the described algorithm is working. In fact the size reduction with one HB is lightly lower than the case of 2 or 3 HB.

10.6 Discussion and Conclusions

The main aim of this work consists in testing and validating different methods focused on interpretability capabilities. In particular, hyperbox classifiers have been investigated for the detection and classification of different types of heartbeats in the ECG, which is of major importance in the diagnosis of cardiac dysfunctions. The learning capacity and the classification ability for normal beats (N) and premature ventricular contractions (PVC) have been tested, with particular interest in the aspect of the interpretability of the results. The MIT-BIH arrhythmia database, consisting of 48 half-hour excerpts of two-channel ambulatory ECG recordings, has been used for testing and validating the proposed methods.

This approach is described for the classification of multidimensional data with the presence of two classes or groups. Multiclass problems can be split into a family of two-class problems, which can be solved in an appropriate sequence. Moreover, in the framework of Genetic Algorithms, the use of particular accuracy and optimization algorithms may help cope with the multiclass case.

The identification of the "optimal" hyperboxes or hyperellipsoids in the feature space was developed using two strong approaches of pattern recognition: the fuzzy c-means and the genetic algorithms. In particular the following three methods have been tested:

FCM-GA, where the fuzzy c-means and the genetic algorithm optimize the hyperboxes
GA-HB, where the hyperboxes have been optimized by genetic algorithms
GA-HE, where the genetic algorithm perform an optimization of a class of hyperellipsoids.

The FCM-GA method represents a more linear learning procedure, because first the prototypes of the clusters are determined, and consequently the genetic algorithm performs the optimization of the hyperboxes in a delimited search region. The GA-HB technique represents a powerful and direct method for providing the optimal hyperboxes, increasing the interpretability of the results.

Finally the GA-HE method introduces a very general family of hyperellipsoids, characterized by a differentiable and well-defined analytical expression, with a light decrease of the interpretation capability. All the three methods obtained a good performance in the classification of N/PVC beats, obtaining a mean accuracy of 97.7–98.2% with FCM-GA, 99.2–99.4% with GA-HB, and 99.5% with the GA-HE algorithm, using one or more hyperboxes/hyperellipsdoids. In general the number of hyperboxes/hyperellipsoids is not a critical point, and increasing their number does not necessarily provide a better accuracy. This means that a limited number of hyperboxes or hyperellipsoids is sufficient to produce classifiers with high interpretation capabilities, without a significant reduction of the accuracy.

The last experiment is consisting in determining the minimal number and size of the hyperboxes/hyperellipsoids, which performed a simplification of the visual interpretation and this corresponds to an implicit selection of the more meaningful hyperboxes.

The results showed that hyperbox classifiers are very intuitive, whereas the hyperellipsoids possess a very well-defined analytical expression, and both obtain good classification accuracies.

References

AAMI.: Testing and reporting performance results of cardiac rhythm and ST-segment measurement algorithms. Ansi/AAMI EC57:1998/(R)2008. Association for the Advancement of Medical Instrumentation (2008)

Bezdek, J.C.: Pattern Recognition with Fuzzy Objective Function. Plenum, New York (1981)

Bortolan, G. and Pedrycz, W.: Fuzzy descriptive models: an interactive framework of information granulation. IEEE Trans. Fuzzy Sets. **10**, 743–755 (2002a)

Bortolan, G., Pedrycz, W.: An interactive framework for an analysis of ECG signals. Artif. Intell. Med. **24**, 109–132 (2002b)

Bortolan, G., Pedrycz, W.: Hyperbox classifier for arrhythmia classification. Kybernetes. **36**, 531–547 (2007)

Bortolan, G., Willems, J.L.: Diagnostic ECG classification based on neural networks. J. Electrocardiol. **26**, 75–79 (1994)

Bortolan, G., Brohet, C. Fusaro, S.: Possibilities of using neural networks for diagnostic ECG classification. J. Electrocardiol. **29**, 10–16 (1996)

Bortolan, G., Jekova, I., Christov, I.: Comparison of four methods for premature Ventricular Contraction and normal beat clustering. IEEE Comp. Cardiol. **32**, 921–924 (2005)

Bortolan, G., Christov, I., Pedrycz, W.: Hyperbox classifiers for ECG beat analysis. IEEE Comp. Cardiol . **34**, 145–148 (2007)

Christov, I., Bortolan, G.: Ranking of pattern recognition parameters for premature ventricular contractions classification by neural networks. Physiological Measurement, **24**, 1281–1290 (2004)

Christov, I., Jekova, I., Bortolan, G.: Premature ventricular contraction classification by the Kth nearest-neighbours rule. Physiol. Meas. **26**, 123–130 (2005)

Christov, I., Gómez-Herrero, G., Krasteva, V., Jekova, I., Gotchev, A., Egiazarian, K.: Comparative study of morphological and time-frequency ECG descriptors for heartbeat classification. Med. Eng. Phys. **28**, 876–887 (2006)

Conn, A.R., Gould, N.I.M., Toint, P.L.: A globally convergent augmented Lagrangian pattern search algorithm for optimization with general constraints and simple bounds. SIAM J. Numer. Anal. **28**, 545–572 (1991)

Daskalov, I.K., Christov, I.: Electrocardiogram signal preprocessing for automatic detection of QRS boundaries. Med. Eng. Phys. **21**, 37–44 (1999)

Daskalov, I., Dotsinsky, I., Christov, I.: Developments in ECG acquisition, preprocessing, parameter measurement and recording. IEEE Eng. Med. Biol. **17**, 50–58 (1998)

Gabrys, B., Bargiela, A.: General fuzzy min-max neural network for clustering and classification. IEEE Trans. Neural Netw. **11**, 769–783 (2001)

Gómez-Herrero, G., Gotchev, A., Christov, I., Egiazarian, K.: Feature extraction for heartbeat classification using independent component analysis and matching pursuits. In: International Conference on Acoustics, Speech and Signal Processing, ICASSP2005, pp. 725–728, Philadelphia (2005)

Gómez-Herrero, G., Jekova, I., Krasteva, V., Christov, I., Gotchev, A., Egiazarian, K.: Relative estimation of the Karhunen-Loève transform basis functions for detection of ventricular ectopic beats. IEEE Comp. Cardiol. **33**, 569–572 (2006)

Jaklic, A., Leonardis, A., Solina, F.: Segmentation and Recovery of Superquadrics. Kluwer Academic, London (2000)

Jekova, I., Bortolan, G., Christov, I.: Pattern recognition and optimal parameter selection in premature ventricular contraction classification. IEEE Comp. Cardiol. **31**, 357–360 (2004)

Jekova, I., Bortolan, G., Christov, I.: Assessment and comparison of different classification methods for heart beat clustering. Med. Eng. Phys. **30**, 248–257 (2008)

Mark, R., Moody, G.: MIT-BIH Arrhythmia Data Base Directory. Massachusetts Institute of Technology, Cambridge (1988)

Silipo, R., Bortolan, G., Marchesi, C.: Design of hybrid architectures based on neural classifier and RBF pre-processing for ECG analysis. Int. J. Approx Reason. **21**, 177–196 (1999)

Simpson, P.K.: Fuzzy min-max neural networks: 1. Classification. IEEE Trans. Neural Netw. **3**, 776–586 (1992)

Chapter 11
Evolutionary Optimization of ECG Feature Extraction Methods: Applications to the Monitoring of Adult Myocardial Ischemia and Neonatal Apnea Bradycardia Events

A.I. Hernández, J. Dumont, M. Altuve, A. Beuchée, and G. Carrault

11.1 Introduction

Since the first recordings by Einthoven, more than a century ago (Einthoven 1902), the electrocardiogram (ECG) has emerged as an irreplaceable exploration tool of the cardiac electrical activity. ECG signals can be acquired easily, by the application of simple, inexpensive, and safe medical devices, either in acute, ambulatory, or telemedical contexts. Compared to other methods of observation of the cardiac activity, the ECG is the first and sometimes the only indicator of changes occurring at different scales, from the molecular level to the whole organ level. In this sense, it constitutes an essential diagnostic tool for common diseases such as myocardial ischemia, arrhythmia, or rare diseases such as heart muscle dystrophies. It has also been used as a window to explore other physiological processes of the

A.I. Hernández (✉) · G. Carrault
INSERM, U642, Rennes, F-35000, France and Université de Rennes 1, LTSI, Rennes, F-35000, France
e-mail: alfredo.hernandez@inserm.fr; guy.carrault@univ-rennes1.fr

J. Dumont
INSERM, U642, Rennes, F-35000, France, Université de Rennes 1, LTSI, Rennes, F-35000, France and SORIN Group CRM, Clamart, France
e-mail: jerome.dumont@univ-rennes1.fr

M. Altuve
Department of Industrial Technology, Simon Bolivar University, Caracas 1080, Venezuela, INSERM, U642, Rennes, F-35000, France and Université de Rennes 1, LTSI, Rennes, F-35000, France
e-mail: miguel.altuve@univ-rennes1.fr

A. Beuchée
INSERM, U642, Rennes, F-35000, France, Université de Rennes 1, LTSI, Rennes, F-35000, France, and Département de Pédiatrie, Pavillon Le Chartier, CHU, Rennes, France
e-mail: alain.beuchee@chu-rennes.fr

A. Gacek and W. Pedrycz (eds.), *ECG Signal Processing, Classification and Interpretation: A Comprehensive Framework of Computational Intelligence*, DOI 10.1007/978-0-85729-868-3_11, cardiovascular system, such as the short-term autonomic regulation, by means of the analysis of the heart rate variability (van Ravenswaaij-Arts et al. 1993). Current research is focused on a better exploration of ECG signals to

- Extract even more information from each ECG beat
- Combine the information obtained from the available ECG channels of a given patient (12 channels in standard ECG, 3 orthogonal channels on vectorcardiography, etc.)
- Study the temporal dynamics of the different features extracted
- Analyze large-scale ECG databases in order to derive new knowledge that may be useful to improve diagnosis and therapeutic actions

The first and second points require the application of robust, automated signal processing and modeling methods for the detection of individual beats from ECG signals and for their segmentation and characterization. Several contributions have been proposed in the literature (Sörnmo et al. 2005); however, their optimal application on clinical data is a complex problem for several reasons.

- Despite the application of different data preprocessing techniques, biomedical data often exhibits a low signal-to-noise ratio.
- There is a significant intra- and inter-patient variability of the main signal components, even among healthy subjects.
- Knowledge of the underlying physiological processes is often incomplete and the final detection or classification stages are based on heuristics, often represented by a set of rules.

Moreover, the typical signal processing chains currently proposed for the detection, segmentation, and classification of ECG signals are complex and require a significant number or parameters (filter cutoff frequencies, thresholds, etc.) that may be difficult to optimize for a given application.

In the next section of this chapter, we present a brief state of the art on current ECG segmentation methods and propose a complete signal processing chain, adapted to the detection and segmentation of ECG signals. Section 3 is dedicated to the complex problem of the optimization of the different parameters characterizing this signal processing chain, by means of an original approach based on evolutionary computing methods. This approach is applied in Sects. 11.4 and 11.5 to the optimal detection and segmentation of ECG signals acquired from adults and newborn infants, respectively.

11.2 Overview of ECG Segmentation Methods and Proposed Approach

As in most data-processing applications, a preprocessing step is necessary to detect the events of interest from the raw data and to extract features that may be useful for the classification and interpretation steps. In the clinical context, this feature extraction is typically performed by a clinician in any analysis of the ECG of a patient. However, its automation is important in order to handle large volumes of data, while improving repeatability. Several applications are concerned, such as the follow-up of patients suffering from cardiovascular diseases, drug evaluation, estimation of the physiological response of the autonomic nervous system, and so on. Within this ECG processing step, the segmentation of individual waves on each beat remains probably the most complex issue, especially for P and T waves. The purpose of this section is thus to present a brief recall of the main components of a typical signal processing chain for the detection and segmentation of the main ECG waves and to propose a particular approach, based on a wavelet transform decomposition.

11.2.1 Main ECG Processing Steps

In general, the automatic segmentation of the ECG is preceded by the following steps: (1) preprocessing and filtering of the raw ECG signal, (2) QRS complex detection, and, eventually, (3) beat alignment and averaging. A representative example of applying these processing and segmentation steps on a real ECG is shown in Figure 11.1. A brief description and bibliography for each one of these steps is proposed in the following paragraphs.

The main objective of the preprocessing step is to minimize the noise that contaminates the ECG signal (50/60 Hz noise, electrode motion artifacts, baseline drifts, and so on). The rejection of interference at 50/60 Hz has been the subject of numerous publications and a review by Levkov et al. (2005) lists a large number of methods. Methods based on adaptive filtering are often chosen because they can track changes in phase and amplitude of the interference (Thakor and Zhu 2002; Ziarani and Konrad 2002; Islam et al. 2010). Baseline drifts are low-frequency and high-amplitude noises that are mainly related to patient movement and breathing. Many methods have been proposed to minimize their effect, including the application of spline interpolations (Jane et al. 1992; Yang et al. 2010), filter banks (Shusterman et al. 2000; Leski and Henzel 2005), and Kalman filters (Mneimneh et al. 2008).

The localization of each beat from the ECG signal is performed by detecting the most prominent set of waves (the QRS complex). A review of QRS detection methods can be found in Kohler et al. (2002), and current methods provide satisfactory results in most of the cases. However, a study conducted in our laboratory showed that current QRS detection methods show distinct behaviors with respect to the presence of noise and variations in QRS morphology and that an interesting gain in performance can be obtained by combining (or fusing) the output obtained from a set of heterogeneous QRS detectors (Portet et al. 2005). Individual beats are then extracted by applying a fixed or adaptive-width time window, defined around each QRS detection instant. In order to obtain an average beat, a preliminary step of beat correlation with respect to a set of beat prototypes is often performed.

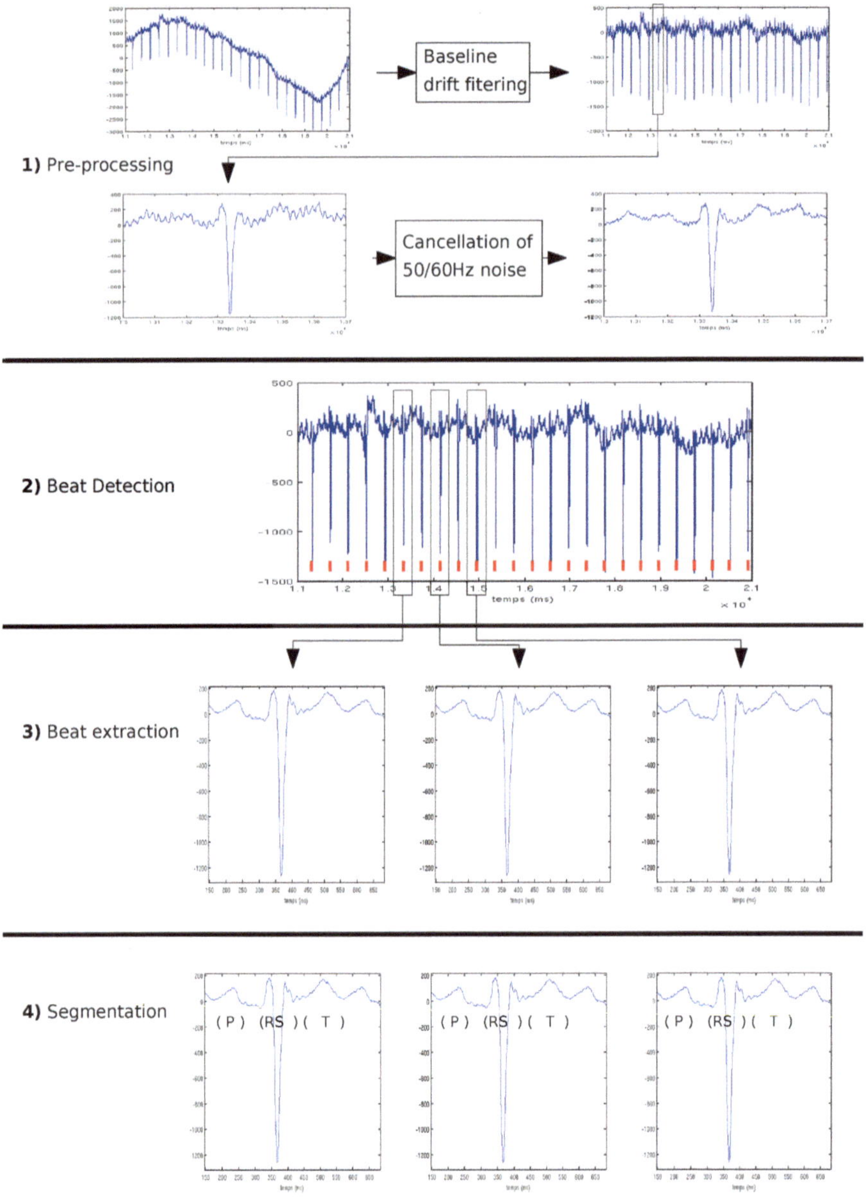

Fig. 11.1 Diagram representing the main ECG signal processing steps with examples from a record of the QT database from Physionet

Each detected beat is thus averaged out with a predefined number of preceding beats, highly correlated with the same beat prototype. This is done for each beat, except when no heartbeat prototype does provide a measure of correlation above a given threshold. In that case, the current beat itself becomes a new prototype (Dumont et al. 2010b).

Finally, beat segmentation (or delineation) can be applied to these isolated beats. This segmentation usually provides an estimation of the main ECG wave positions: P wave start (Pon), peak of the P wave (Ppeak), P wave end (Poff), beginning and end of the QRS complex (QRSon and QRoff, respectively), peak of the R wave (Rpeak), T wave peak (Tpeak), T wave start (Ton), and the T wave end (Toff). Once this segmentation is performed, it is easy to extract other useful indicators, such as the energy of each wave, the level and slope of the ST segment or QRS slopes. A detailed presentation of the main ECG segmentation methods is proposed in the next section.

11.2.2 State of the Art on ECG Segmentation Methods

The precise segmentation of each ECG wave is a difficult task, even for experimented cardiologists (CSE 1985). These difficulties are mainly related to the low signal-to-noise ratio often observed in ECG signals, the wide variety of wave morphologies that exists, even among healthy subjects, the lack of a universal definition of the ending instants of some waves (especially for the QRS complex and the T wave), and the fact that the spectral components of these different waves overlap. A number of works have addressed this segmentation problem in the literature, based on filtering and derivation, adaptive filtering, dynamic programming, Markov models, or wavelet decomposition.

11.2.2.1 Filtering and Derivation

The method proposed by Laguna et al. (1994) is based on the application of a low-pass filter and a differentiator. A simple technique based on thresholds and time windows is then used to determine the significant slopes characterizing the QRS complex. For the detection of P and T waves, a second low-pass filter is applied. As for the QRS, time windows are set to detect significant slopes. However, for the T wave, a heart rate–dependent time window is used. Wave peaks are defined as the zero-crossing instants of the differentiated signals and then the wave limits are sought by setting thresholds on the significant slope values. This approach shows that it is interesting to analyze the QRS complex and the P and T waves with at least two distinct filtering resolutions. Although this segmentation method is rather simple, the results obtained from its application on the Physionet QTDB database (Laguna et al. 1994), presented in Table 11.1, show interesting segmentation results.

Table 11.1 Segmentation results obtained by Laguna on the QTDB from Physionet

Pon	Poff	QRSon	QRSoff	Tpeak	Toff
10.4 ± 12.5	-3.7 ± 11.4	-4.1 ± 9.0	-1.0 ± 8.4	-8.0 ± 15.0	11.6 ± 28.2

Results represented by average $\pm$ standard deviation

11.2.2.2 Adaptive Filtering

The method suggested by Soria-Olivas et al. (1998) combines a simple filter and an adaptive filter. It includes a semiautomatic learning step, as cardiologists perform manually the detection of the T wave, following their personal criterion. This allows for the estimation of a constant adjustment, introduced in the adaptive filter. Subsequently, the ECG is filtered by a static and then an adaptive filter. A local minimum of the filtered ECG appears at the end of each T wave and this feature is used for T wave segmentation. The results of this algorithm are satisfactory but it is important to recall that it cannot be used without a prescreening by a cardiologist. Moreover, the authors have not performed quantitative tests on ECG databases. It is therefore difficult to assess accurately the differences in performance with a fully automatic method.

11.2.2.3 Beat Segmentation by Realignment Using Dynamic Programming

Dynamic time warping (DTW) has been initially defined as a distance measure between time series that is insensitive to time expansion and compression. This method is based on a sample-by-sample realignment of a given series, with respect to another series (taken as reference), by minimizing a cumulative distance calculated from all available samples. Its adaptation to beat segmentation fully exploits this realignment property of the DTW: each detected beat is compared and realigned with a previously segmented beat, either manually or based on one of the previous methods. Different ECG segmentation methods integrating a DTW estimation have been proposed, with distinct preprocessing approaches: piecewise linear approximations (Vullings et al. 1998) or adaptive piecewise constant approximations (Zifan et al. 2006). However, this algorithm is naturally highly dependent on the set of pre-segmented beats used as reference and may be difficult to apply in real-time applications.

11.2.2.4 Markovian Modeling

Markov models have received special attention for the analysis of time series, particularly in the context of speech processing. The first applications in modeling of the ECG signal were introduced by Doerschuck (1985) and were focused on the simulation of arrhythmia. Later, Coast et al. (1990) proposed a Markov model for detecting a sequence of ECG waves, including the presence or absence of

P-waves, for the detection of supraventricular arrhythmia. The first application to the segmentation of the QRS complex was presented in Coast (1993) and generalized later on by Thoraval (1995) for the segmentation of all ECG waves.

Other models, such as that of Koski (1996), for the simulation of ECG signals, or the works from Clavier and Boucher (1996), for the early detection of atrial fibrillation after segmentation and classification or P-waves, integrate, within the model states, information about the slope, amplitude, or duration of ECG segments in order to differentiate each wave. More recently, the application of two concurrent models was proposed: the first model is similar to those of Koski and Clavier, with parameters retrieved from a linear regression on the ECG signal; the second model is based on the analysis of the coefficients of a wavelet decomposition (Hughes et al. 2003). Significantly better results are obtained when integrating the wavelet decomposition (e.g., a higher detection rate of P-waves). These results provide a better performance than those reported in Graja and Boucher (2003) and Laguna et al. (1994).

A wavelet decomposition has also been proposed by Thoraval (1995), integrating other parameters extracted from the ECG (frequency, amplitude, and so on) within semi-Markovian models; by Lepage et al. (2001) with specific Markov models for each decomposition level, or more recently, by Graja and Boucher (2005), which proposed a tree-like Markovian model where interstate connectivity only exists between the wavelet coefficients of neighboring levels.

Although many refinements have been proposed since the first models by Coast and Doerschuk to improve the segmentation results, their application to large databases is uncommon. This is partly due to the difficulty inoptimizing the choice of features to be modeled, and the large amounts of annotated data needed for the model learning step.

11.2.2.5 Wavelet-Based Beat Segmentation

Since the pioneering works of Senhadji et al. (2002), multiscale methods have shown a growing importance on the processing of ECG signals. These methods, which permit noise reduction at rough scales and then to refine the research of wave positions with the help of finer scales, provide robust segmentation procedures when compared to other methods. Algorithms based on a wavelet transform (WT) decomposition have been proposed in the literature in this sense (Li et al. 1995; Bahoura et al. 1997; Martinez et al. 2004). In most of the cases, the mother wavelet employed $\psi(t)$, from which are derived the approximation $H(z)$ and detail $G(z)$ filters is a quadratic spline, with the following Fourier transform:

$$\Psi(\omega) = j\omega \left(\frac{\sin(\frac{\omega}{4})}{\frac{\omega}{4}} \right)^4 \tag{11.1}$$

This wavelet can be seen as the derivative of a low-pass function. It is thus interesting to analyze the slope of the different decomposition levels around the wave boundaries, to derive rules for the segmentation of each wave. In the works

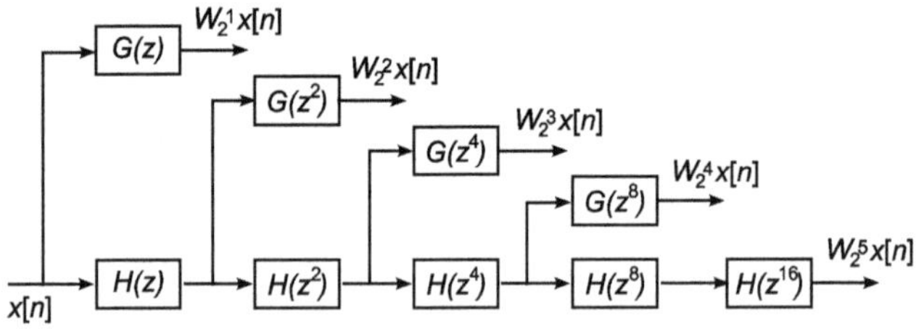

Fig. 11.2 Filter bank of the wavelet decomposition (without decimation). $G(z)$ and $H(z)$ are the high-pass and low-pass filters, respectively. $W_2^k x[n]$ are the outputs of filters at scales 2^k ($k \in 1, 2, \ldots, 5$) to beat $x[n]$

of Li et al. (1995) and Martinez et al. (2004), this approach has been retained by processing the original ECG signal $x[n]$ using a five-level WT dyadic decomposition ($W_2^1 x[n]$ to $W_2^5 x[n]$) implemented as a typical octave filter bank, but keeping a high temporal resolution at every scale by suppressing the decimators usually employed, as shown in Fig. 11.2. The main differences between these two works are in the rules used to identify each wave boundary. More recently, these rules have been optimized by Dumont et al. (2010b).

In the literature, the numerous parameters characterizing these detection and segmentation methods are often adjusted manually and empirically, without knowing whether their multiple interactions lead to a better segmentation performance (Li et al. 1995; Martinez et al. 2004). Performance improvements with respect to previous works can thus be expected by optimizing these parameters. This problem was our main motivation for proposing a generic and automatic methodology to optimize parameters and thresholds of such complex signal processing chains.

11.3 Optimal Beat Detection and Segmentation Based on Evolutionary Computing

This section presents an evolutionary approach to jointly optimize the parameters of the proposed detection and segmentation methods. The optimization procedure aims to define parameter values for the whole signal processing chain leading to a beat segmentation as close as possible to those proposed as a reference in annotated databases. In other words, the objective is to propose optimal parameter values that minimize an error function defined between the output of the segmentation algorithm and a set of annotations. This procedure, which is depicted in Fig. 11.3, integrates a priori knowledge only by means of the manual annotations performed by the cardiologists when defining the learning database and by the definition of the limits of the parameter search space. However, the large dimension of the search space, which may contain multiple local minima, and the fact that the segmentation algorithm is composed of different thresholds (which means that the cost function is

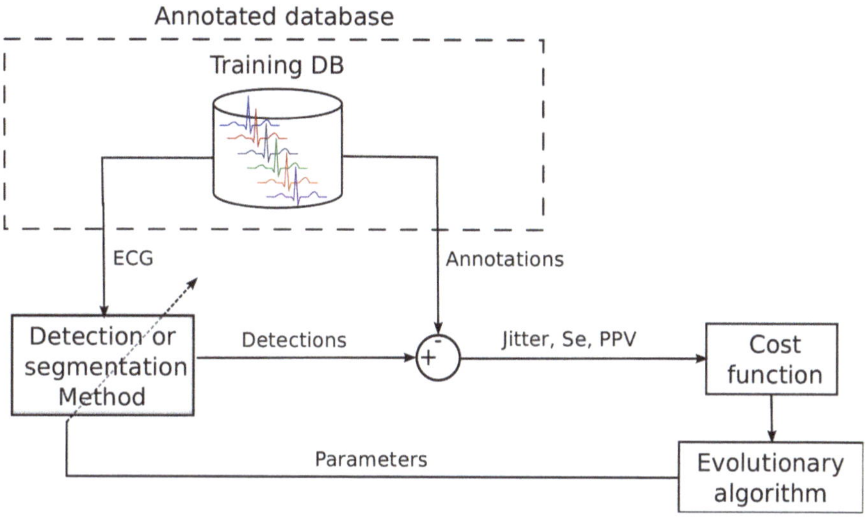

Fig. 11.3 Diagram representing the training phase of the proposed parameter optimization method. An annotated ECG database, usually obtained as a subset of a larger database, is used for this training phase. The evolutionary algorithm is configured to minimize an error function which integrates the sensitivity (Se), the positive predictive value (PPV), and the detection jitter provided by the method being optimized for a given set of parameters

discontinuous in the parameter space) imply the application of robust optimization methods. These constraints are not compatible with the use of classical optimization methods based on gradient estimation or the simplex method. On the other hand, stochastic optimization methods, such as evolutionary algorithms, are particularly suited for this type of problems.

Evolutionary algorithms (EA) are optimization techniques, inspired on the theories of evolution and natural selection, which can be employed to find an optimal configuration for a given system within specific constraints (Michalewicz 1996). In these algorithms, each individual of a population is characterized by a set of parameters to be optimized (or chromosome). An initial population is created, usually from a set of random chromosomes, and this population will evolve, improving its global performance, by means of an iterative process. During this process, each individual is evaluated by means of a "fitness function" (which can be defined as a negative cost function), representing how its chromosome configuration can be a good solution for the given problem. A new generation is produced by applying mutation and crossover operators, with probabilities p_m and p_c, respectively, on selected individuals presenting low values on their cost functions.

11.3.1 Proposed Evolutionary Algorithm Configuration

EA have been applied in several biomedical applications to estimate a large set of parameters and have provided interesting results (Eichler West et al. 1999; Hernández et al. 2002). Convergence and robustness properties of EA have been largely studied in the literature (Michalewicz 1996). These properties depend on (1) an adequate individual coding, (2) the proper definition of the fitness (or cost) function, and (3) the appropriate definition of a selection method and genetic operators for crossover and mutation. The definitions of these components for the specific evolutionary algorithm proposed in this work are detailed in the next subsections.

11.3.1.1 Individual Coding

In the original definition of genetic algorithms (GA) by Holland (1992), chromosomes were designed as strings of G parameters (G genes), each one coded with b bits. An extension of this coding to real values has been proposed by Michalewicz (1996). This representation is often accompanied by a matrix of maximum and minimum values for each gene to restrain the search space to valid solutions and also accelerate the convergence to the optimal solution. This real-value coding has been compared experimentally with the binary representations and has demonstrated faster convergence times and an improved accuracy and higher reproducibility of the estimated solutions (Janikow and Michalewicz 1991). A real-value coding was thus selected for this problem. The upper and lower bounds of each gene are defined differently for time windows and for thresholds. Values for time windows are taken from extreme durations of each wave, based on physiological knowledge. Concerning threshold values, the parameters obtained from the bibliography were augmented or decreased in a tenfold manner.

11.3.1.2 Cost Function

The segmentation algorithm proposed in this chapter provides an estimation of the ECG wave positions previously defined: Pon, Ppeak, Poff, QRSon, QRoff, Rpeak, Tpeak, and Toff. The proposed cost function evaluates several performance criteria for each one of these estimations. These criteria are

- Probability of detection error, defined as

$$Perr_p = \sqrt{(1 - Se_p)^2 + (1 - PPV_p)^2} \tag{11.2}$$

  where Se_p and PPV_p are, respectively, the sensitivity and positive predictive values obtained for wave position p ($p \in$ {Pon, Ppeak ... Tpeak, Toff }).

This probability is calculated as the distance between the detection point obtained (Se_p, PPV_p) and the optimal detection point ($Se = 1$ and $PPV = 1$).

- Mean detection jitter $\overline{\varepsilon_p}$, computed as the average jitter committed between the annotation (Ann_p) and the detection (Det_p), over all M records and all N_m beats of each record:

$$\overline{\varepsilon_p} = \frac{1}{M} \sum_{m=1}^{M} \frac{\sum_{n=1}^{N_m} |Ann_p^m(n) - Det_p^m(n)|}{N_m}. \tag{11.3}$$

- Standard deviation of the detection jitter σ_p, calculated as the mean of the standard deviation of the detection jitter for each record (σ_p^m):

$$\sigma_p = \frac{\sum_m^M \sigma_p^m}{M}. \tag{11.4}$$

These three criteria are evaluated for all p and should be jointly minimized. This kind of multi-objective optimization can be approached as a single-objective problem, with a cost function defined as a weighted average of the different criteria

$$O = \sum_{p=1}^{P} \left(\frac{Perr_p}{a_p} + \frac{\overline{\varepsilon_p}}{b_p} + \frac{\sigma_p}{c_p} \right) \tag{11.5}$$

where a_p, b_p, and c_p can be defined as the best results retrieved from the literature (Martinez et al. 2004; Laguna et al. 1994) for $Perr_p$, $\overline{\varepsilon_p}$, and σ_p, respectively. Qualitatively, this cost function evaluates the improvement ratio between our results ($Perr_p, \overline{\varepsilon_p}$, and σ_p) and the corresponding best results reported in the literature (a_p, b_p, and c_p). It is the result of this cost function that is minimized by the optimization algorithm.

11.3.1.3 Selection Method and Genetic Operators

Each new generation of individuals is created randomly from the individuals of the current generation through a selection process that favors the evolution of individuals presenting the lowest values on their cost function. Several criteria for assigning the selection probability have been proposed in the literature. The most common are the "roulette" method (introduced by Holland 1992) and the "ranking" method. In the case of the ranking method, the values of the selection probability p_l are calculated according to the rank of the individual l, when individuals are sorted in descending order of their performance. The probabilities are thus given by

$$p_l = \frac{q * (1-q)^{r_l - 1}}{1 - (1-q)^P} \tag{11.6}$$

where q is the probability of drawing the individual of rank 1, r_l is the rank of individual l, and P is the total number of individuals. Other selection methods such as the "tournament" or elitist methods can be used, but they are particular cases of the ranking procedure. The ranking method was used in this work for individual selection, with parameter q fixed at 0.08 as proposed in Houck et al. (1995).

Several crossover operators have been proposed in the literature, initially for the binary representation and then extended to the real-value representation. In this work, the simple, arithmetic, and heuristic crossovers are applied. The mutation operators affect a single individual, by randomly modifying one or more of its genes. Two types of mutation were used in this work, based on uniform or nonuniform distributions. More details on the definition of these genetic operators can be found elsewhere (Holland 1992; Michalewicz 1996).

11.3.2 Application of the Evolutionary Algorithm

Two different applications of the proposed segmentation algorithm, combined with the optimization methodology, will be presented in this chapter: (1) the segmentation of adult ECG recordings for the analysis of ischemic episodes (Sect. 11.4) and (2) the detection and segmentation of the QRS complex on ECG records acquired from preterm infants in newborn intensive care units, to perform an early detection of apnea-bradycardia events (Sect. 11.5).

11.4 Optimal Segmentation of Adult ECG Recordings for Myocardial Ischemia Monitoring

Myocardial ischemia remains a major public health problem. The accurate detection and characterization of ischemic episodes is crucial, as it reduces the delay between the appearance of the first symptoms and the application of an adapted reperfusion therapy, thus improving the survival rate (McGinn et al. 2005). It is also useful for the analysis of transient ischemic episodes, because their frequency is a useful indicator for risk stratification of patients suffering from cardiovascular diseases (Touzé et al. 2005). Although the analysis of the ST-segment remains the most common electrocardiographic method used to characterize myocardial ischemia, it suffers from a poor specificity (Smrdel and Jager 2004). It is thus currently admitted that a way to overcome this low specificity is to combine the information from the ST segment with other indicators extracted from each beat (Langer and Armstrong 1998).

This section is organized in three subsections, covering the main aspects of a complete data processing application for the detection of ischemic episodes. The proposed wavelet-based beat segmentation method is presented in Sect. 11.4.1.

Section 11.4.2 covers the optimization of this segmentation method and presents the resulting optimal parameters. Finally, Sect. 11.4.3 proposes a multivariate analysis of the features extracted from the beat segmentation phase, in order to improve the detection of ischemic episodes.

11.4.1 Proposed Beat Segmentation Method

In this section, ECG wave positions are computed through the four-stage process described in Sect. 11.2.1. Algorithms taken from the literature were used for the first two stages: 50/60 Hz rejection (Thakor and Zhu 2002) and baseline drift cancellation (Shusterman et al. 2000), and the Pan and Tompkins algorithm (Pan and Tompkins 1985) was chosen for QRS detection.

The segmentation stage is based on a WT decomposition and is inspired from the works of Martinez et al. (2004) (see Sect. 11.2.2.5). Each beat is extracted from the ECG signal and delimited into a small temporal support to form the signal $x[n]$ (or W_2^0) to be decomposed. This approach is implemented as represented in Fig. 11.2. Once the WT decomposition is performed, first the R wave, then the Q and S waves, and finally the P and T waves are segmented by applying a set of rules. The global procedure is as follows:

- The R wave is detected by analyzing W_2^2, by looking for the two largest peaks of opposite sign, and then by searching the zero crossing on W_2^1 between these slopes. If several zero crossings appear, the one associated with the highest signal amplitude on W_2^0 is retained. Two parameters (R1 and R2) define the left and right boundaries of the temporal support for the R wave search.
- The isoelectric level is determined with the method proposed by Smrdel and Jager (2004).
- The Q and S waves, as well as QRSon and QRSoff, are retrieved by analyzing the local maxima on the first two scales, W_2^1 and W_2^2, which have a quite high frequency content, as in Martinez et al. (2004). The thresholds γ_{QRSpre} and $\gamma_{QRSpost}$ are proportional to the maximum slope of the R wave and are used to identify the other significant slopes of the Q and S waves. Temporal supports for searching these waves are defined by the parameters QRS_Qlim and QRS_Slim.
- The P and T waves are delimited by analyzing scales W_2^4 or W_2^5: if these waves are not found at W_2^4, W_2^5 is also analyzed. Their peaks are found on the immediate lower scale (i.e., W_2^3 or W_2^4). The thresholds for wave detection are $\varepsilon_{(P)}$ and $\varepsilon_{(T)}$ and are relative to the power at scales W_2^4 or W_2^5. The significant slopes are identified with respect to thresholds γ_T and γ_P. Time windows for P-wave and T wave detection depend on the previous RR interval (thresholds P_RR and T_RR). T1•/P1• are the left boundaries of these windows and T2•/P2• are the right boundaries, • is the index that changes in function of the RR interval.

- The wave onset and offset (for S, Q, P, and T waves) are detected with respect to the thresholds $\xi_{(QRSon,QRSend,Ton,Tend,Pon,Pend)}$ relative to the amplitude of the first or last significant slope.

Compared to the work of Martinez et al. (2004), an additional test is performed to check if the peaks are further away from the isoelectric level than the wave onset or offset. If not, it is considered that the current delineation is wrong and the temporal support is redefined. This test is applied successively, starting from a large temporal support and reducing it progressively.

Obviously, the performance of this approach depends on the appropriate definition of temporal analysis windows, but also on the identification of appropriate decision thresholds that will detect significant slopes and the boundaries of each waves. However, this is a difficult task, involving a large number of parameters (30 parameters for the proposed segmentation method) having multiple interactions. The evolutionary approach described in the previous section will be thus applied in Sect. 11.4.2 to optimize these parameters.

11.4.2 Optimization of the Beat Segmentation Method

11.4.2.1 Data Selection

In order to optimize the beat segmentation method, the annotated QTDB database from Physionet was used for training and evaluation purposes (Goldberger et al. 2000). The QTDB provides a total of 105 ECG records, presenting a wide variety of pathologies, each record containing two ECG channels sampled at 250 Hz. Compared to other databases, it contains a large number of annotated beats per record (30 annotated beats per record instead of a single beat on the CSE database). Annotations are also particularly complete, with all positions of the points Pon, Ppeak, Poff, QRSon, QRSoff, Tpeak, Toff. Moreover, this database has been used to evaluate other ECG segmentation methods in the literature and, thus, provides an interesting corpus for performance comparison.

The learning and test sets were constructed from the whole QTDB, using the following procedure: (1) every record on the QTDB is divided into three segments of the same duration, called sub-records; (2) two-thirds of all sub-records are randomly selected and assigned to the training set. The remaining sub-records are assigned to the test set. A total of 13 different learning/test sets are generated so as to learn and evaluate 13 instances of the optimal parameters and analyze their dependence on the training/test set used.

11.4.2.2 Evolutionary Algorithm Configuration and Optimization Results

The global optimization procedure is defined by the consecutive application of two evolutionary algorithms, so as to reduce the size of each search space.

- In the first EA (EA1), parameters associated with the segmentation of the P wave and QRS complex are optimized in a joint manner.
- In the second EA (EA2), parameters associated with the T wave are optimized by reusing the best parameters obtained at the end of EA1.

This decomposition is possible because the temporal support for the research of the T wave is related to the detection of the S wave, and it is considered that the detection of T wave will be optimal when the S wave detection has been previously optimized.

For both EA1 and EA2, 80 generations with 60 individuals were used. The probability of crossover, p_c, is set at 0.7. The mutation probability, p_m, is adapted during the learning phase, starting with a high value during the early generations to ensure research throughout the state space, and decreasing its value toward the end to facilitate convergence to a reliable minimum. Back's equation for the adaptive calculation of p_m (Back and Schutz 1996) was chosen because of its interesting convergence properties (Sebag et al. 1997; Thierens 2002). Back's equation is defined as follows:

$$p_m = \left(2 + \frac{(n_P - 2)}{Maxgen - 1} * gen\right)^{-1} \quad (11.7)$$

with n_P the number of parameters, $Maxgen$ the maximum number of generations, and gen the number of the current generation.

The whole optimization procedure (EA1+EA2) was applied 13 times using different learning and test sets and different initial populations in order to evaluate their sensitivity to the learning/test data and the robustness of the obtained optimal parameters. Table 11.2 presents the optimized parameters (with their means and standard deviations) obtained from EA1, and Table 11.3 presents the optimized parameters obtained from EA2.

Some parameter values show small standard deviations, such as the time windows used for searching the P, Q, S, and T waves, or the thresholds that define the onset and offset of P and T waves. These results indicate a high sensitivity of the segmentation algorithm to these parameters and, also, the fact that the proposed parameter values have been correctly estimated. On the other hand, the time windows used to locate the R wave, or the thresholds that define the beginning and the end of the QRS complex, show significant variations among the different training sets. These results indicate the lower sensitivity of the segmentation algorithm to these parameters. Indeed, a wide range of values for these parameters gives approximately the same results. It is important to underline that the proposed approach is not only useful for adjusting the settings but also to analyze the sensitivity of each parameter with respect to the results of segmentation.

11.4.2.3 Performance Evaluation of the Optimal Segmentation Method

Jane et al. (1997) proposed an analytical framework for the evaluation of segmentation algorithms, based on annotated ECG databases, similar to the QTDB. To

Table 11.2 Parameters used by the segmentation algorithm with their optimal values

Parameter	Value
P11	278±31
P12	240±17
P21	88±14
P22	99±27
R1	118±34
R2	111±37
P_{RR}	664±182
ε_P	0.12±0.05
γ_P	0.4±0.09
ξ_{Pon}	0.41±0.08
ξ_{Pend}	0.76±0.05
γ_{QRSpre}	0.09±0.03
$\gamma_{QRSpost}$	0.11±0.03
$\xi_{QRSonpos}$	0.07±0.04
$\xi_{QRSonneg}$	0.07±0.04
$\xi_{QRSendpos}$	0.21±0.12
$\xi_{QRSendneg}$	0.23±0.11
QRS_{Qlim}	88±22
QRS_{Slim}	154±32

Represented by average ± standard deviation, obtained after EA1

Table 11.3 Parameters used by the segmentation algorithm with their optimal values

Parameter	Value
ε_T	0.24±0.06
γ_T	0.28±0.07
ξ_{Ton}	0.17±0.09
ξ_{Tend}	0.36±0.07
T11	111±24
T21	441±75
T12	90±16
T22	0.6±0.08
T23	581±94
T_{RR1}	705±155
T_{RR2}	1231±70

Represented by average ± standard deviation, obtained after EA2

validate our method and the optimization procedure, the same analytical framework is applied. A comparison with the algorithms proposed by Martinez et al. (2004) and Laguna et al. (1994) is thus possible.

The mean detection jitter (Eq. 11.3) and its standard deviation (Eq. 11.4) are weighted by the number of beats per record and averaged over the records in the test set. The probability of detection error ($Perr_p$) is derived from the sensitivity and positive predictivity, as calculated in Martinez et al. (2004). These three criteria (mean detection jitter, its standard deviation, and the probability of detection error) are estimated for all the extracted features. Figure 11.4 shows the distributions of our results using different test sets. The crosses (+) and stars (*) are respectively the results from Martinez et al. (2004) and Laguna et al. (1994), presented in these references. The right column is the average of all indicators. Some comments may be made on each criterion:

- Concerning the mean detection jitter (or deviation), the median value of the proposed method is closer to zero than the other two methods, for the points Pon, Ppeak, and QRSon. It is also better than Martinez et al. (2004) for Poff and better than Laguna et al. (1994) for QRSoff, Tpeak, and Toff.
- Concerning the standard deviation of the detection jitter, the median is lower for Pon, Peak, Poff, QRSon, and Tpeak, but is higher than Martinez et al. (2004) and Laguna et al. (1994) for QRSoff and higher than Martinez et al. (2004) for Toff.
- The probability of detection error is significantly lower for the P wave, but slightly worst results are obtained for the T wave. Nevertheless, this criterion is more difficult to analyze than the others because only a limited set of beats were annotated from the whole QTDB and differences may exist on the way each work evaluated non-annotated beats.
- Finally, when these three criteria are evaluated in a global manner (for all the features extracted), the proposed approach delivers the best performance in all cases. This is the more powerful feature of the proposed optimization approach. Coefficients a_p, b_p, and c_p in Eq. 11.5 can be adjusted if more importance should be given to a particular set of features.

In order to verify that the proposed method optimized the error detection probability, an additional test was performed. Receiver operating characteristic (ROC) curves were calculated for the detection of P and T waves, for each test set, by varying the main parameters. Figure 11.5 shows one instance of these ROC curves for the detection of the P wave, which varies depending on the parameter ε_P (range 0 to 0.43 in steps of 0.01). The point minimizing the probability of detection error is found to be $\varepsilon_P = 0.17$ from the analysis of the ROC curve, while the optimization algorithm has set this parameter to 0.15 during the learning process. Similar results are obtained for the T wave.

11.4.3 Detection of Ischemic Events

In order to detect myocardial ischemia events, the optimized segmentation algorithm presented above has been applied to estimate the position of the beginning and the end of the QRS complex, the T wave end, and the position of the extrema of the Q, R, S, and T waves from records extracted from the STAFF3 database. The

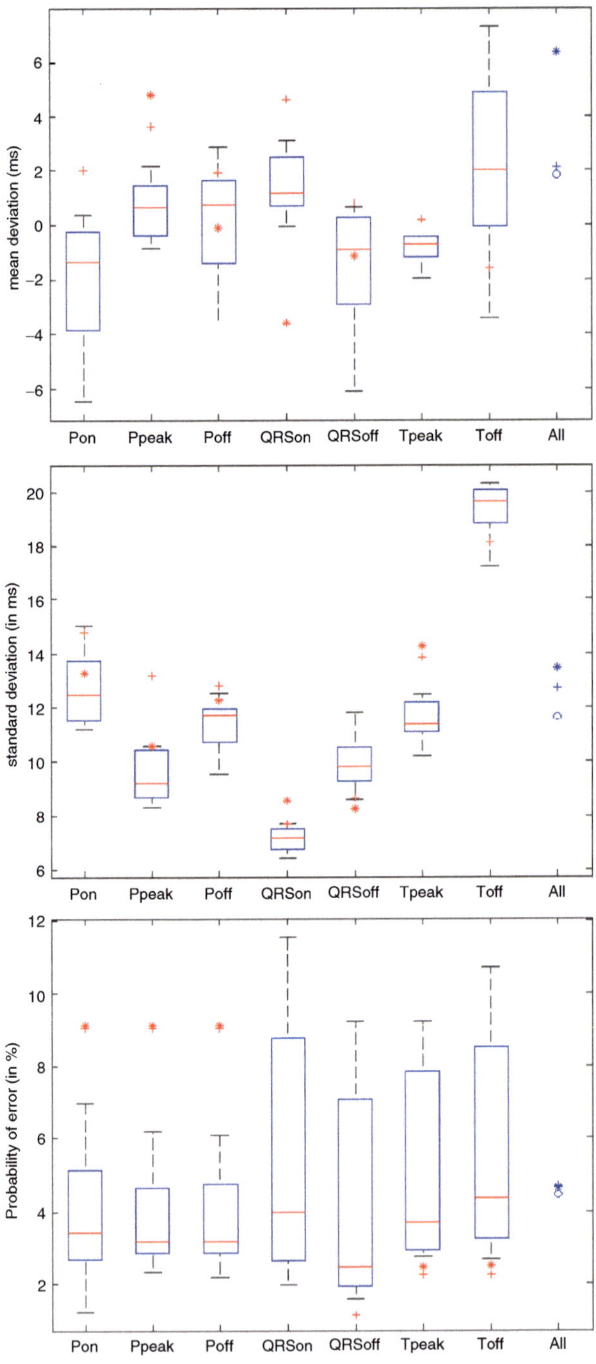

Fig. 11.4 Boxplots of the results of the segmentation procedure showing the three performance evaluation criteria (mean and standard deviation of the detection jitter and the probability of detection error). Values are obtained from the application of the optimization procedure for 13 different learning and test sets, for all the features Extracted

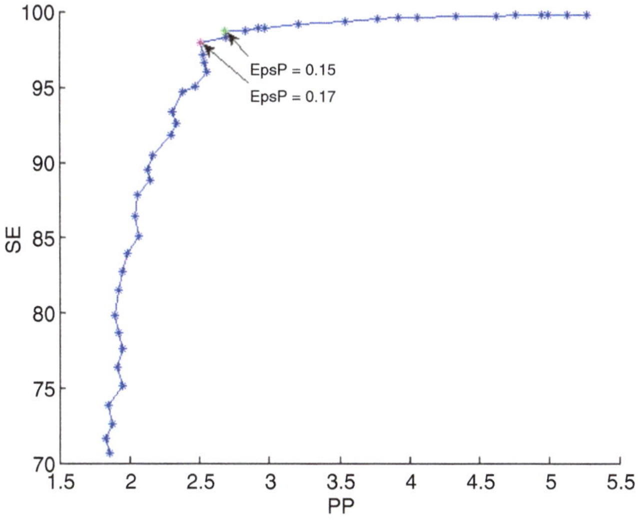

Fig. 11.5 ROC curve to evaluate the detection of the P wave for different values of parameter ε_P

STAFF3 database has been designed to study new indicators that may be useful for the detection of ischemic episodes induced by balloon inflation (PTCA) and accurately annotated. Studies published in the literature on this subject (Pueyo et al. 2008; Castro et al. 2004; Pettersson et al. 2000; Martinez et al. 2006; Garcia et al. 2000) reveal the major electrocardiographic modifications occurring during ischemia, such as changes in the high frequencies or duration of the QRS, or changes in T wave shape. However, these changes are based on the application of a threshold on the instantaneous values of these series to detect the ischemia, without taking into consideration their dynamics. In this case, noise spikes can, for example, provide false alarms. The correlation between the indicators is also underexploited. To improve this detection, it then appears important to take into consideration the temporal evolution of these indicators and, if possible, their joint evolution.

We have recently proposed the application of Hidden Semi-Markovian models to analyze the evolution of such kind of electrocardiographic features, in order to improve the detection of ischemic events (Dumont et al. 2010a). This section briefly presents the electrocardiographic features extracted for this clinical application, the proposed detection approach, and a quantitative evaluation of its performance, based on the STAFF3 database.

11.4.3.1 Extracted Electrocardiographic Features

The optimal beat detection and segmentation method presented in Sect. 11.4.2 has been applied to the STAFF3 database. This database contains records from 108 patients. For this study, only 68 patients without previous history of myocardial

Table 11.4 Extracted features

Amplitudes	Q, R, S, and T waves, ST level
Intervals	RR, QRSd (duration of the QRS complex), QT, and RT

infarction are considered and four records had to be removed because of lead disconnections. Concerning the records, there are at least, for each patient, (1) one 12-leads ECG recorded during the PTCA, with accurate annotation on the beginning and end of the inflation, and (2) one 12-leads ECG recorded before the operation. An additional preprocessing step of beat orthogonalization, based on a principal component analysis, was thus applied in order to reduce the number of leads per record (from 12 to 2 in our case).

After the application of this signal processing chain, the indicators presented in Table 11.4 are extracted and time series of these features are constructed and re-sampled to 1 Hz. Two examples of these time series are presented in Fig. 11.6.

11.4.3.2 HSMM-Based Ischemia Event Detection

The proposed ischemia detector is based on the analysis of the dynamics of the extracted time series, by means of a Hidden Semi-Markovian Model (HSMM), described in detail in Dumont et al. (2010a). Briefly, a reference HSMM (Mod_{Ref}) and an ischemic HSMM (Mod_{PTCA}) are learned by analyzing the time series extracted from a "reference" and an "ischemic" training sets. Both models are then applied to the extracted time series from a test set, and then the log-likelihood of each model is computed. A detection rule is applied by evaluating the difference of the log-likelihood of both models and comparing it with a threshold.

The training and evaluation of these models was performed as follows:

- The reference and ischemic training sets are extracted from half of the patients on the STAFF3 database, randomly selected. For Mod_{Ref}, the pre-inflation period is used in priority. If the record does not contain pre-inflation data, the pre-operation ECG is used instead. For Mod_{PTCA}, the data between the beginning and the end of the inflation procedure is exploited.
- The HSMM ischemic detector is applied on pre-operation records (to evaluate specificity) and inflation records (to evaluate sensitivity) of the second half of the STAFF3 database patients. The time series of the records to test are extracted and the log-likelihoods for the two models are computed;
- The proposed HSMM method was also compared to a more classical approach proposed by Langley, based on the classical ST level parameter.

ROC curves presenting ischemia detection performance for different combinations of electrocardiographic features and for different threshold values are shown in Fig. 11.7. The classical ST-level-based ichemia detector proposed by Langley is also shown as reference. The analysis of the ROC curves clearlydemonstrates

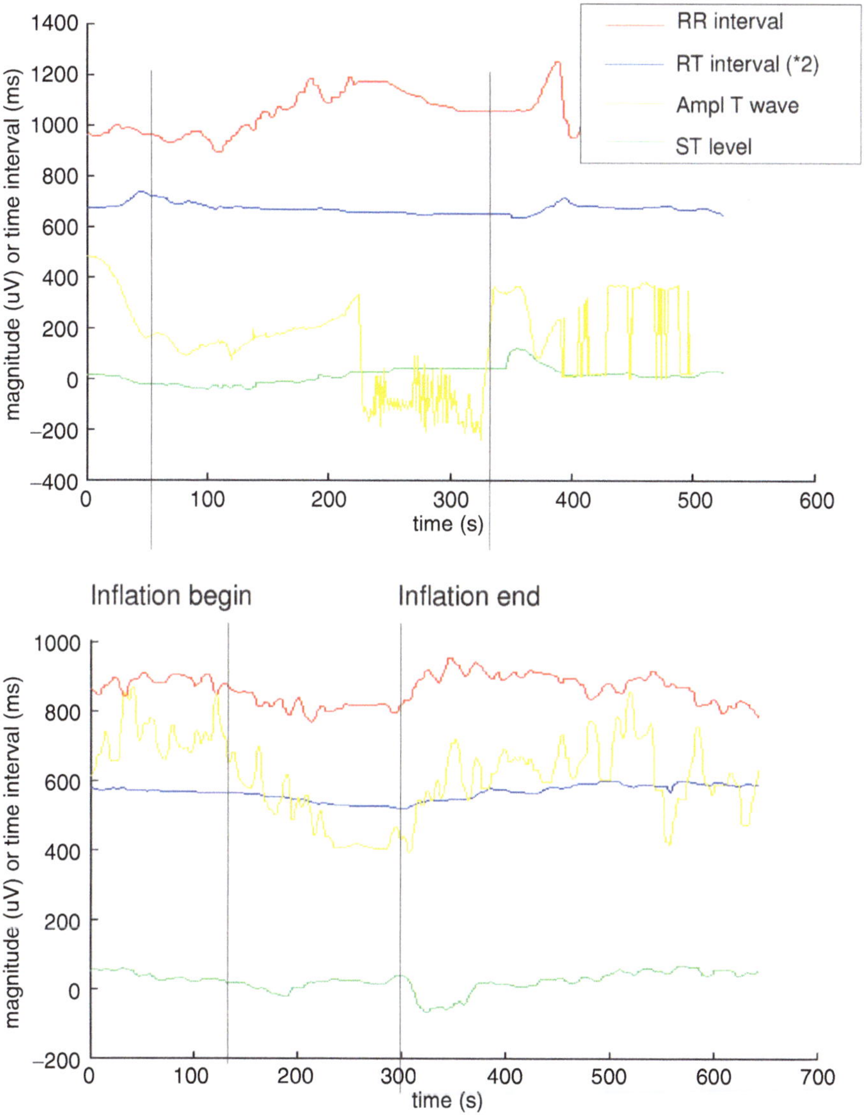

Fig. 11.6 Two examples of time series obtained from the STAFF3 database, with annotations concerning the inflation periods

the interest of the HSMM approach and confirms the benefit of a multidimensional analysis of an ischemic event. The areas under the ROC curves were also computed and are shown in Table 11.5. The scores confirm that the HMM approach appears as a pertinent method and the RT parameter contains relevant information for ischemia detection.

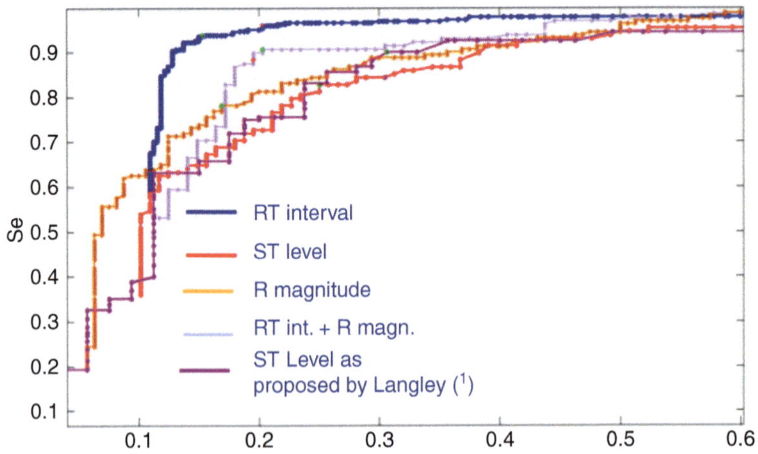

Fig. 11.7 ROC curves for the detection of the ischemic event from different sets of electrocardiographic features

Table 11.5 Areas under the ROC curves for several parameters

Parameter	Value
HMM and RT	0.865
HMM and R	0.85
HMM and RT and R	0.834
Langley and ST	0.834
HMM and ST	0.826

As a summary, results obtained with percutaneous transluminal coronary angioplasty (PTCA) records of the STAFF3 database, when adjusted to the optimal detection point, show an improved detection rate (96% of sensibility and 80% of specificity) with respect to other methods applied on the same database.

11.5 Optimal Segmentation of Preterm Newborn ECG Recordings for the Detection of Apnea-Bradycardia Episodes

Apnea and bradycardia episodes in preterm infants may compromise oxygenation and tissue perfusion, leading to neurological morbidity or even infant death. For these reasons, in neonatal intensive care units (NICU), preterm infants undergo continuous cardiorespiratory monitoring through polygraphic recordings, to detect these apnea-bradycardia episodes and to initiate quick nursing actions, such as manual stimulation, mask ventilation, intubation, etc. Current research in this field is oriented toward a better understanding of the initiation of apnea-bradycardia episodes and the prediction or early detection of these episodes in order to decrease the intervention delay, reduce the consequences associated with apnea, and improve the quality of life of preterm newborns.

Most of the works in the literature are based on the analysis of the heart rate signal alone (Poets et al. 1993). The objective of this section is to study the information content of other features derived from the ECG (namely, the R-wave amplitude and the QRS complex duration) before, during, and after apnea-bradycardia episodes, in order to eventually integrate them in a new early detection approach. In order to achieve this objective, two major steps must be followed: (1) the accurate detection of each beat from the newborn's ECG and (2) the segmentation of each QRS complex, in order to derive the features of interest. However, to our knowledge, published QRS detection and ECG segmentation methods have been developed for the adult ECG and none of them have been adapted to the specific characteristics of the newborn's ECG (higher HR than adults, shorter QRS complex duration, and so on). The evolutionary approach presented in Sect. 11.3 is thus applied in this section to the optimization of the QRS detection and segmentation methods (proposed in Sect. 11.4) to the specific properties of preterm newborns.

11.5.1 Data Selection

Data were obtained from a population of 32 preterm infants hospitalized in the NICU at the University Hospital of Rennes from June 2003 to June 2004, who presented more than one bradycardia per hour or the need for bag-and-mask resuscitation. At the moment of the recording, the median birth weight was 1,235 g, the median age was 31.2 weeks, and the postnatal age was 12.1 days. More details on the clinical protocol are available in Beuchée (2005). Each record of this database contains one ECG lead acquired during 1 h at 400 Hz. Bradycardia events were annotated by analyzing the cardiac cycle length (RR interval) series, using the standard definition proposed by Poets et al. (1993). Two database subsets were constructed to carry out the different studies on this section.

- DB1: This dataset is used to optimize and test the beat detector; therefore, the positions of the R waves have been annotated for each beat. This subset is composed of 50 ECG segments, defined from 5 min before the beginning of a bradycardia episode until 2 min after the end, and containing only one bradycardia event during this period. DB1 is constituted of 51,655 beats (1032.83 $\pm$ 82.69 mean beats per record) and a mean RR interval of 420.77 $\pm$ 58.31 ms.
- DB2: This dataset is used to optimize and test the QRS segmentation process; therefore, the position of the R wave, QRSon, QRSoff, and the isoelectric level have been annotated for each beat. DB2 is composed of 93 ECG segments, randomly chosen from the entire database, and with at least one ECG segment per patient. The ECG segments are characterized by a normal HR and by one or more bradycardia episodes per segment. This dataset is composed of 4,463 beats (48 beats per record) and a mean RR interval of 421.76 $\pm$ 22.43 ms.

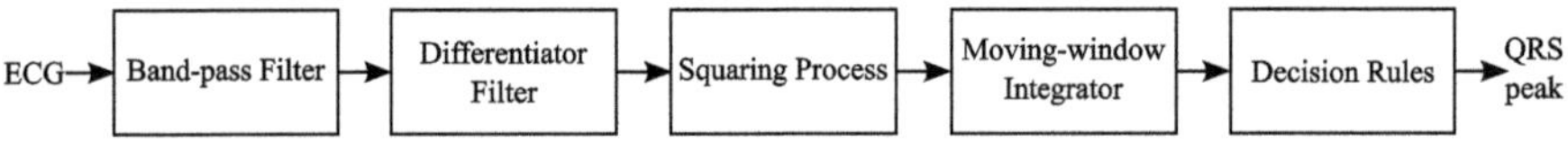

Fig. 11.8 QRS detection method

11.5.2 QRS Detection Method

A real-time QRS detection algorithm represented synthetically in Fig. 11.8 was implemented. The four first steps are analogous to those proposed by Pan and Tompkins (1985), where the ECG signal is processed by a band-pass filter (cascade of low-pass and high-pass filters) followed by a differentiator filter, an amplitude squaring process, and a moving-window integrator of length MWI. However, the last step is different from the approach proposed by Pan and Tompkins and is based on an adaptive threshold which tracks the amplitude modifications on the transformed ECG signal. This threshold is continually adjusted by a set of heuristic rules defined as follows.

The adaptive threshold (THR) is calculated by using

$$THR = \overline{Npeak} + \delta(\overline{Speak} - \overline{Npeak}) \tag{11.8}$$

where δ is a constant, $\overline{Speak}$ is the average of the NP peaks greater than THR ($Speak$), and $\overline{Npeak}$ is the average of the NP peaks lower than THR ($Npeak$). $\overline{Speak}$ and $\overline{Npeak}$ are determined by using

$$\overline{Speak} = \frac{\sum_{i=1}^{NP} Speak_i}{NP} \tag{11.9}$$

$$\overline{Npeak} = \frac{\sum_{i=1}^{NP} Npeak_i}{NP} \tag{11.10}$$

Peaks greater than THR are classified as a QRS complex. Finally, a blanking period (*Refr*) and a search window (*SW*) are applied to the band-pass-filtered signal to find the instant corresponding to the peak value (fiducial point). If a QRS complex is not detected during *RRlim*, the parameters are reset and a new QRS detection process begins from the last QRS correctly detected. Table 11.6 summarizes the parameters of the QRS detector to be optimized.

Table 11.6 Parameters of the QRS detection method and its values before and after the application of the optimization process

		Value		
Parameter	Description	Before	After	Units
fc_{Low}	Cutoff frequency of low-pass filter	15	20.71	Hz
fc_{High}	Cutoff frequency of high-pass filter	5	9.49	Hz
MWI	Window size for moving-average integration process	150	78.41	ms
NP	Numbers of peaks used to determine the mean of the peaks	5	7	Peaks
δ	Constant for determining the adaptive threshold	0.31	0.1485	
$Refr$	Length of the blanking period	200	233.54	ms
SW	Window size for QRS peak detection	20	30.75	ms
$RRlim$	Time limit for reinitializing QRS detection	1500	1959.46	ms

11.5.3 QRS Segmentation Method

After the detection phase, the QRS complex segmentation method proposed in Sect. 11.4 was applied to find the Q, R, and S waves and the onset and offset of the QRS complex (QRSon and QRSoff). Only scales $W2^1$ and $W2^2$ were analyzed as scales $W2^3$ to $W2^5$ are used for P and T wave segmentation, which are not estimated in this application. The detection of the isoelectric level is an important constraint as the PQ segment is shorter in preterm infants. Therefore, two different parameters have been defined: $ISO1$ to search the isoelectric level and $ISO2$ as the size of the flattest waveform window.

To cope with the wide HR variations observed in preterm infants, parameters $(R1, R2, QRS_Qlim, QRS_Slim, ISO1, ISO2)$ were redefined as scaled versions of the instantaneous RR interval

$$T_i = m_i RR \tag{11.11}$$

where $i \in \{R1, R2, Qlim, Slim, ISO1, ISO2\}$ and m_i are the scale factors to be optimized (Altuve et al. 2009).

11.5.4 Configuration of the Optimization Algorithm

As in the previous application, two independent evolutionary algorithms, namely EA1 and EA2, were sequentially applied: EA1 optimizes the parameters of the QRS detector and EA2 optimizes the parameters of the QRS segmentation method. This separation can be done as an optimal ECG wave segmentation can be obtained only if the QRS detection phase has been previously optimized.

Learning and test sets, containing QRS complexes with different morphologies, were constructed as follows:

- EA1 learning set (used for the optimization of the beat detector): This dataset is composed of 2,500 beats (50 beats per record) obtained from DB1. The first 25 ECG records do not present any bradycardia Episodes (RR $= 400.89 \pm 13.02$ ms). They were extracted from the first part of each ECG record. The other 25 ECG records present bradycardia episodes (RR $= 584.38 \pm 161.79$ ms).
- EA2 learning set (used for the optimization of the QRS segmentation method): It is composed of 2,256 beats from 47 ECG records obtained from DB2. In this set, 34 ECG records (1,632 beats) present a normal HR (RR $= 402.39 \pm 6.06$ ms) and 13 ECG records (624 beats) contain bradycardia episodes (RR $= 534.02 \pm 115.14$ ms).
- EA1 test set (used during the test phase of the QRS detector): This dataset is composed of the entire DB1.
- EA2 test set (used during the test phase of the QRS segmentation process): This dataset is composed of 2,207 beats from the rest of the 46 ECG records obtained from DB2. This set presents a normal HR (RR $= 404.19 \pm 8.34$).

As in the previous example, a cost function integrating the probability of detection error (Eq. 11.2), the mean detection jitter (Eq. 11.3), and the standard deviation of the detection jitter (Eq. 11.4) will be minimized in this application. The QRS detection method provides the position of the fiducial point (FP) and the segmentation algorithm the position of QRSon, QRoff, Rpeak, and isoelectric level (ISO). In this section, the cost function is defined as

$$O = Perr_p + \overline{\varepsilon_p} + \sigma_p \tag{11.12}$$

for EA1 and for $p =$ FP and as

$$O = \sum_{p=1}^{P} (Perr_p + \overline{\varepsilon_p} + \sigma_p) \tag{11.13}$$

for EA2 and for $p \in \{\text{QRSon, QRoff, Rpeak, ISO}\}$.

To create the initial population of EA1, the parameters to be optimized were largely increased and decreased from the values proposed by Pan and Tompkins (1985). In the same way for EA2, the scaled parameters related to temporal search windows were defined from possible extreme positions and durations of each wave, and the scaled parameters related to thresholds were largely increased and decreased from the values proposed in Dumont et al. (2010b).

The ranking selection and standard genetic operators for real-valued chromosomes (simple, arithmetic, and heuristic crossover, multi-nonuniform and nonuniform mutation) were used in both EA. Twenty parameters were optimized: eight from the QRS detector and twelve from the QRS segmentation process. Both EA were driven over 80 generations with 200 individuals. The probability of crossover p_c was 0.7 and the probability of mutation p_m according to Eq. 11.7. The best individuals of the last generation, obtained from five different instances of the whole EA optimization process, were chosen as the optimal parameters. The performance quantification of the optimized QRS detection and QRS segmentation methods

Table 11.7 Optimal parameter values obtained from EA2 for the QRS segmentation algorithm

Parameter	Value
m_{R1}	0.1211
m_{R2}	0.0990
m_{Qlim}	0.1003
m_{Slim}	0.1170
γ_{QRSpre}	0.1241
$\gamma_{QRSpost}$	0.0909
$\xi_{QRSonpos}$	0.0486
$\xi_{QRSonneg}$	0.0800
$\xi_{QRSendpos}$	0.1635
$\xi_{QRSendneg}$	0.6995
m_{ISO1}	0.1192
m_{ISO2}	0.0149

was made by evaluating the sensitivity, the PPV, the mean detection jitter, and the standard deviation of the detection jitter on the first and second test sets, respectively, before and after the optimization of both processes.

11.5.5 Results

Results are presented in two parts. First, the evaluation of QRS detection and segmentation methods, with their optimal parameters, is presented. Then, an analysis of the QRS complex variations before and during apnea-bradycardia is proposed.

11.5.5.1 Beat Detection and Segmentation Performance

A description of the parameters of the QRS detector to be optimized and its values, before and after the application of the proposed optimization methodology, are presented in Table 11.6. The optimal cutoff frequencies of the low-pass and high-pass filters were higher than those used in adults by Pan and Tompkins (1985). This result is confirmed by the fact that, compared to the QRS observed in adults, the QRS of preterm infants is generally thinner and is higher frequency content. The decreased time support of the moving-average integration can also be explained by the higher frequency content of the QRS complex in newborns.

The optimal parameters of the QRS segmentation process are shown in Table 11.7. An example of these optimal parameter values, for a typical RR interval of 400 ms, is illustrated in Table 11.8. The obtained results show a decreased length for all the search windows, increased thresholds for γ_{QRSpre}, $\xi_{QRSonneg}$, and $\xi_{QRSendneg}$ and a decrease in thresholds $\gamma_{QRSpost}$, $\xi_{QRSonpos}$, and $\xi_{QRSendpos}$.

Table 11.8 Example of the optimal values for the different search windows and thresholds optimized in EA2, for an instantaneous RR of 400 ms

Parameter	Results from EA2	Other approaches
T_{R1}	48.44 ms	118 ms
T_{R2}	39.6 ms	111 ms
T_{Qlim}	40.12 ms	88 ms
T_{Slim}	46.8 ms	154 ms
γ_{QRSpre}	0.1241	0.09
$\gamma_{QRSpost}$	0.0909	0.11
$\xi_{QRSonpos}$	0.0486	0.07
$\xi_{QRSonneg}$	0.0800	0.07
$\xi_{QRSendpos}$	0.1635	0.21
$\xi_{QRSendneg}$	0.6995	0.23
T_{ISO1}	47.68 ms	108 ms
T_{ISO2}	5.96 ms	20 ms

Table 11.9 Performance of the QRS detection and segmentation methods, before and after the optimization process

	Sen (%)		PPV (%)		$\overline{\varepsilon}$ (ms)		σ (ms)	
Indicator	Before	After	Before	After	Before	After	Before	After
FP	91.20	97.74	92.22	98.03	3.51	1.18	15.60	10.23
Rpeak	98.46	98.46	98.46	98.46	1.39	1.69	1.44	0.66
QRSon	40.33	90.21	40.33	90.21	43.48	3.07	11.61	1.27
QRSoff	77.07	80.24	77.07	80.24	7.81	4.49	5.64	2.64
ISO	0	80.61	0	80.61	48.88	4.29	2.61	2.29

The performance of the QRS detection and segmentation methods is shown in Table 11.9. Parameters obtained from the optimization method increased the sensitivity and the positive predictive value of the fiducial point, QRS onset, QRS offset, and isoelectric level. Additionally, a significant decrease in the mean and standard deviation of the detection jitter was obtained for QRS onset, QRS offset. and the isoelectric level. Optimal parameters of the WT segmentation method did not significantly modify the R wave detection performance. Although the standard deviation of the detection jitter was improved, the mean detection jitter was slightly higher.

The next section shows how these beat detection and segmentation algorithms, using the obtained optimal parameters, have been applied to a series of ECG signals acquired from preterm newborns in order to better characterize the onset of apnea-bradycardia events.

11.5.5.2 Characterization of Apnea-Bradycardia Episodes from the Analysis of the QRS Complex

Changes in the intrathoracic pressure during normal respiration or apnea may reflect changes in the ECG waves (Penzel et al. 2006). This fact motivated us to study the modifications of the QRS complex morphology during apnea-bradycardia episodes

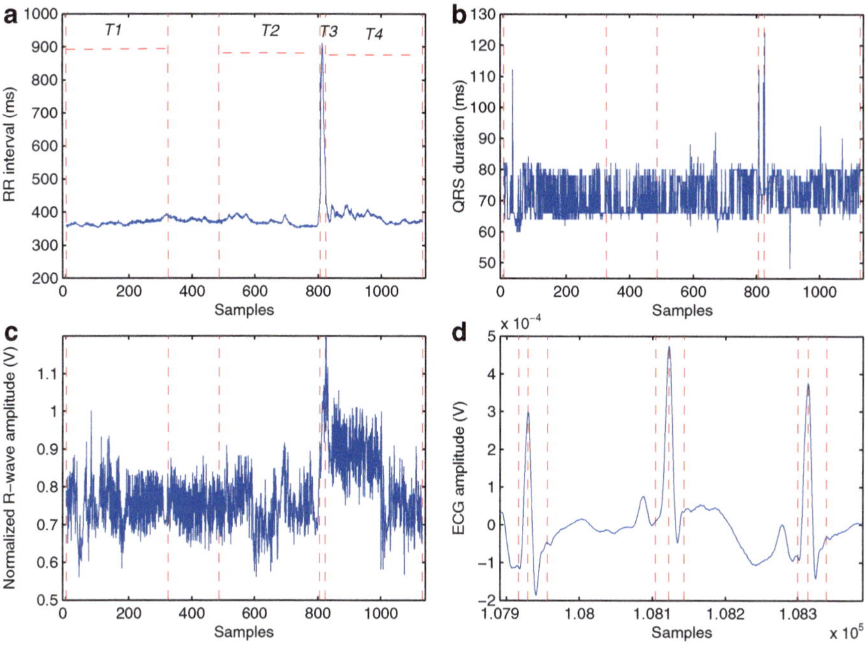

Fig. 11.9 Segment with small differences between T1 and the other intervals. (**a**) Time series RR, (**b**) time series QRSd, (**c**) time series Ramp, and (**d**) QRS complex segmentation results for this segment. In (**a**)–(**c**) the *vertical dashed lines* delimit the intervals. In (**d**) the *vertical dashed lines* show QRSon, R wave, and QRSoff obtained from the segmentation

in preterm infants. Time series representing RR, R wave amplitude, and QRS duration were thus extracted from DB1 (see Sect. 11.5.1) and further analyzed. These series were analyzed during the following time intervals:

- T1: defined with a temporal support of 2 min, starting from the beginning of the ECG segment (5 min before the bradycardia). There are no apnea-bradycardia events in T1 and the heart rate is mostly around its mean rest value.
- T2: is defined from the third to the fifth minute. In T2 there are no bradycardia events but the apnea episode has already begun. We are interested in finding some relevant information during this interval, just before the bradycardia event.
- T3: is defined with a variable temporal support, covering the entire bradycardia event. Both apnea and bradycardia are present in T3.
- T4: is defined from the end of the bradycardia until the end of the ECG segment, with a temporal support of 2 min. Heart rate usually returns to its baseline value during T4.

Additionally, time series corresponding to the R wave amplitude were normalized with respect to the highest value found in T1. Two examples of the extracted time series, indicating the T1–T4 periods are presented in Figs. 11.9 and 11.10. In order to find significant variations between the interval T1 (considered

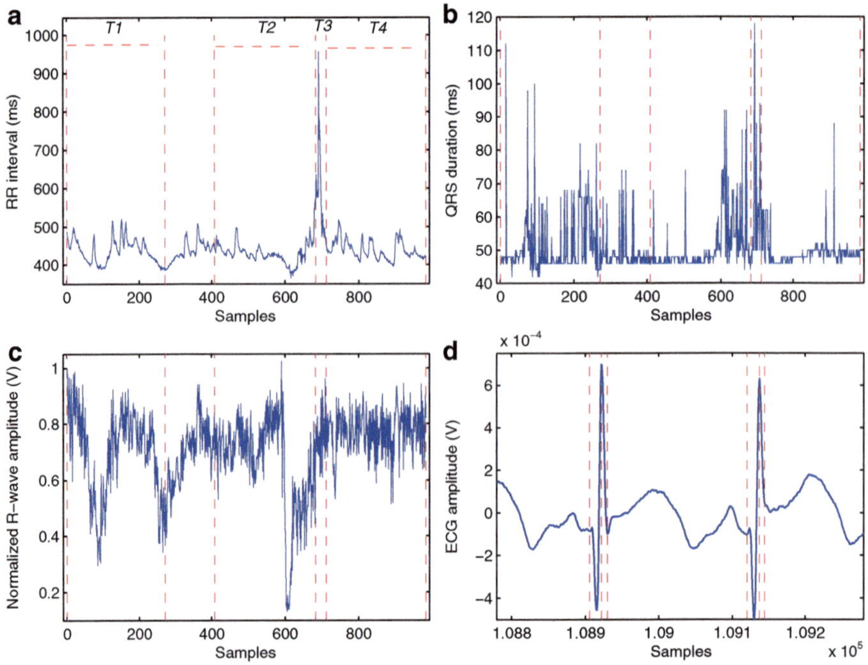

Fig. 11.10 Segment with big differences between T1 and the other intervals. (**a**) Time series RR, (**b**) time series QRSd, (**c**) time series Ramp, and (**d**) QRS complex segmentation results for this segment. In (**a**)–(**c**) the *vertical dashed lines* delimit the intervals. In (**d**) the *vertical dashed lines* show QRSon, R wave, and QRSoff obtained from the segmentation

as reference) and the other intervals (T2, T3, and T4) for all time series $TS \in \{RR, Ramp, QRSd\}$, four criteria were evaluated:

- Weighted mean ($w\mu$): is the average of the mean of each record m ($\overline{TS}_m^{Ti}$, $\forall Ti \in \{T1, T2, T3, T4\}$) which are weighted according to their number of beats per record (Nm):

$$w\mu_{Ti} = \frac{\sum_{m=1}^{M} N_m \overline{TS}_m^{Ti}}{\sum_{m=1}^{M} N_m}. \tag{11.14}$$

- Weighted standard deviation ($w\sigma$): is the average of the standard deviation of each record m (σTS_m^{Ti}, $\forall Ti \in \{T1, T2, T3, T4\}$) which are weighted according to their number of beats per record:

$$w\sigma_{Ti} = \frac{\sum_{m=1}^{M} N_m \sigma TS_m^{Ti}}{\sum_{m=1}^{M} N_m}. \tag{11.15}$$

Table 11.10 Weighted mean and weighted standard deviation ($w\mu \pm w\sigma$) of the time series analyzed with respect to the different temporal supports of interest (T1,...,T4)

Time series	T1	T2	T3	T4
RR	407.90 ± 14.60	414.58 ± 28.43	712.01 ± 147.94	413.89 ± 19.72
Ramp	0.8233 ± 0.0605	0.8187 ± 0.0638	0.8155 ± 0.0754	0.8293 ± 0.0661
QRSd	61.03 ± 5.887	61.58 ± 6.22	66.35 ± 15.06	61.43 ± 7.08

- Mean of the absolute difference (μAD): is the average of the absolute difference between the mean of the interval T1 ($\overline{TS}_m^{T1}$) and the mean of the other intervals ($\overline{TS}_m^{Ti}$, $\forall Ti \in \{T1, T2, T3, T4\}$), over all records ($M$):

$$\mu AD_{T1-Ti} = \frac{\sum_{m=1}^{M} |\overline{TS}_m^{T1} - \overline{TS}_m^{Ti}|}{M}. \tag{11.16}$$

- Standard deviation of the absolute difference (σAD): is the average of the absolute difference between the standard deviation of the interval T1 (σTS_m^{T1}) and the standard deviation of the other intervals (σTS_m^{Ti}, $\forall Ti \in \{T2, T3, T4\}$), over all records ($M$):

$$\sigma AD_{T1-Ti} = \frac{\sum_{m=1}^{M} |\sigma TS_m^{T1} - \sigma TS_m^{Ti}|}{M}. \tag{11.17}$$

The statistical hypothesis test of Mann-Whitney U was used to analyze the variations of these criteria between different intervals. A p-value of $p < 0.05$ is considered significant. Results for $w\mu$ and $w\sigma$ are shown in Table 11.10. It can be noticed that the highest values of RR and QRSd were obtained for T3 (during the bradycardia event), followed by T2, and the lowest values were obtained for T1. Results for Ramp are particularly interesting: the lowest value of $w\mu$ and the highest value for $w\sigma$ were obtained in T3. From T1 to T3, a decrease of $w\mu$ and an increase of $w\sigma$ was observed and the highest value of $w\mu$ was obtained in T4.

Table 11.11 shows the results of the absolute differences $\mu AD_{T1-Ti} \pm \sigma AD_{T1-Ti}$ for time series RR, Ramp, and QRSd. In this table, the highest value is observed for $T1 - T3$ for all time series. Finally, Table 11.12 shows the results from the Mann-Whitney U hypothesis test, computed for the mean of each time series (RR, Ramp, and QRSd) during different intervals. For the RR time series, significant differences were obtained between intervals T1 and T3, as expected. Also, significant differences were observed for all time series when comparing T1–T2 vs. T1–T3 and T1–T3 vs. T1–T4.

Two segments presenting significant differences between T1 and the other intervals are shown in Figs. 11.9 and 11.10. Bradycardia episodes can be easily

Table 11.11 Mean and standard deviation of the absolute difference ($\mu AD_{T1-Ti} \pm \sigma AD_{T1-Ti}$) of the time series analyzed

Time serie	T1–T2	T1–T3	T1–T4
RR	11.26 ± 15.31	285.06 ± 123.24	13.93 ± 8.76
Ramp	0.0442 ± 0.0192	0.0966 ± 0.0388	0.0585 ± 0.0238
QRSd	2.02 ± 1.66	10.17 ± 9.38	2.57 ± 2.17

Table 11.12 Hypothesis test for the mean of the time series analyzed

Interval	*p*(*RR*)	*p*(*Rmap*)	*p*(*QRSd*)
T1 vs T2	0.29312	0.71741	0.8713
T1 vs T3	<0.0001[a]	0.60754	0.10448
T1 vs T4	0.26556	0.40614	0.68167
T1–T2 vs T1–T3	<0.0001[a]	0.00028[a]	<0.0001[a]
T1–T2 vs T1–T4	0.30923	0.09732	0.5602
T1–T3 vs T1–T4	<0.0001[a]	0.02311[a]	<0.0001[a]

[a]Statistically significant

identified from the RR series in Figs. 11.9a and 11.10a. Changes in Ramp are clearly observed in Figs. 11.9c and 11.10c, particularly during T2. Some errors from the automatic QRS segmentation process are observed in subfigures (d) (QRSon and QRSoff are not always correctly detected) and in subfigures (b) (time series QRS duration shows several artifacts).

Finally, boxplots of the difference in the mean value between T1 and the other intervals for the time series Ramp are shown in Fig. 11.11. The circle "•" represents the case shown in Fig. 11.9 and the square "■" corresponds to the segment shown in Fig. 11.10. The highest difference in the mean is observed between T1 and T3.

Results presented in this section suggest that the early detection of apnea-bradycardia episodes can be improved by a multivariate method combining the traditional analysis of RR series with the characterization of other electrophysiological features extracted from the ECG. In particular, the variabilities of the R-wave amplitude and QRS durations seem to provide pertinent information that can be exploited for monitoring purposes. It is important to note that, in this application, the most interesting results were obtained when comparing the differences between different time intervals (e.g., T1–T2 vs T1–T3) and not their instantaneous values. This fact underlines the importance of the analysis of the *dynamics* of these time series, by means of appropriate modeling methods. Current work is directed to (1) the study of other features derived from the ECG of preterm infants such as the PR interval, the P wave morphology and the QT interval (2) their optimal combination and (3) the analysis of the dynamics of these series by means of semi-makovian models.

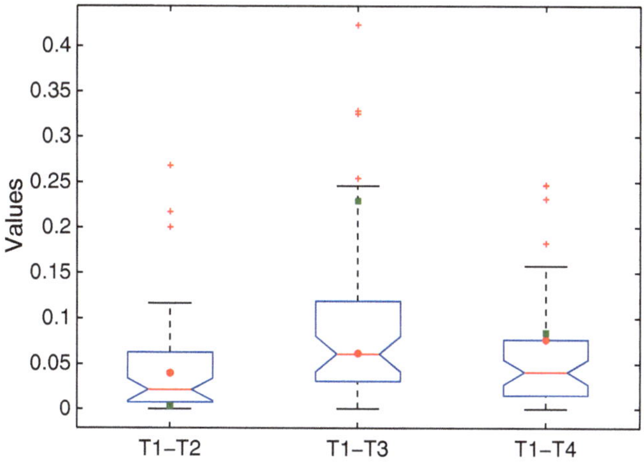

Fig. 11.11 Boxplots of the difference in the mean between T1 and the other intervals for the time series Ramp. The circle "•" represents the case shown in Fig. 11.9 and the square "■" the one illustrated in Fig. 11.10

11.6 Conclusions and Perspectives

This chapter presented a brief overview of the main signal processing methods for the detection and segmentation of ECG beats. The performance of all of these methods strongly depends on the definition of a set of parameters (filter cutoff frequencies, thresholds, etc.), which may be specific to a given patient population. The optimization of these parameters, in order to maximize the detection and segmentation performance on clinical data, is a complex task that is usually performed manually, on a subset of the available parameters and based on a single criterion. In this sense, an evolutionary optimization approach is proposed, which minimizes a multi-objective error function, defined between the output of these detection and/or segmentation methods and the annotations obtained from specific clinical ECG databases. This error function takes into account not only the error detection probability, but also the mean and standard deviation of the detection jitter.

Two example applications, focusing on concrete clinical problems, have been presented: the detection of myocardial ischemia episodes on adult patients and the characterization of apnea-bradycardia events on preterm infants. Three distinct analysis phases were applied for each application: (1) an initial optimization of the detection and segmentation methods, which is specific for the targeted population, (2) a characterization phase, based on the processing of beat-to-beat time series constituted from the different features extracted from the segmentation phase, and (3) a quantitative evaluation and comparison phase, intended to validate and compare the proposed approach to other methods from the literature. For both clinical applications, significant performance improvements have been achieved by using the optimal parameters obtained from the proposed evolutionary approach and by combining the different extracted features into multivariate detection schemes. However, despite the higher performances obtained, the segmentation methods can be still improved, particularly for the QRSoff and Toff instants. Further work is directed to the extension of these methods to a multi-lead ECG analysis system, which would be helpful in this sense.

References

Altuve, M., Carrault, G., Cruz, J., Beuchée, A., Pladys, P., Hernández, A.: Analysis of the QRS complex for apnea-bradycardia characterization in preterm infants. In: Engineering in Medicine and Biology Society, 2009. EMBC 2009. Annual International Conference of the IEEE, pp. 946–949. IEEE, Minneapolis (2009)

Back, T., Schutz, M.: Intelligent mutation rate control in canonical genetic algorithms: foundations of intelligent systems. In: Ras, Z., Michalewicz, M. (eds.) Proceedings of the International Symposium on Methodologies for Intelligent Systems, *Lect. Notes Comput. Sci.* **1079**, 158–167. National Technical Information Service, Springer Berlin/Heidelberg (1996)

Bahoura, M., Hassani, M., Hubin, M.: Dsp implementation of wavelet transform for real time ecg wave forms detection and heart analysis. Comput. Meth. Programs Biomed. **52**, 35–44 (1997)

Beuchée, A.: Intérêt de l'analyse de la variabilité du rythme cardiaque en néonatalogie. comportement des systèmes de régulation cardiovasculaire dans le syndrome apnée/bradycardie du nouveau-né, vol. 1, PhD. thesis, Université de Rennes (2005)

Castro, N., Gomis, P., Wagner, G.: Assessment of myocardial ischemia through high frequency energy estimation over the time-frequency plane using wavelets. Comput. Cardiol. **30**, 517–520 (2004)

Clavier, L., Boucher, J.: Segmentation of electrocardiograms using a hidden Markov model. In: Engineering in Medicine and Biology Society, 1996. Bridging Disciplines for Biomedicine. Proceedings of the 18th Annual International Conference of the IEEE, vol. 4, pp. 1409–1410. IEEE, Piscataway (1996)

Coast, D.: Segmentation of high-resolution ECGs using hidden Markov models. Acoustic. Speech Signal Process. ICASSP-93 **1**, 67–70 (1993)

Coast, D., Stern, R., Cano, G., Briller, S.: An approach to cardiac arrhythmia analysis using hidden Markov models. IEEE Trans. Biomed. Eng. **37**(9), 826–836 (1990)

CSE: Recommandations for measurement standards in quantitative electrocardiography. Eur. Heart J.: The CSE Working Party **6** 815–825 (1985)

Doerschuck, P.: A Markov Chain Approach to Electrocardiogram Modeling and Analysis. PhD. thesis, Massachusetts Institute of Technology, Boston, Massachussetts, USA (1985)

Dumont, J., Carrault, G., Gomis, P., Wagner, G., Hernandez, A.: Detection of myocardial ischemia with hidden Semi-Markovian models. In: Computers in Cardiology, 2009, pp. 121–124. IEEE, Park City (2010a)

Dumont, J., Hernández, A.I., Carrault, G.: Improving ecg beats delineation with an evolutionary optimization process., IEEE Trans. Biomed. Eng. **57**(3), 607–15 (2010b)

Eichler West, R., de Schutter, E., Wilcox, G.: Using evolutionary algorithms to search for control parameters in a nonlinear partial differential equation. Ima Vol. Math. Appl. **111**, 33–64 (1999)

Einthoven, W.: Galvanometrische registratie van het menschilijk electrocardiogram. In: Herinneringsbundel Professor SS Rosenstein, pp. 101–107. Eduard Ijdo, Leiden (1902)

Garcia, J., Wagner, G., Sörnmo, L., Olmos, S., Lander, P., Laguna, P.: Temporal evolution of traditional versus transformed ECG-Based indexes in patients with induced myocardial ischemia. J. Electrocardiol. **33**, 37–47 (2000)

Goldberger, A.L., Amaral, L.A.N., Glass, L., Hausdorff, J.M., Ivanov, P.C., Mark, R.G., Mietus, J.E., Moody, G.B., Peng, C.-K., Stanley, H.E.: Physiobank, physiotoolkit, and physionet: components of a new research resource for complex physiologic signals. Circulation **101**(23), e215–e220 (2000)

Graja, S., Boucher, J.: Multiscale hidden Markov model applied to ECG segmentation, In: IEEE International Symposium on Intelligent Signal Processing, 2003, pp. 105–109. IEEE Computer Society, Tokyo (2003)

Graja, S., Boucher, S.: Hidden markov tree model applied to ECG delineation. IEEE Trans. Instrum. Meas. **54**, 2163–2168 (2005)

Hernández, A.I., Carrault, G., Mora, F., Bardou, A.: Model-based interpretation of cardiac beats by evolutionary algorithms: signal and model interaction. Artif. Intell. Med. **26**(3), 211–235 (2002)

Holland, J.H.: Genetic algorithms. Sci. Am. **267**(1), 66–72 (1992)

Houck, C., Joines, J., Kay, M.: A genetic algorithm for function optimization: A Matlab implementation, NCSU-IE TR 95-09 (1995)

Hughes, N., Tarassenko, L., Roberts, S.: Markov models for automated ECG interval analysis. In: Proceedings NIPS, vol. 16, pp. 611–618. MIT Press, Cambridge, MA (2003)

Islam, S., Jidin, R., Ali, M.: Performance study of adaptive filtering algorithms for noise cancellation of ECG signal. In: 7th International Conference on Information, Communications and Signal Processing, 2009. ICICS 2009, pp. 1–5. IEEE, Macau (2010)

Jane, R., Laguna, P., Thakor, N., Caminal, P.: Adaptive baseline wander removal in the ECG: comparative analysis with cubic spline technique. Comput. Cardiol. **18**, 143–146 (1992)

Jane, R., Blasi, A., Garcia, J., Laguna, P.: Evaluation of an automatic threshold based detector of waveform limits in Holter ECG with the QT database. In: Computers in Cardiology, pp. 295–298. IEEE Computer Society, Long Beach (1997)

Janikow, C., Michalewicz, Z.: An experimental comparison of binary and floating point representations in genetic algorithms. In: Proceedings of the Fourth International Conference on Genetic Algorithms, pp. 31–36. Morgan Kaufmann Publishers, San Mateo (1991)

Kohler, B., Hennig, C., Orglmeister, R.: The principles of software QRS detection, IEEE Eng. Med. Biol. Mag. **21**(1), 42–57 (2002)

Koski, A.: Modelling ECG signals with hidden Markov models. Artif. Intell. Med. **8**(5), 453–471 (1996)

Laguna, P., Jane, R., Caminal, R.: Automatic detection of wave boundaries in multi-lead ecg signals: validation with the cse data-base. Comput. Biomed. Res. **27** 45–60 (1994)

Langer, A., Armstrong, P.: ST segment monitoring in patients with acute ischemic syndromes: Past and future revue. J. Thromb. Thrombolysis **5**, S119–S123 (1998)

Lepage, R., Boucher, J., Blanc, J., Cornilly, J.: ECG segmentation and P-wave feature extraction: application to patients prone to atrial fibrillation. In: Engineering in Medicine and Biology Society. Proceedings of the 23rd Annual International Conference of the IEEE, vol. 1, pp. 298–301 Istanbul (2001)

Leski, J., Henzel, N.: ECG baseline wander and powerline interference reduction using nonlinear filter bank. Signal Process. **85**(4), (2005) 781–793

Levkov, C., Mihov, G., Ivanov, R., Daskalov, I., Ivaylo, C., Dotsinsky, I.: Removal of power-line interference from the ECG: a review of the subtraction procedure. Biomed. Eng. Online **4**, 50 (2005)

Li, C., Zheng, C., Tai, C.: Detection of ECG characteristic points using wavelet transforms. IEEE Trans. Biomed. Eng. **42**(1), 21–28 (1995)

Martinez, J.P., Almeida, R., Olmos, S., Rocha, A.P., Laguna, P.: A wavelet-based ecg delineator: evaluation on standard databases. IEEE Trans. Biomed. Eng. **51**, 570–581 (2004)

Martinez, J., Olmos, S., Wagner, G., Laguna, P.: Characterization of repolarization alternans during ischemia: time-course and spatial analysis. IEEE Trans. Biomed. Eng. **53**, 701–11 (2006)

McGinn, A., Rosamond, W., Goff, D., et al.: Trends in prehospital delay time and use of emergency medical services for acute myocardial infarction: experience in 4 US communities from 1987–2000. Am. Heart J. **150**(3), 392–400 (2005)

Michalewicz, Z.: Genetic Algorithms + Data Structures = Evolution Programs, 3rd edn. Springer, Berlin/Heidelberg (1996)

Mneimneh, M., Yaz, E., Johnson, M., Povinelli, R.: An adaptive Kalman filter for removing baseline wandering in ECG signals. In: Computers in Cardiology, 2006, pp. 253–256. IEEE, Valencia (2008)

Pan, J., Tompkins, W.: A real-time QRS detection algorithm. IEEE Trans. Biomed. Eng. **32** 230–236 (1985)

Penzel, T., Nottrott, M., Canisius, S., Greulich, T., Becker, H.F., Vogelmeier, C. P428 ecg morphology changes improves detection of obstructive sleep apnea. Sleep Med. **7**(Suppl 2), S101–S102 (2006)

Pettersson, J., Pahlm, O., Carro, E., Edenbrandt, L., Ringborn, M., Sörnmo, L., Warren, S.G., Wagner, G.S.: Changes in high-frequency QRS components are more sensitive than ST-segment deviation for detecting acute coronary artery occlusion. J. Am. Coll. Cardiol. **36**, 1827–1834 (2000)

Poets, C.F., Stebbens, V.A., Samuels, M.P., Southall, D.P.: The relationship between bradycardia, apnea, and hypoxemia in preterm infants. Pediatr. Res. **34**(2), 144–147 (1993)

Portet, F., Hernandez, A., Carrault, G., Evaluation of real-time QRS detection algorithms in variable contexts. Med. Biol. Eng. Comput. **43**(3), 379–385 (2005)

Pueyo, E., Sörnmo, L., Laguna, P.: QRS slopes for detection and characterization of myocardial ischemia. IEEE Trans. Biomed. Eng. **55**, 468–477 (2008)

Sörnmo, L., Laguna, P.: Bioelectrical Signal Processing in Cardiac and Neurological Applications. Elsevier Academic Press, Amsterdam/Boston (2005)

Sebag, M., Schoenauer, M., Ravise, C.: Toward civilized evolution: developing inhibitions. In: Bäck, T. (ed.) Proceedings of the Seventh International Conference on Genetic Algorithms, pp. 291–298. Morgan Kaufmann, San Francisco (1997)

Senhadji, L., Carrault, G., Bellanger, J., Passariello, G.: Comparing wavelet transforms for recognizing cardiac patterns. Eng. Med. Biol. Mag. IEEE **14**(2), 167–173 (2002)

Shusterman, V., Shah, S.I., Beigel, A., Anderson, K.P.: Enhancing the precision of ECG baseline correction: selective filtering and removal of residual error. Comput. Biomed. Res. **33**(2), 144–160 (2000)

Smrdel, A., Jager, F.: Automated detection of transient ST-segment episodes in 24h electrocardiograms. Med. Biol. Eng. Comput. **42**(3), 303–311 (2004)

Soria-Olivas, E., Martínez-Sober, M., Calpe-Maravilla, J., Guerrero-Martínez, J.F., Chorro-Gascó, J., Espí-López, J.: Application of adaptive signal processing for determining the limits of P and T waves in an ECG. IEEE Trans. Biomed. Eng. **45**(8), 1077–1080 (1998)

Thakor, N., Zhu, Y.: Applications of adaptive filtering to ECG analysis: noise cancellation and arrhythmia detection. IEEE Trans. Biomed. Eng. **38**(8), 785–794 (2002)

Thierens, D.: Adaptive mutation rate control schemes in genetic algorithms. In: Proceedings of the 2002 Congress on Evolutionary Computation, vol. 1, pp. 980–985. Barcelona (2002)

Thoraval, L.: Analyse statistique de signaux électrocardiographiques par modèles de markov cachés. PhD. thesis, Université de Rennes (1995)

Touzé, E., Varenne, O., Chatellier, G., Peyrard, S., Rothwell, P., Mas, J.-L.: Risk of myocardial infarction and vascular death after transient ischemic attack and ischemic stroke: a systematic review and meta-analysis. Stroke **36**, 2748 (2005)

van Ravenswaaij-Arts, C., Kollee, L., Hopman, J., Stoelinga, G., van Geijn, H.: Heart rate variability. Ann. Intern. Med. **118**(6), 436 (1993)

Vullings, H., Verhaegen, M., Verbruggen, H.: Automated ECG segmentation with dynamic time warping. In: Engineering in Medicine and Biology Society, 1998. Proceedings of the 20th Annual International Conference of the IEEE, vol. 1, pp. 163–166. IEEE Service Center, Picatway (1998)

Yang, L., Zhang, S., Li, X., Yang, Y.: Removal of pulse waveform baseline drift using cubic spline interpolation. In: 4th International Conference on Bioinformatics and Biomedical Engineering (iCBBE), 2010, pp. 1–3. IEEE, Shenzhen (2010)

Ziarani, A.K., Konrad, A.: A nonlinear adaptive method of elimination of power line interference in ECG signals. IEEE Trans. Biomed. Eng. **49**(6), 540–547 (2002)

Zifan, A., Saberi, S., Moradi, M.H., Towhidkhah, F.: Automated ECG segmentation using piecewise derivative dynamic time warping. Int. J. Biomed. Sci. **1**(3), 181–185 (2006)

Index

A. Gacek and W. Pedrycz (eds.), *ECG Signal Processing, Classification and Interpretation: A Comprehensive Framework of Computational Intelligence*, DOI 10.1007/978-0-85729-868-3, © Springer-Verlag London Limited 2012

MIX
Papier aus verantwortungsvollen Quellen
Paper from responsible sources
FSC® C105338

If you have any concerns about our products,
you can contact us on
ProductSafety@springernature.com

In case Publisher is established outside the EU,
the EU authorized representative is:
Springer Nature Customer Service Center GmbH
Europaplatz 3, 69115 Heidelberg, Germany

Printed by Libri Plureos GmbH
in Hamburg, Germany